Electrophysiology: The Basics

A Companion Guide for the Cardiology Fellow during the EP Rotation

Jonathan S. Steinberg, MD

Chief, Division of Cardiology
Al-Sabah Endowed Director of the Arrhythmia Institute
St. Luke's and Roosevelt Hospitals
Professor of Medicine
Columbia University College of Physicians and Surgeons
New York, New York

Suneet Mittal, MD

Director, Electrophysiology Laboratory
St. Luke's and Roosevelt Hospitals
Associate Professor of Medicine
Columbia University College of Physicians and Surgeons
New York, New York

Wolters Kluwer | Lippincott Williams & Wilkins
Health
Philadelphia • Baltimore • New York • London
Buenos Aires • Hong Kong • Sydney • Tokyo

Acquisitions Editor: Frances DeStefano
Product Manager: Leanne McMillan
Production Manager: Bridgett Dougherty
Senior Manufacturing Manager: Benjamin Rivera
Marketing Manager: Kimberly Schonberger
Design Coordinator: Teresa Mallon
Production Service: SPi Technologies

530 Walnut Street
Philadelphia, PA 19106 USA
LWW.com

Printed in China

Library of Congress Cataloging-in-Publication Data
Introductory guide to electrophysiology / [edited by] Jonathan S. Steinberg, Suneet Mittal.
p. ; cm.
Includes bibliographical references and index.
ISBN-13: 978–1–60547–343–7
ISBN-10: 1–60547–343–X
1. Arrhythmia. 2. Heart—Electric properties. 3. Electrophysiology. I. Steinberg, Jonathan S. II. Mittal, Suneet.
[DNLM: 1. Electrophysiologic Techniques, Cardiac—methods. WG 141.5.F9 I613 2010]
RC685.A65I593 2010
616.1'280645—dc22

2009025944

To purchase additional copies of this book, call our customer service department at (800) 638-3030 or fax orders to (301) 223-2320. International customers should call (301) 223-2300.

Visit Lippincott Williams & Wilkins on the Internet: at LWW.com. Lippincott Williams & Wilkins customer service representatives are available from 8:30 am to 6 pm, EST.

RRS0908

10 9 8 7 6 5 4 3 2 1

To Alice, Rachel and Josh, for their support and encouragement.
JSS

To my wife Deepti and daughters Sonia and Priya for their patience and support.
SM

CONTRIBUTORS

Aysha Arshad, MD

Director, ECG Laboratory and Attending Physician
Al-Sabah Arrhythmia Institute
St. Luke's and Roosevelt Hospitals
Assistant Professor of Medicine
Columbia University College of Physicians and Surgeons
New York, New York

Nitish Badhwar, MBBS

Assistant Professor of Medicine
Department of Cardiac Electrophysiology
University of California
San Francisco, California

Deepak Bhakta, MD

Assistant Professor of Clinical Medicine
Department of Medicine
Indiana University School of Medicine
Staff Cardiac Electrophysiologist
Clarian Health System
Krannert Institute of Cardiology
Indianapolis, Indiana

Noel G. Boyle, MD, PhD

Professor of Medicine
Director, EP Labs
UCLA Cardiac Arrhythmia Center
David Geffen School of Medicine at UCLA
Los Angeles, California

Eric Buch, MD

Director, Specialized Program for Atrial Fibrillation
UCLA Cardiac Arrhythmia Center
David Geffen School of Medicine at UCLA
Los Angeles, California

David J. Callans, MD

Professor
Department of Medicine
University of Pennsylvania
Associate Director of Electrophysiology
University of Pennsylvania Health System
Department of Medicine
Hospital of the University of Pennsylvania
Electrophysiology, Founders 9129
Philadelphia, Pennsylvania

Aman Chugh, MD

Assistant Professor
Department of Internal Medicine—Electrophysiology
University of Michigan
Ann Arbor, Michigan

Andrea Corrado, MD

Cardiovascular Department
Dell'Angelo Hospital
Via Pallagnella
Mestre, Venezia, Italy

Iwona Cygankiewicz, MD, PhD

Visiting Assistant Professor
Heart Research Follow-up Program
Cardiology Division
University of Rochester Medical Center
Rochester, New York
Associate Professor in Medicine
Department of Electrocardiology
Medical University of Lodz, Poland

Marc Dubuc, MD

Associate Professor of Medicine
Université de Montréal
Montreal Heart Institute
Quebec, Canada

Katia Dyrda, MD, MSc, PEng

Electrophysiology Fellow
Montreal Heart Institute
Université de Montréal
Quebec, Canada

Kenneth Ellenbogen, MD

Kontos Professor of Medicine
Vice Chair, Division of Cardiology
Director, Cardiac Electrophysiology
Department of Internal Medicine
Virginia Commonwealth University
Richmond, Virginia

Gianni Gasparini, MD

Cardiovascular Department
Dell'Angelo Hospital
Via Pallagnella
Mestre, Venezia, Italy

Peter G. Guerra, MD

Assistant Professor of Clinical Medicine
Université de Montréal
Head of Clinical Electrophysiology
Montreal Heart Institute
Quebec, Canada

Lorne J. Gula, MD, MS

Professor
Division of Cardiology
University of Western Ontario
Cardiologist
London Health Sciences Center
London, Ontario, Canada

Gautham Kalahasty, MD

Assistant Professor of Medicine
Department of Internal Medicine
Virginia Commonwealth University
Staff Physician Department of Medicine
Medical College of Virginia Hospitals of Virginia Commonwealth University
Richmond, Virginia

Paul Khairy, MD, PhD

Associate Professor of Medicine
Université de Montréal
Montreal Heart Institute
Quebec, Canada

George J. Klein, MD

Professor
Division of Cardiology
University of Western Ontario
Cardiologist
London Health Sciences Center
London, Ontario, Canada

Andrew D. Krahn, MD

Professor
Division of Cardiology
University of Western Ontario
Cardiologist
London Health Sciences Center
London, Ontario, Canada

Shuaib Latif, MD

Electrophysiology Fellow
Hospital of the University of Pennsylvania
Philadelphia, Pennsylvania

Ken W. Lee, MD

Electrophysiologist
Department of Cardiac Electrophysiology
Mt Carmel Columbus Cardiology Consultants
Mt Carmel Hospital and Clinics
Columbus, Ohio

Charles J. Love, MD

Professor of Medicine
Director, Cardiac Rhythm Device Services
Division of Cardiovascular Medicine
The Ohio State University
President, International Board of Heart Rhythm Examiners, Inc.
(Formerly NASPExAM, Inc.)
Columbus, Ohio

Laurent Macle, MD

Associate Professor of Clinical Medicine
Université de Montréal
Montreal Heart Institute
Quebec, Canada

Jaimie Manlucu, MD

Cardiology Fellow
Division of Cardiology
University of Western Ontario
London Health Sciences Center
London, Ontario, Canada

John M. Miller, MD

Professor of Medicine
Department of Medicine
Indiana University School of Medicine
Director, Clinical Cardiac Electrophysiology
Clarian Health System
Krannert Institute of Cardiology
Indianapolis, Indiana

Suneet Mittal, MD

Director, Electrophysiology Laboratory
St. Luke's and Roosevelt Hospitals
Associate Professor of Medicine
Columbia University College of Physicians and Surgeons
New York, New York

Fred Morady, MD

Professor of Internal Medicine
Department of Internal Medicine – Electrophysiology
University of Michigan Ann Arbor, Michigan

Stanley Nattel, MD

Professor of Medicine
Université de Montréal
Head of Electrophysiology Research
Montreal Heart Institute
Quebec, Canada

Mark W. Preminger, MD, FACC

Director, Implantable Device Section
Al-Sabah Arrhythmia Institute
Division of Cardiology
St. Luke's and Roosevelt Hospitals
New York, New York

Antonio Raviele, MD

Chief Cardiovascular Department
Dell'Angelo Hospital
Via Pallagnella
Mestre, Venezia, Italy

Denis Roy, MD

Professor and Executive Vice-Dean of Medicine
Université de Montréal
Montreal Heart Institute
Quebec, Canada

Melvin M. Scheinman, MD

Professor of Medicine
Department of Cardiac Electrophysiology
University of California
San Francisco, California

John A. Scherschel, MD

Senior Fellow in Electrophysiology
Department of Medicine
Indiana University School of Medicine
Senior Cardiac Electrophysiology Fellow
Clarian Health System
Krannert Institute of Cardiology
Indianapolis, Indiana

Kalyanam Shivkumar, MD, PhD

Professor of Medicine and Radiology
Director, UCLA Cardiac Arrhythmia Center
David Geffen School of Medicine at UCLA
Los Angeles, California

Tina Sichrovsky, MD

Attending Physician
Al-Sabah Arrhythmia Institute
St. Luke's and Roosevelt Hospitals
Assistant Professor of Medicine
Columbia University College of Physicians and Surgeons
New York, New York

Allan C. Skanes, MD

Professor
Division of Cardiology
University of Western Ontario
Cardiologist
London Health Sciences Center
London, Ontario, Canada

Jonathan S. Steinberg, MD

Chief, Division of Cardiology
Al-Sabah Endowed Director of Arrhythmia Institute
St. Luke's and Roosevelt Hospitals
Professor of Medicine
Columbia University College of Physicians and Surgeons
New York, New York

Mario Talajic, MD

Professor and Chair of Medicine
Université de Montréal
Montreal Heart Institute
Quebec, Canada

Bernard Thibault, MD

Associate Professor of Clinical Medicine
Université de Montréal
Montreal Heart Institute
Quebec, Canada

Anil V. Yadav, MD

Assistant Professor of Clinical Medicine
Department of Medicine
Indiana University School of Medicine
Staff Cardiac Electrophysiologist
Clarian Health System
Krannert Institute of Cardiology
Indianapolis, Indiana

Raymond Yee, MD

Professor
Division of Cardiology
University of Western Ontario
Cardiologist
London Health Sciences Center
London, Ontario, Canada

Wojciech Zareba, MD, PhD

Professor of Medicine (Cardiology)
Director, Heart Research Follow-up Program
Cardiology Division
University of Rochester Medical Center
Rochester, New York

PREFACE

Cardiac electrophysiology has emerged as a highly specialized and complex segment of cardiovascular care, such that it requires additional focused training, often extending 2 years beyond traditional cardiology fellowship. The reasons for this are multiple and include a need to develop an ability to interpret complex electrophysiologic patterns, master the technical skills necessary for device implantation and catheter ablation, and incorporate a vast array of indications for treatment of a variety of arrhythmic conditions. This substantial knowledge base and skill set can become an intimidating barrier to acquisition of the more modest goals of the cardiology fellow, a basic understanding of arrhythmic mechanisms and clinical presentations, comfort of knowing which patient to refer or not refer for arrhythmia procedures and why, and an ability to interpret and weigh the recommendations of electrophysiology specialists. This is further compounded by the fact that the current training guidelines in the United States require only 2 months of electrophysiology experience, far too little to reach even modest training goals. In addition, the classic textbooks in electrophysiology are far too dense and complex for the noninitiated or for those interested only in a nonelectrophysiology career. Hence, we have designed a textbook specifically for the cardiology fellow faced with these predicaments, deliberately providing material appropriate for the trainee who will pursue a career in general cardiology or one of the nonelectrophysiology cardiology specialties. The topics mirror official training requirements and the text is written for a very well defined target audience who will have to advance through certification examinations. The book is meant to be read and its material mastered during the rotations undertaken by cardiology trainees, or for other interested professionals. The contributors are universally recognized for expertise in their subject matter and have enthusiastically joined in an effort to educate future cardiologists.

Jonathan S. Steinberg, MD
Suneet Mittal, MD

CONTENTS

Contributors iv
Preface viii

SECTION I EVALUATION AND MANAGEMENT

1 Bradycardia 1
Andrea Corrado, Gianni Gasparini, and Antonio Raviele

2 Supraventricular Tachycardia: AVNRT, AVRT 10
Nitish Badhwar, Ken W. Lee, and Melvin M. Scheinman

3 Atrial Arrhythmias 36
Jonathan S. Steinberg, Aysha Arshad, and Tina Sichrovsky

4 Ventricular Tachycardia 65
Shuaib Latif and David J. Callans

5 Syncope 74
Suneet Mittal

6 Sudden Cardiac Death and the Cardiac Arrest Survivor 82
Jaimie Manlucu, Raymond Yee, Lorne J. Gula, George J. Klein, Allan C. Skanes, and Andrew D. Krahn

SECTION II THE ELECTROPHYSIOLOGY LABORATORY

7 Electrophysiology Equipment 95
Mark W. Preminger

8 Electrophysiologic Testing: Indications and Limitations 109
Aman Chugh and Fred Morady

9 Principles of Mapping and Ablation 125
Eric Buch, Noel G. Boyle, and Kalyanam Shivkumar

10 Indications for Cardiac Rhythm Management Devices 137
Gautham Kalahasty and Kenneth Ellenbogen

11 Miscellaneous Procedures 154
Aysha Arshad and Suneet Mittal

SECTION III THE PACEMAKER AND DEFIBRILLATOR CLINIC

12 Device Interrogations and Utilization of Diagnostic Data 169
Charles J. Love

SECTION IV MISCELLANEOUS TOPICS

13 Approach to the Patient with Wide Complex Tachycardia 186
John M. Miller, Deepak Bhakta, John A. Scherschel, and Anil V. Yadav

14 Antiarrhythmic Medications. 195
Katia Dyrda, Paul Khairy, Stanley Nattel, Mario Talajic, Peter G. Guerra, Bernard Thibault, Marc Dubuc, Laurent Macle, and Denis Roy

15 Channelopathies. 210
Iwona Cygankiewicz and Wojciech Zareba

Index 225

SECTION I

Evaluation and Management

CHAPTER 1

Bradycardia

Andrea Corrado, Gianni Gasparini, and Antonio Raviele

SINUS RHYTHM

The electrical activation of the heart originates spontaneously from the cells of the sinoatrial node (SAN), which is situated at the junction between the right atrium and the superior vena cava and has a frequency between 60 and 100 bpm. For this reason, the normal rhythm of the heart is called *sinus rhythm*. If the frequency of the sinus rhythm is lower than 60 or higher than 100 bpm, the term *sinus bradycardia* or *sinus tachycardia* is used (Fig. 1-1).

SINUS BRADYCARDIA

Sinus bradycardia is often a physiological phenomenon, particularly in vagotonic subjects (e.g., athletes). Sometimes it is secondary to the action of pharmaceutical drugs (digitalis, beta-blockers, or calcium antagonists). In some subjects, it may be a manifestation of SAN dysfunction. In the latter case, the bradycardia is more marked (<50 bpm) and is associated with other electrocardiographic expressions of SAN disease, such as sinoatrial block and/or atrial tachyarrhythmia (atrial fibrillation or flutter).

AUTONOMIC BLOCKADE

In order to distinguish sinus bradycardia due to SAN dysfunction from sinus bradycardia due to vagal hypertonia, it may be useful to elicit a so-called autonomic blockade, which involves evaluating the heart rate during the simultaneous administration of a beta-blocker (propranolol 0.2 mg/kg) and atropine (0.04 mg/kg). The objective is to “block” the influence of the autonomic system (sympathetic and parasympathetic) on the heart rate, thereby uncovering the “intrinsic” SAN frequency. The following formula enables us to calculate the heart rate (X) that can be regarded as normal during autonomic blockade:

$$118.1 - (0.57 \times \text{age}) = X \pm 14\% \text{ (normal heart rate)}$$

A heart rate below this value in patients aged less than 45 years (or ±18% in patients >45 years) is indicative of SAN dysfunction.

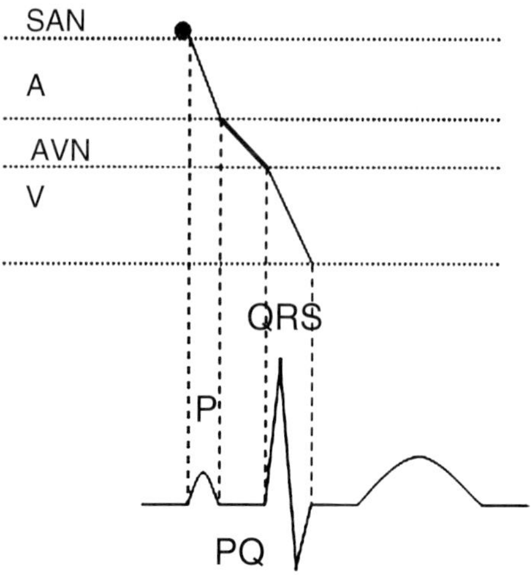

FIGURE 1-1. From the SAN, the impulse travels along preferential pathways made up of specialized fibrous cells to the atria (A), AVN, His bundle and its branches, and finally to the ventricular myocardium (V). This sequence of electrical activation occurs in little more than 200 ms; on the surface ECG, it generates the P wave, the PR interval, and the QRS complex in succession.

SINOATRIAL BLOCK

Sinoatrial block is defined as the lack of transmission to the atria of the impulses generated by the SAN. There are various degrees of sinoatrial block.

***First-degree sinoatrial block*:** Delayed propagation of the impulse from the SAN to the atria (this condition is not recognizable on surface ECG).

***Second-degree Wenckebach sinoatrial block*:** (see Fig. 1-2). In the presence of a "typical" Wenckebach sinoatrial block, three characteristic phenomena can be observed:

- the PP intervals are progressively reduced prior to the pause,
- the pause is less than twice the interval that precedes it, and
- the PP interval following the pause is longer than the PP interval that precedes it.

***Second-degree Mobitz sinoatrial block*:** (see Fig. 1-3). Unlike second-degree Wenckebach sinoatrial block, in this case,

- the PP intervals are not progressively reduced since the pause,
- the pause is equal to twice the interval that precedes it, and
- the PP interval following the pause is not longer than the PP interval that precedes it.

2:1 *sinoatrial block*: (see Fig. 1-4).

***Third-degree sinoatrial block*:** (see Fig. 1-5).

***Sinus arrest*:** The lack of formation of the sinus impulse is a very rare condition. Indeed, it is very unlikely that none of the cells which make up the SAN will be able to generate an electrical impulse. Electrocardiographically, this form is indistinguishable from third-degree sinoatrial block.

SINUS NODE–CORRECTED RECOVERY TIME AND SINOATRIAL CONDUCTION TIME

In patients with clinical and electrocardiographic signs of suspected SAN dysfunction, it may be useful to perform an endocavitary electrophysiological study in order to calculate the corrected sinus node recovery time (CSNRT) and the sinoatrial conduction time (SACT).

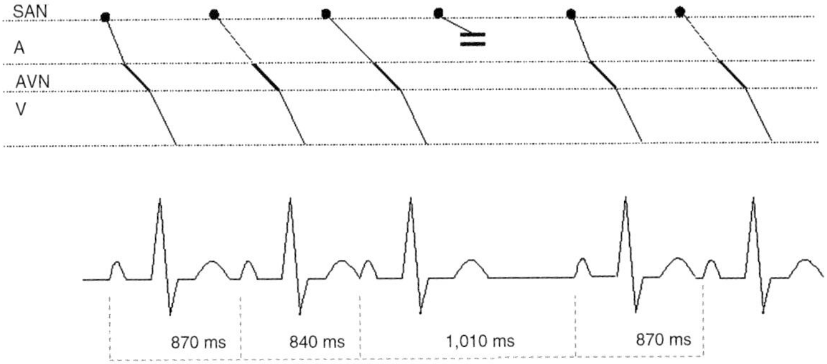

FIGURE 1-2. Second-degree Wenckebach sinoatrial block. Propagation of the impulse from the SAN to the atria progressively slows down and is finally interrupted.

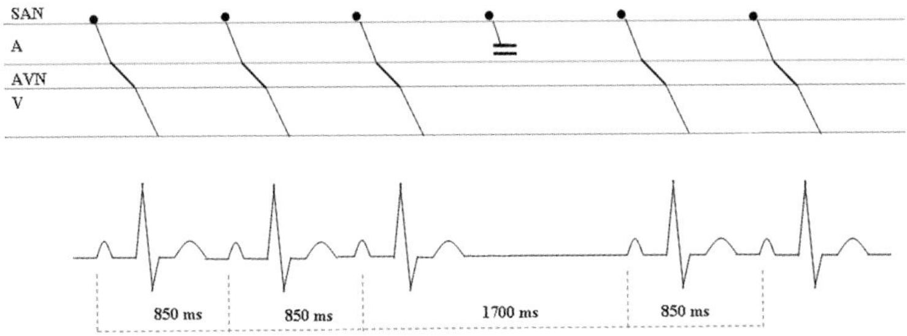

FIGURE 1-3. Second-degree Mobitz sinoatrial block. Sudden lack of conduction of a sinus impulse without progressive lengthening of conduction time.

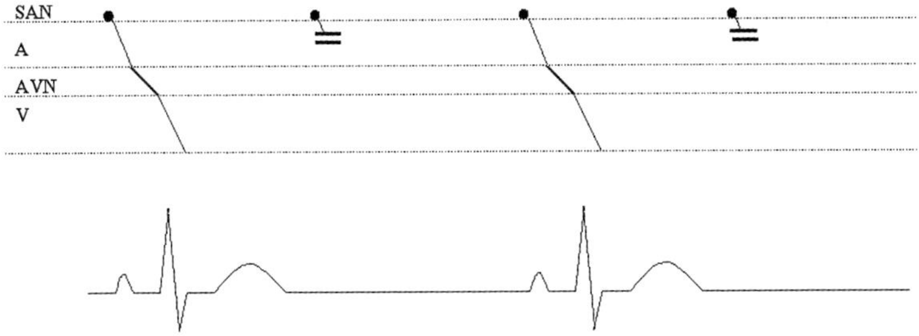

FIGURE 1-4. 2:1 sinoatrial block is characterized by the lack of conduction to the atria of each alternate impulse (on surface ECG, bradycardia is indistinguishable from sinus bradycardia due to reduced SAN automaticity).

***CSNRT*:** (see Fig. 1-6A). The postpacing pause represents the sinus node recovery time (SNRT). This interval is then "corrected" on the basis of the spontaneous rhythm according to the following formula:

SNRT – PP interval during spontaneous rhythm = CSNRT

Therefore in our example: 1470 – 870 ms = 600 ms.

A CSNRT greater than 550 ms is indicative of sinus dysfunction and a CSNRT greater than 1,000 ms is a definitive indication for pacemaker implantation. Moreover, it is advisable to check for the presence of significant pauses in the first ten postpacing beats (so-called secondary pauses), as this finding is also indicative of SAN dysfunction.

SACT**:** (see Fig. 1-6B). The SACT is calculated by applying the following formula:

(postpacing PP return interval – postreturn PP interval)/2 = SACT

Therefore, in our example: (950 – 800 ms)/2 = 75 ms.

An SACT greater than 120 ms is indicative of sinus dysfunction.

Moreover, if SNCRT or SACT is not clearly pathological, a more than 50% increase in these times during provocative testing with ajmaline (1 mg/kg) or flecainide (2 mg/kg) is indicative of SAN dysfunction.

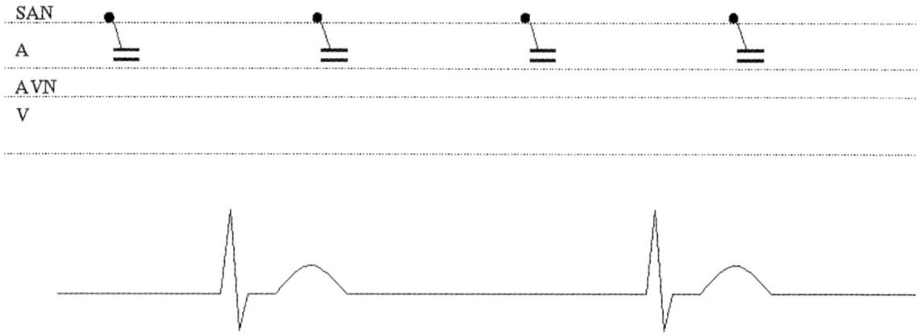

FIGURE 1-5. Third-degree sinoatrial block. In this condition, no sinus impulse is conducted to the atria. In such cases, a junctional escape rhythm generally emerges.

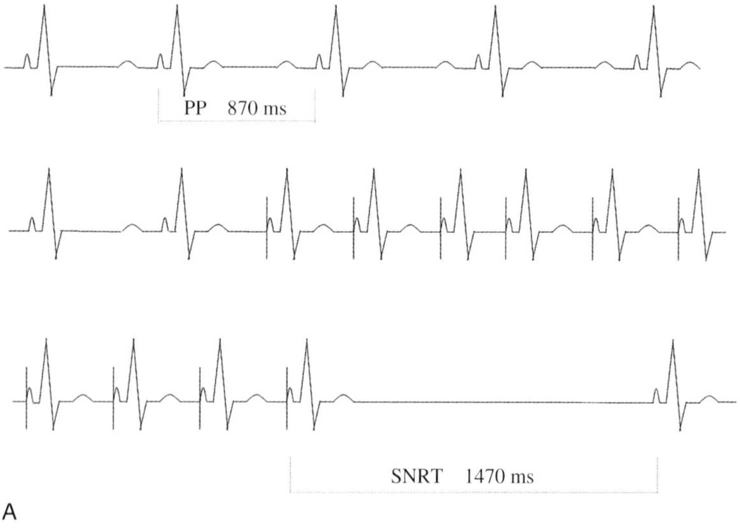

FIGURE 1-6. A: The study protocol for CSNRT evaluation involves applying atrial stimulations programmed at increasing pacing rates (up to max. 170 bpm) for 60 s.

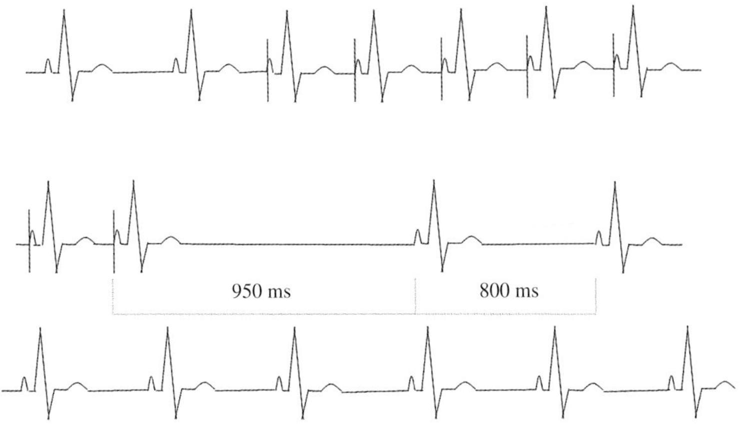

B

FIGURE 1-6. B: There are various protocols for the evaluation of the SACT. According to our studies, the one which is considered most reliable involves continuous atrial stimulation for 8 beats at a frequency of about 10 bpm higher than that of the spontaneous rhythm.

ATRIOVENTRICULAR JUNCTION

The system of atrioventricular conduction is contained within the so-called Koch triangle, which is delimited by the tendon of Todaro, the septal flap of the tricuspid valve, and the ostium of the coronary sinus. The apex of the triangle is constituted by the His bundle. The atrioventricular node (AVN) is located inside this triangle.

ATRIOVENTRICULAR BLOCK

There are different types of atrioventricular block (AVB).

***First-degree AVB*:** This is characterized by a less than 0.20 s lengthening of the PR interval on surface ECG. Strictly speaking, the term "block" is inexact, since in reality it is only a conduction delay.

***Second-degree Wenckebach* AVB:** (see Fig. 1-7).

***Second-degree Mobitz AVB*:** (see Fig. 1-8).

2:1 *AVB*: (see Fig. 1-9).

***Third-degree AVB*:** (see Fig. 1-10).

NODAL BLOCK AND INTRA- OR INFRA-HISIAN BLOCK

AVB may occur in the area of the AVN (*nodal block*, Fig. 1-11) or in the area of the His bundle (*intra- or infra-hisian block*, Fig. 1-12). This is a very important distinction, as there are considerable differences with regard to prognosis and therapy. On surface ECG, a range of findings can suggest the site of the block:

A nodal site is suggested by

– the presence of a narrow QRS,
– the presence of second-degree Wenckebach AVB,
– progression of the degree of block during carotid sinus massage, and
– reduction of the degree of block during atropine infusion or physical exercise.

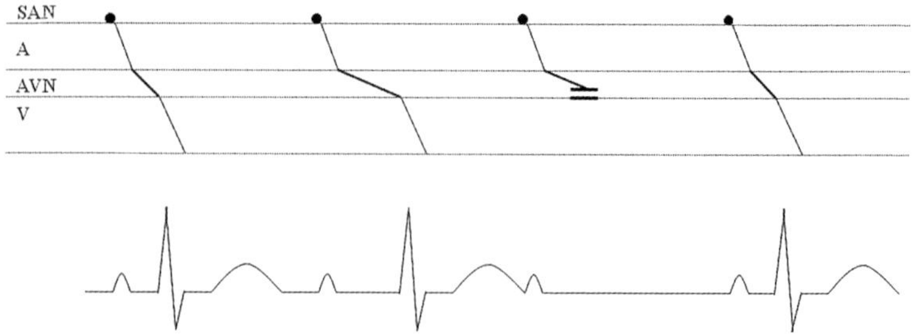

FIGURE 1-7. Second-degree Wenckebach AVB. In this condition, the PR progressively lengthens until a P wave is not followed by a QRS complex and a pause occurs. The sinus impulse that follows the pause is again conducted with a relatively short PR.

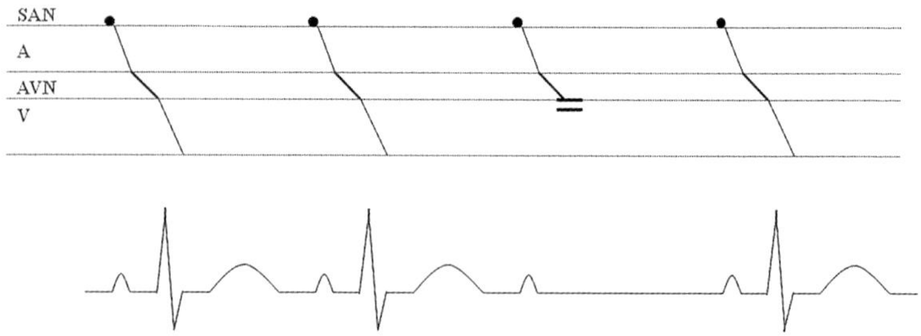

FIGURE 1-8. Second-degree Mobitz AVB. Unlike second-degree Wenckebach AVB, this form exhibits a sudden lack of conduction of a sinus impulse to the ventricles, without previous progressive lengthening of the PR interval.

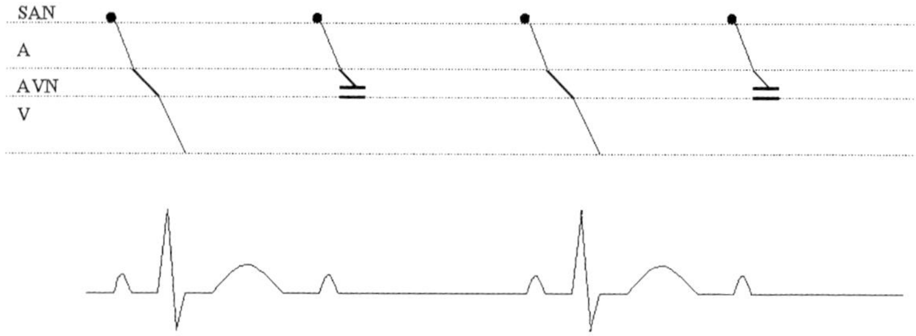

FIGURE 1-9. 2:1 AVB. The sinus impulses are alternately conducted or blocked; only one out of every two P waves is followed by a QRS.

An intra- or infra-hisian site is suggested by

– the presence of a wide QRS (>0.12 s),
– the presence of phases of second-degree Mobitz AVB,
– reduction of the degree of block during carotid sinus massage, and
– progression of the degree of block during atropine infusion or physical exercise.

Accurate location of the site of the block requires endocavitary recording of the hisian electrogram (Fig. 1-13).

The following conduction times are regarded as normal:

AH less than 130 ms
H duration less than 30 ms

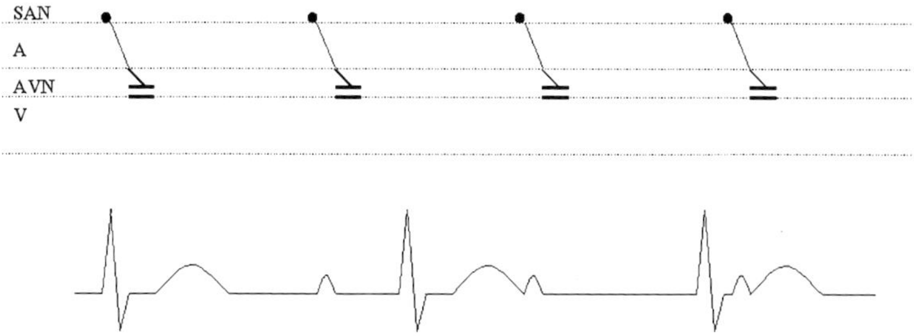

FIGURE 1-10. Third-degree AVB. This is characterized by the lack of conduction of all sinus impulses to the ventricles. In these cases, an escape rhythm emerges, which originates from the atrioventricular junction.

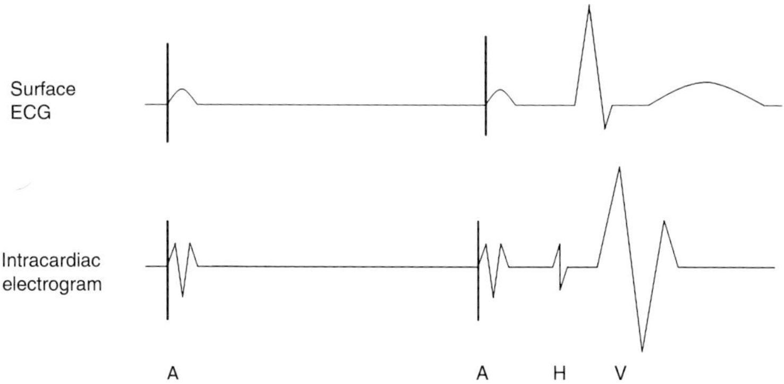

FIGURE 1-11. Nodal AVB.

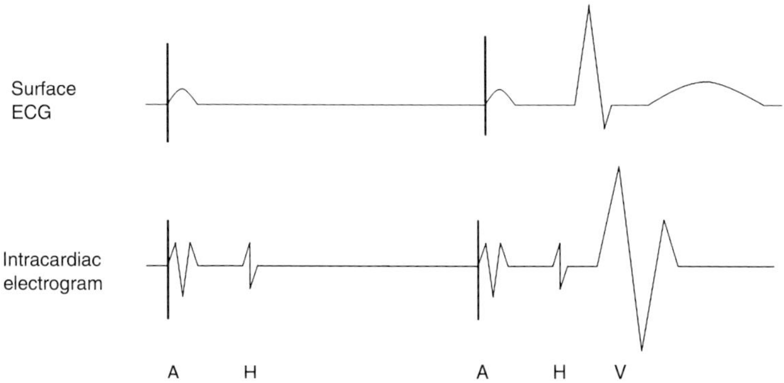

FIGURE 1-12. Intra- or infra-hisian block.

HV less than 55 ms

HV conduction, even if basically normal, can also be investigated during endocavitary electrophysiological study by means of

- incremental atrial pacing up to 2:1 AVB,
- provocative testing with IV ajmaline, IV flecainide, or
- other class I antiarrhythmic drugs.

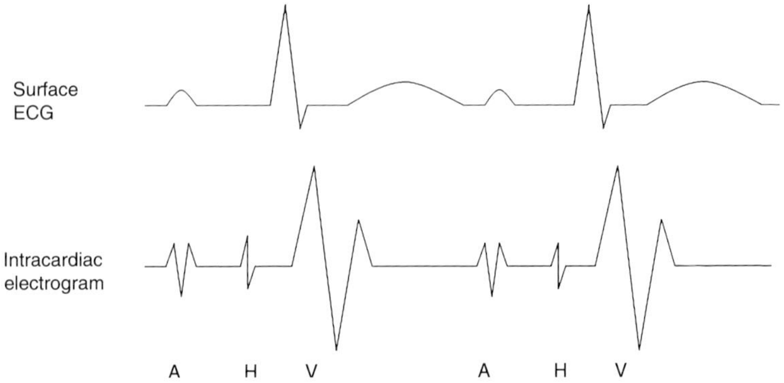

FIGURE 1-13. His-bundle electrogram. Recording from the His-bundle shows a rapid-inscription deflection between the atrium (A) and ventricle (V), which corresponds to the electrical activation of the His (H) bundle. The following conduction times are regarded as normal: AH less than 130 ms, H duration less than 30 ms, HV less than 55 ms.

The finding of pathological intra- or infra-hisian conduction has a great impact on the prognosis and therapy of AVBs. In particular, the presence of an HV greater than 100 ms or the appearance of an intra- or infra-hisian AVB during atrial pacing or during the infusion of class I antiarrhythmic drugs is an indication for pacemaker implantation.

COMMENT REGARDING PREDICTIVE VALUE OF PROVOCATIVE TEST FOR DISCLOSING PATIENTS WITH UNEARTHING SINUS NODE OR ATRIOVENTRICULAR NODE DYSFUNCTION

Predictive value of provocative test as a means of identifying patients at increased risk of future severe sinus node dysfunction or AV block is controversial.

Results of our studies indicate that ajmaline test is a useful provocative test for disclosing patients who will develop severe sinus node dysfunction and for selecting those who need pacemaker implantation. In fact, in our studies the predictive accuracy of ajmaline test, after a mean follow-up of 46 months, was 93%.

Nonphysiological intra- or infra-hisian block induced by atrial pacing or ajmaline test during electrophysiological study is generally considered an indication for pacing. However, failure to induce distal block cannot be taken as evidence that the patient will not develop AV block in the future.

For a more detailed discussion of the indications for pacemaker implantation, the reader should refer to the specific chapter (Chapters 8 and 10).

KEY POINTS

1. **Sinus bradycardia** is often a physiological phenomenon, particularly in vagotonic subjects.
2. In order to distinguish sinus bradycardia due to sinus atrial disfunction from **sinus bradycardia due to vagal hypertonia**, it may be useful to evaluate heart rate during the simultaneous administration of a beta-blocker and atropine (**autonomic blockade**).

(Continued)

3. In order to disclose patients with **unearthing sinus node dysfunction,** it may be useful to perform endocavitary electrophysiological study by means of calculating the **CSNRT and the SACT**.
4. **Sinoatrial block** is defined as the lack of transmission to the atria of the impulses generated by the sinus atrial node. **AVB** is defined as the lack of transmission of the impulses between atria and ventricles. Both have various degrees of block.
5. AVB may occur in the area of the AVN **(nodal AVB)** or in the area of the His bundle **(intra- or infra-hisian AVB)**. On surface ECG, a range of findings can suggest the site of the block. This is a very important distinction, as there are **considerable differences with regard to the prognosis and therapy**.
6. An accurate location of the site of the AVB requires endocavitary recording of the **hisian conduction interval**. The presence of a hisian conduction interval greater than 100 ms is an indication for pacemaker implantation.
7. Even if hisian conduction interval is basically normal, the appearance of an intra- or infra-hisian AVB during **provocative testing with incremental atrial pacing or with class I antiarrhythmic drugs** is an indication for pacemaker implantation.

SUGGESTED READINGS

Bonow L, Zipes M. *Braunwald's Heart Disease: A Textbook of Cardiovascular Medicine*. 8th Ed. Saunders; 2008.

Brignole M, Giada F, Raviele A, et al. Pacing for syncope: What role? Which perspective? *Eur Heart J*. 2007;9:137–143.

Epstein AE, DiMarco JP, Ellenbogen KA, et al. ACC/AHA/HRS 2008 Guidelines for Device-based Therapy of Cardiac Rhythm Abnormalities: A report of the American College of Cardiology/American Heart Association Task Force on Practice Guidelines. *J Am Coll Cardiol*. 2008;27;51(21):e1–e62.

Fuster V, O'Rourke RA, Walsh RA, et al. *Hurst's the Heart*. 8th Ed. McGraw-Hill; 2008.

Josephson ME. *Clinical Cardiac Electrophysiology: Techniques and Interpretations*. 6th Ed. Lippincott Williams & Wilkins; 2008.

Narula OS. *Cardiac Arrhythmias: Electrophysiology, Diagnosis and Management*. Baltimore-London: Williams & Wilkins; 1979.

Raviele A, D'Este D, Sartori F, et al. The reliability of Narula's technique for the evaluation of sino-atrial conduction time. Comparison with Strauss' technique and proposal of a new equation. *G Ital Cardiol*. 1980;10:290–300.

Raviele A, Di Pede F, Callegari E, et al. Ajmaline test for the evaluation of sinus node function in man. *G Ital Cardiol*. 1981;11:1669–1683.

Raviele A, Di Pede F, Zanocco A, et al. Predictive value of ajmaline test in sinus node dysfunctions. A four-year prospective follow-up of 77 cases. *G Ital Cardiol*. 1985;15:751–760.

Raviele A, Di Pede F, Zuin G, et al. Clinical significance of corrected sinus node recovery time and natural and unnatural history of sinus node dysfunctions. A four-year prospective follow-up of 101 cases. *G Ital Cardiol*. 1982;12:563–574.

Raviele A, Sartori F, D'Este D, et al. Clinical value of sino-atrial conduction time. *G Ital Cardiol*. 1979;9:344–357.

CHAPTER 2

Supraventricular Tachycardia: AVNRT, AVRT

Nitish Badhwar, Ken W. Lee, and Melvin M. Scheinman

Supraventricular tachycardias (SVTs) denote all tachyarrhythmias that originate from the supraventricular tissue or require it to be a part of the reentrant circuit. *Paroxysmal* supraventricular tachycardia (PSVT) denotes a clinical syndrome characterized by a rapid tachycardia with an abrupt onset and termination. These arrhythmias are frequently encountered in otherwise healthy patients without structural heart disease. Recognition, identification, and differentiation of the various SVTs are of great importance in formulating an optimal treatment strategy.

While much of the early knowledge of SVTs was derived from surface ECG recordings, it was the monumental works of Coumel, Durrer, Josephson, Jackman, Scherlag, and Wellens that yielded important mechanistic and therapeutic insights into these rhythm disturbances. Some of the seminal developments in this field include the introduction of reliable intracardiac His bundle recording and programmed electrical stimulation in the 1960s, the first successful surgical ablation of an accessory pathway (AP) in a patient in 1968, the first catheter-based ablation of an arrhythmia in a human being in 1981, and the development of radiofrequency catheter ablation (RFCA) in 1986.

The mechanism responsible for the majority of arrhythmias including SVTs is reentry, while a small proportion is due to triggered activity or abnormal automaticity. Reentry requires two distinct pathways that have different speeds of conduction (slow and fast) and varying recovery times (refractoriness). Extra, early beats, such as premature atrial or ventricular contractions (PACs or PVCs), may fail to conduct down the normal (fast conducting but slow to recover) pathway but can travel down the fast recovering but slow conducting pathway. At the distal junction of the two pathways, the arriving slow impulse then returns in a retrograde fashion up the now recovered fast normal pathway. This completes the circuit with activation of the myocardial tissue at each end of the pathway. RFCA successfully eliminates the extra pathway by the application of thermal energy typically leaving only normal conduction.

EPIDEMIOLOGY

The prevalence of SVT is estimated to be 570,000 in the US population with about 89,000 new cases diagnosed annually. Based on data from the Marshfield Epidemiologic Study Area (MESA) study, the average age of onset of SVT is 57 years (range: infancy to 90 years old). The three most common causes of PSVT include atrioventricular nodal reentrant tachycardia (AVNRT) (56%), followed by atrioventricular reentrant tachycardia (AVRT) (27%) and atrial tachycardia (AT) (17%).

Mechanism of SVT also appears to be influenced by age and gender. SVT using APs (73%) are most common in the pediatric population. The age of onset of symptoms in patients with AVNRT is almost a decade later than those with AP-mediated tachycardias. Studies have shown that the incidence and prevalence of SVTs increases with advancing age, patients ≥65 years old are five times more likely to develop symptomatic SVT than those less than 65 years old. For all age groups, women are twice more likely to develop SVT than men. Wolff-Parkinson-White (WPW) syndrome tends to be more frequent in males than females, although the difference is reduced with increasing age due to the loss of pre-excitation. It is also known that patients with WPW who have concomitant atrial and ventricular fibrillation were more likely to be male. In contrast, both AVNRT and AT are more frequent in females than males.

CLINICAL PRESENTATION

SVT is usually regular with a heart rate of 160 to 200 bpm, but the rate can range from 80 to 240 bpm. Tachycardias are usually not life threatening and are associated with an aborted sudden death rate of 2% to 4.5%. However, they are responsible for a wide spectrum of symptoms including palpitations, dyspnea, chest pain, anxiety, and syncope. Patients with a SVT rate ≥170 bpm were more likely to have presyncope and syncope. Although most SVTs occur in patients without organic heart disease, they may also occur in patients with ischemic heart disease, valvular stenosis, or reduced left ventricular function. In these instances, the tachycardia episode can precipitate myocardial ischemia and heart failure. In rare instances, paroxysmal SVT may result in cardiac arrest in which the culprit tachyarrhythmia (usually atrial fibrillation or atrial flutter) conducts rapidly over an AP. When incessant, SVT may cause cardiomyopathy, although the cardiomyopathy may be reversible when the tachyarrhythmia is treated expeditiously. Paroxysmal SVT symptoms may at times be triggered by physical or psychological stress.

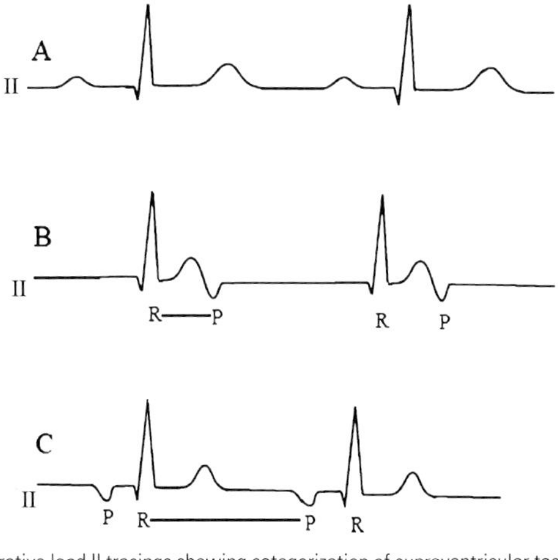

FIGURE 2-1. Illustrative lead II tracings showing categorization of supraventricular tachycardias into short RP (tracing **B**, RP < PR) versus long RP tachycardias (tracing **C**, RP > PR). Tracing **A** shows normal sinus rhythm. (Reprinted from Lee KW, Badhwar N, Scheinman MM. Supraventricular tachycardia-I. *Curr Probl Cardiol.* Sep 2008;33(9):467–546, Copyright (2008).)

In premenopausal women, attacks may be related to menses. Physical findings during paroxysmal SVT usually include a rapid, regular pulse.

Resting 12-lead ECG should be examined for rhythm disturbances, P wave morphologies, premature supraventricular complexes, PR interval abnormalities (e.g., very short, or a sudden prolongation in the presence of a premature supraventricular complex), delta waves, ST-segment/T wave abnormalities, and any evidence of structural heart disease. The presence of overt pre-excitation implicates AVRT as the culprit tachycardia. The 12-lead ECG during SVT provides important diagnostic information and should be obtained as long as hemodynamic stability is not compromised. If the ECG is not available, a rhythm strip can be helpful. While most SVTs present as a narrow-complex (QRS $\leq$ 120 ms) tachycardia, they can also present as a wide-complex (QRS > 120 ms) tachycardia as a result of (i) functional or preexisting bundle branch block or (ii) pre-excitation, either from a bystander pathway or as part of the circuit in the case of an antidromic tachycardia. Both the regularity of the QRS complexes and the relationship of the P waves to the onset of QRS complexes during the tachycardia provide important diagnostic information. Figure 2-1 illustrates the relationship of the visible P waves to the QRS complexes as a SVT discriminator (long vs. short RP). Table 2-1 provides a categorization of SVTs based on the regularity of the tachycardia and the RP versus PR relationship.

Evaluation methods such as history, physical examination, and ECG provide a diagnosis in only 50% of patients with symptoms such as palpitations, presyncope, and syncope. If exercise consistently triggers the arrhythmia, exercise stress testing may be needed to elicit the rhythm abnormality. Ambulatory ECG recordings and cardiac electrophysiologic (EP) studies may be needed to obtain additional diagnostic information. Depending on the frequency of symptoms, specific ambulatory and implantable ECG recording devices can be used for arrhythmia detection. Patients with frequent symptoms (approx. three to four times per week) can be monitored with a 24- or 48-h Holter recording. Those with less frequent symptoms (approx. three to four times per month) can be monitored with a continuous loop event recorder. Finally, patients with rare (a few times per year) or unpredictable symptoms, or those with potential hemodynamic instability during an episode, can be monitored with a subcutaneously implantable loop recorder.

TABLE 2-1 Categorization of Narrow-complex Supraventricular Tachycardias Based on Regularity of QRS Complexes and RP versus PR Relationship on the ECG

Regular QRS Complexes	Irregular QRS Complexes
Short RP:	Atrial tachycardia with variable AV conduction
Typical (slow-fast) AVNRT	Multifocal atrial tachycardia
Orthodromic AVRT	Atrial flutter with variable AV conduction
Atypical (slow-slow) AVNRT (rare)	Atrial fibrillation
Junctional tachycardia	
AT (rare)	
Long RP:	
Atrial tachycardia (more common)	
Atypical (fast-slow) AVNRT	
Permanent junctional reciprocating tachycardia	
Sinus tachycardia	

Short RP denotes RP less than PR; long RP denotes RP greater than PR.

Source: Reprinted from Lee KW, Badhwar N, Scheinman MM. Supraventricular tachycardia-I. *Curr Probl Cardiol.* Sep 2008;33(9):467–546, Copyright (2008).

ATRIOVENTRICULAR NODAL REENTRANT TACHYCARDIA

ELECTROPHYSIOLOGY

AVNRT is the most common regular, narrow-complex tachycardia. The compact AV node is 5 to 7 mm in length and 2 to 5 mm in width and is located within the triangle of Koch (bounded by the tendon of Todaro, septal leaflet of the tricuspid valve, and coronary sinus [CS] ostium). At the atrial aspect of the compact node is a zone of transitional cells that are interposed between the compact node and atrial myocardium. Distal to the node are the penetrating bundle of His and bundle branches which are tracts of specialized cells encased by insulating sheaths of fibrous tissue (central fibrous body). Nodelike tissue extends posteriorly both anterior to the CS (right posterior extension) as well as leftward toward the mitral annulus (left posterior extension). There is excellent evidence suggesting that the right posterior nodal extension is involved in the tachycardia circuit (slow pathway). On rare occasions, the tachycardia circuit may involve the left posterior nodal extension in which case a left-sided ablative procedure is required.

A working model used to explain the EP behavior of the AVNRT circuit involves two pathways: one pathway is the so-called *fast pathway* which conducts more rapidly (PR interval 100 to 150 ms) and has a relatively longer refractory period, while the other pathway is the "*slow pathway*" which conducts more slowly (PR interval > 200 ms) and has a relatively shorter refractory period. The fast pathway constitutes the normal, physiological, AV conduction axis. In most patients, the fast pathway is located superiorly and anteriorly in the triangle of Koch, while the slow pathway is located inferiorly and posteriorly and is close to the CS ostium (right posterior nodal extension) (Figs. 2-2 and 2-3).

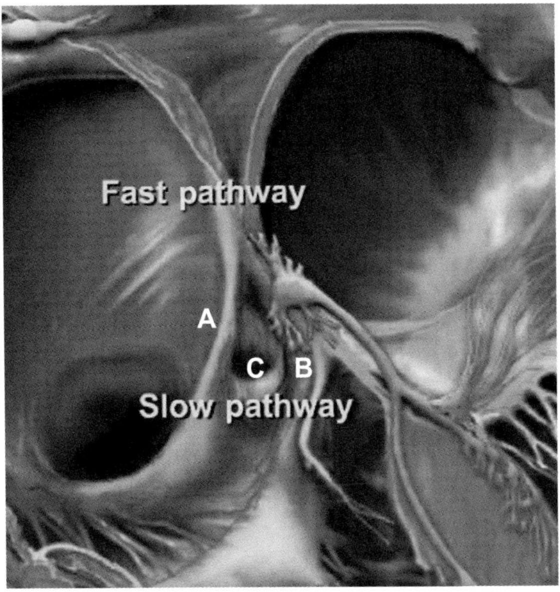

FIGURE 2-2. Anatomy of the AV junction, including landmarks of the triangle of Koch (bounded by the tendon of Todaro [**A**], septal leaflet of the tricuspid valve [**B**], and CS ostium [**C**]). Locations of the fast and slow pathways are labeled. Coronary sinus, CS. (Reproduced with permission from David Criley.)

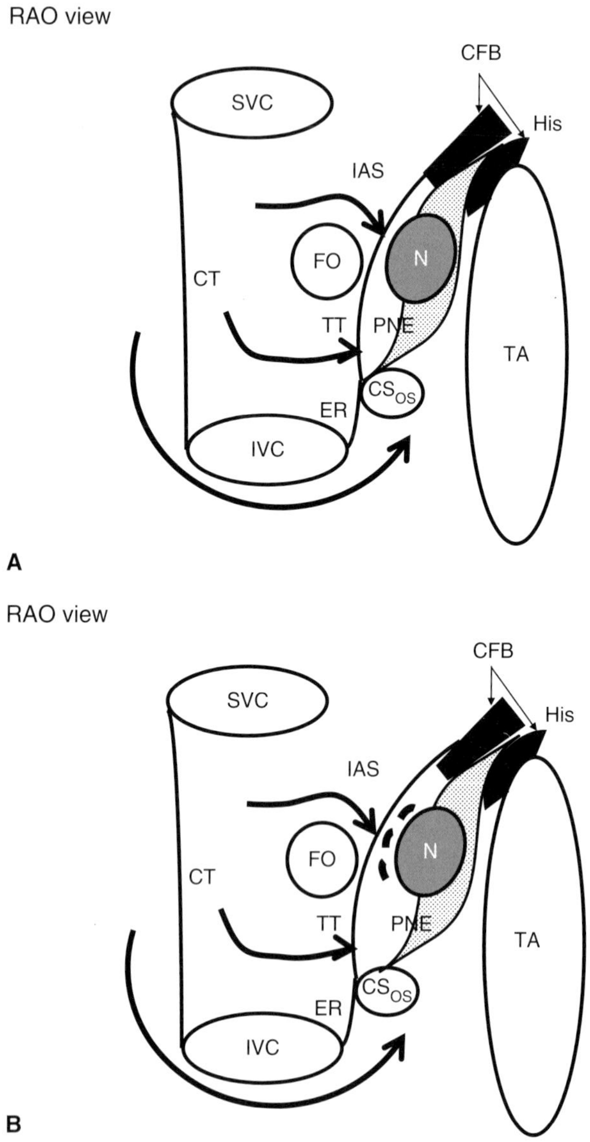

FIGURE 2-3. Diagram of a sinus impulse conducting over the fast and slow pathways **(A)**; a premature atrial complex resulting in conduction block at the fast pathway with conduction solely over the slow pathway **(B)**; atrial echo due to retrograde conduction over the fast pathway **(C)**. Atrial structures: SVC, superior vena cava; CT, crista terminalis; IVC, inferior vena cava; IAS, interatrial septum; FO, fossa ovalis; TT, tendon of Todaro; PNE, posterior nodal extension; CS_{os}, coronary sinus ostium; ER, eustachian ridge; TA, tricuspid ridge; His, bundle of His; N, compact AV node; CFB, central fibrous body. (Reprinted from Lee KW, Badhwar N, Scheinman MM. Supraventricular tachycardia-I. *Curr Probl Cardiol.* Sep 2008;33(9):467–546, Copyright (2008).)

RAO view

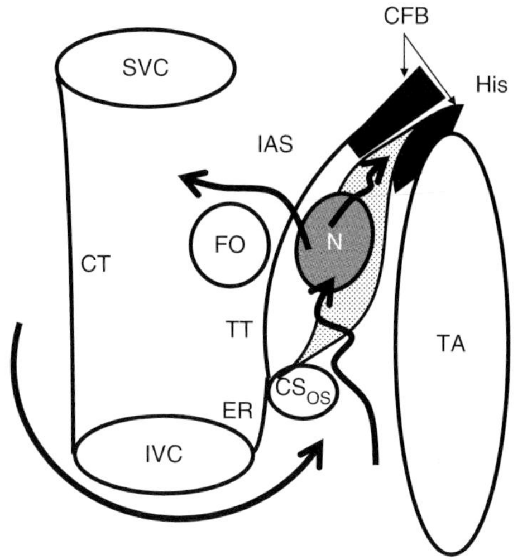

C

FIGURE 2-3. Cont'd.

Dual pathways can be demonstrated in the EP laboratory with delivery of a premature atrial complex that results in a "jump" (>50 ms increase in AH interval with a 10 ms increase in prematurity) in the AH conduction curve. This "jump" is due to antegrade block in the fast pathway with conduction over the slow pathway (Fig. 2-4). On the surface ECG, this "jump" manifests as a sudden prolongation in the PR interval.

Traditionally, AVNRT has been categorized into *typical* or *atypical*. If the retrograde limb of the circuit is the fast pathway, it is deemed *typical*; if it is slow, it is *atypical*. Typical AVNRT is much more common (90%) and involves a slowly conducting antegrade limb with a rapidly conducting retrograde limb (*slow-fast* variant). In contrast, atypical AVNRT is much less common (10%) and includes the *fast-slow* and *slow-slow* variants. Typical AVNRT is usually initiated by a PAC that blocks in the fast pathway and conducts over the slow pathway. If enough time has elapsed such that the fast pathway has recovered excitability, the impulse can conduct retrogradely over the fast pathway, resulting in an echo (Fig. 2-3). If the impulse reenters into the slow pathway, AVNRT may be initiated (Figs. 2-5 and 2-6). Since the atrium and ventricle are activated simultaneously during the tachycardia, the retrograde P wave is either hidden within the QRS or embedded in the terminal portion of the QRS resulting in RP less than PR with *pseudo r'* waves in lead V1 (Fig. 2-7) and *pseudo s'* waves in the inferior leads. In most cases, typical AVNRT can be initiated by single or multiple PACs. On rare occasions, the tachycardia can be initiated by single or multiple PVCs. It is important to note that although typical AVNRT is usually associated with earliest retrograde atrial activation in the His electrogram, earliest retrograde atrial activation at the CS ostium has also been observed due to a posteriorly located fast pathway (8% of cases). Such a transposition of the anatomic locations of the slow and fast pathways has important implications in slow pathway ablation.

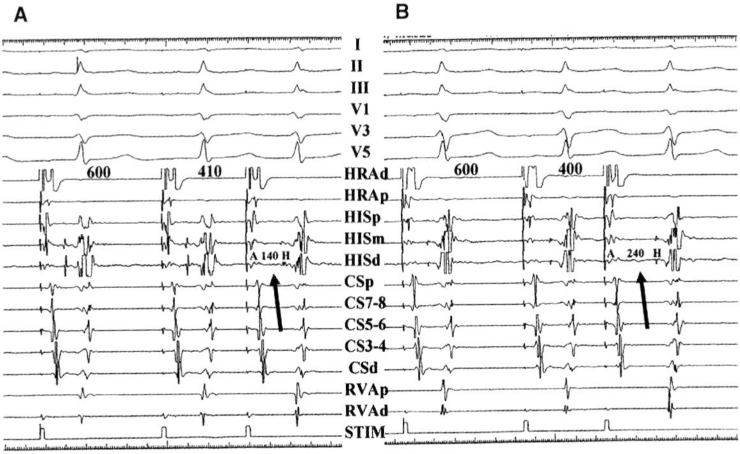

FIGURE 2-4. A patient with dual AV nodal pathways demonstrated by delivery of a single atrial extrastimulus from the distal high right atrium: a 10-ms increase in atrial stimulus prematurity resulted in an AH "jump" greater than 50 ms (140 to 240 ms denoted by *arrows*) **(A, B)**. Surface and intracardiac recording arrangement: ECG leads I, II, III, V1, V3, and V5 on top, followed by intracardiac electrograms distal high right atrium bipole (HRAd), proximal high right atrium (HRAp), proximal His (HISp), middle His (HISm), distal His (HISd), proximal coronary sinus bipole (CSp), seven to eight bipole coronary sinus (CS7 to 8), five to six bipole coronary sinus (CS5 to 6), three to four bipole coronary sinus (CS3 to 4), distal coronary sinus (CSd), proximal right ventricular apex (RVAp), distal right ventricular apex (RVAd), stimulation channel (STIM). (Reprinted from Lee KW, Badhwar N, Scheinman MM. Supraventricular tachycardia-I. *Curr Probl Cardiol*. Sep 2008;33(9):467–546, Copyright (2008).)

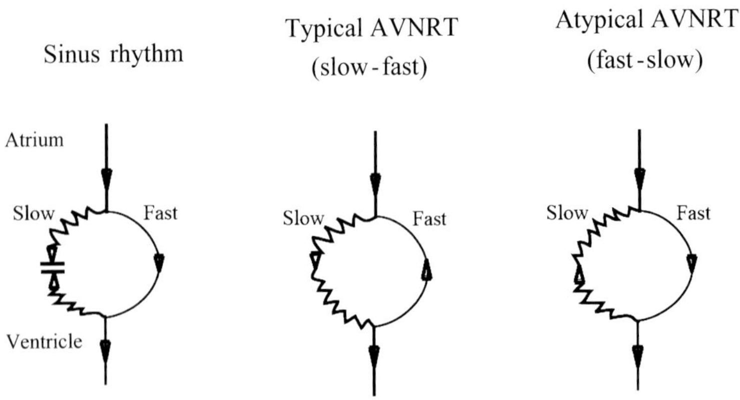

FIGURE 2-5. Simplified schematic diagram of the AVNRT reentrant circuit. During sinus rhythm **(left panel)**, the impulse conducts antegrade over the fast pathway and retrogradely penetrates the slow pathway, concealing antegrade slow pathway conduction. During typical AVNRT **(center panel)**, the impulse finds the fast pathway refractory and conducts over the slow pathway. When the fast pathway has recovered excitability, the impulse is able to rapidly conduct up the fast pathway while also traveling down to activate the ventricle; hence, the atrium and ventricle are activated simultaneously. During atypical AVNRT **(right panel)**, the impulse conducts down the fast pathway and up the slow pathway; here, the atrium is activated after the ventricle. (Reprinted from Lee KW, Badhwar N, Scheinman MM. Supraventricular tachycardia-I. *Curr Probl Cardiol*. Sep 2008;33(9):467–546, Copyright (2008).)

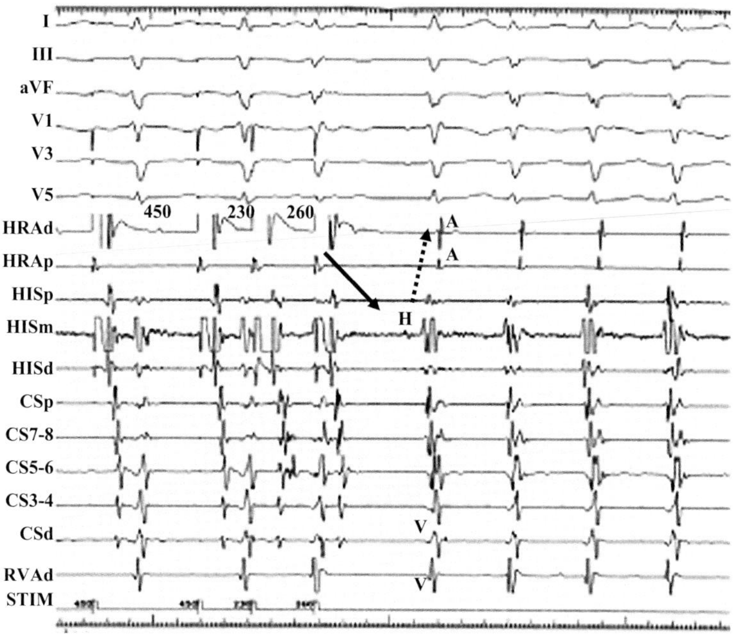

FIGURE 2-6. Typical AVNRT (slow-fast) initiated with double atrial extrastimuli from the distal HRA (450–230–260 ms) resulting in antegrade conduction down the slow pathway (*bold arrow*) and retrograde conduction up the fast pathway (*dashed arrow*). During the tachycardia, the atrium and ventricle are activated simultaneously, resulting in an "A on V" tachycardia. Surface and intracardiac recording arrangement same as Fig. 2-4. (Reprinted from Lee KW, Badhwar N, Scheinman MM. Supraventricular tachycardia-I. *Curr Probl Cardiol*. Sep 2008;33(9):467–546, Copyright (2008).)

Atypical AVNRT may be initiated by a PAC that blocks in the slow pathway and conducts antegrade over the fast pathway with subsequent retrograde conduction over the slow pathway (fast-slow variant, Fig. 2-5). More commonly, the fast-slow variant of atypical AVNRT is initiated by PVC that blocks in the fast pathway; the impulse then conducts to the atrium via the slow pathway, and returns to the ventricle via the fast pathway. Since the atrium is activated late relative to the ventricle, the RP interval is greater than PR. Retrograde P waves are usually discernible and are usually positive in V1 and always negative in inferior leads (Fig. 2-8). In atypical AVNRT, earliest retrograde atrial activation is usually seen in the slow pathway region (posterior septum). However, unusual cases of atypical AVNRT associated with an earliest retrograde atrial activation recorded at the anterior and mid septum (middle type) have been reported.

Sometimes in the EP laboratory, tachycardia may not be readily initiated with programmed stimulation alone in the baseline state and pharmacologic augmentation of autonomic tone may be needed. Drugs commonly used in this situation include isoproterenol, atropine, and phenylephrine. Isoproterenol facilitates initiation of AVNRT by shortening the refractory period of the retrograde fast pathway while prolonging antegrade slow pathway conduction. Isoproterenol can be especially helpful in initiating tachycardia in patients without baseline VA conduction.

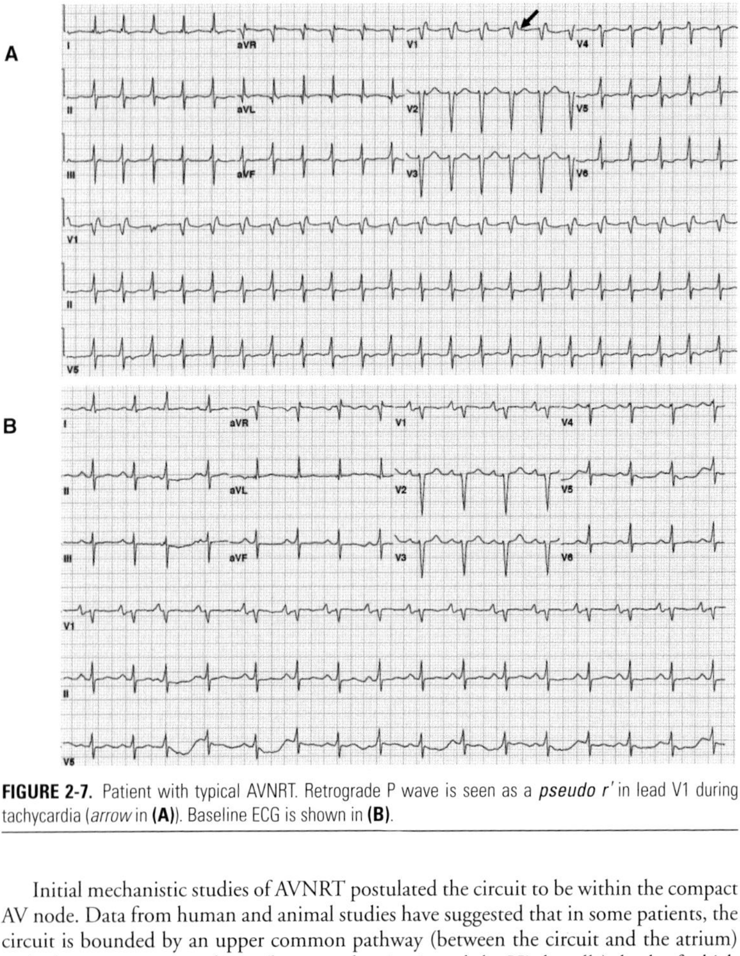

FIGURE 2-7. Patient with typical AVNRT. Retrograde P wave is seen as a ***pseudo** r'* in lead V1 during tachycardia (*arrow* in **(A)**). Baseline ECG is shown in **(B)**.

Initial mechanistic studies of AVNRT postulated the circuit to be within the compact AV node. Data from human and animal studies have suggested that in some patients, the circuit is bounded by an upper common pathway (between the circuit and the atrium) and a lower common pathway (between the circuit and the His bundle), both of which have AV nodal properties. These pathways are believed to gate-keep atrial and ventricular inputs into the circuit. This may explain the finding that in some cases, there is variable success in entrainment of the AVNRT circuit when pacing from various atrial sites, and on rare occasions, neither atrial nor ventricular complexes or extrastimuli are able to penetrate the circuit. More recently, some investigators have accumulated clinical data suggesting the importance of left atrial inputs to the circuit. For either typical or atypical form of AVNRT, antegrade conduction appears to use the right posterior nodal extension, but on rare occasions, the circuit appears to be entirely localized to the LA and can be cured only by ablation within the CS or at the mitral annulus.

PHARMACOLOGIC TREATMENT

Patients with hemodynamic compromise should be electrically cardioverted without delay. In most cases, the tachycardia does not cause significant hemodynamic compromise. Vagal maneuvers can be used to safely and rapidly terminate the tachycardia.

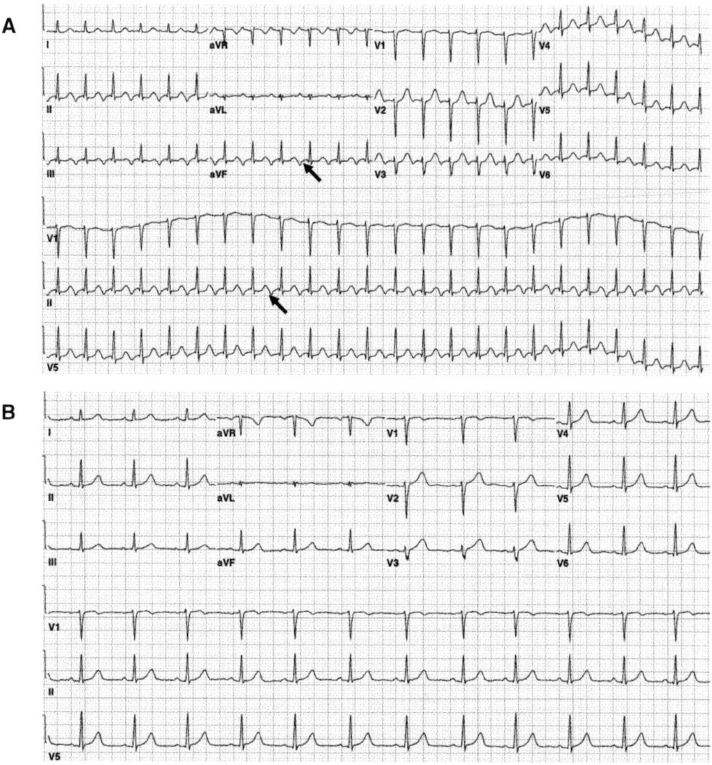

FIGURE 2-8. Patient with atypical (fast-slow) AVNRT. Retrograde P waves are seen in V1 and II, III, aVF during tachycardia (*arrows* in **(A)**). Note the P waves are positive in V1 and negative in the inferior leads. Baseline ECG is shown in **(B)**.

They transiently prolong AV nodal refractoriness and conduction resulting in a block in the antegrade slow pathway in the typical AVNRT circuit or block in either the antegrade or retrograde slow pathway in the atypical AVNRT circuit. Examples of vagal maneuvers include "gag reflex" (finger in the throat), "dive reflex" (facial immersion in cold water), "upside down positive" (legs against the wall), Valsalva maneuver, Müller maneuver, and carotid sinus massage. These maneuvers can be taught to the patient. In the elderly and in those with suspected carotid disease, the carotid sinus massage should be used with caution or avoided altogether.

When vagal maneuvers are ineffective, medications known to prolong refractoriness in the antegrade limb of the AVNRT circuit can be used. These agents include intravenous (IV) calcium-channel blockers (verapamil, diltiazem), beta-blockers (metoprolol, atenolol, propranolol, and esmolol), and adenosine. They should be administered with continuous ECG monitoring. IV adenosine also has a rapid onset of action with an extremely short half-life (1 to 10 s) and is very effective in terminating this tachycardia. Because of its high efficacy and short duration of action, adenosine may be a good option to effect tachycardia termination in patients with impaired left ventricular function.

Caution should be exercised in the use of IV verapamil in patients with impaired left ventricular function and in those with wide-complex tachycardia possibly due to VT. Adenosine usually causes mild adverse effects that are of short duration (<30 s), although in patients with severe reactive airway disease, this drug should be used with caution. Use of digoxin in the acute management of SVT is very limited and is ineffective because of its delayed onset of action, narrow therapeutic window, and interactions with other antiarrhythmic agents, as well as lack of efficacy due to already heightened sympathetic tone in the patient with SVT.

Long-term medical treatment of patients with AVNRT should be individualized. Drug treatment may be deferred in an individual with a first episode of well-tolerated tachycardia. On the other hand, drug treatment should be considered in patients with significant symptoms, coronary artery disease, syncope (even if it is rare), and in those who require emergency room visits or hospital admissions. In the case of typical AVNRT, strategic target of antiarrhythmic drug therapy includes the antegrade limb (slow pathway), retrograde limb (fast pathway), or both limbs. Drugs that mainly affect the antegrade limb include calcium-channel blockers, beta-blockers, digoxin (rarely used), while those that mainly affect the retrograde limb include flecainide, propafenone, procainamide, disopyramide, and quinidine. Class III drugs amiodarone and sotalol affect both limbs. For patients with infrequent tachycardia episodes and mild symptoms, out-of-the hospital administration of oral antiarrhythmic agents, or "pill in the pocket approach," has been reported. Single doses of diltiazem or propranolol have been reported to be efficacious.

CATHETER ABLATION

Factors such as the cost, adverse and potentially proarrhythmic effects, and inconvenience associated with long-term drug treatment of AVNRT combined with the efficacy and safety associated with catheter-based ablation have resulted in increased use of curative ablation for patients with AVNRT. In some patients, catheter ablation is used as a first-line therapy. It is not uncommon that the documented SVT is not inducible in the EP laboratory, despite the administration of isoproterenol and/or atropine. Catheter ablation for AVNRT is highly effective (>95% success rate at >1 year of follow-up) in elimination of SVT in patients with documented but noninducible SVT who are found to have dual AV nodal pathways or single AV nodal echo beats in the EP laboratory.

It is conceivable from the discussion above on the AVNRT circuit that ablation of either the fast or slow pathways may lead to interruption of the circuit and elimination of the arrhythmia. When RFCA was first used to ablate AVNRT, the fast pathway was targeted, and this was associated with a success rate of 80% to 90% but a risk of AV block as high as 20%. Today, fast pathway ablation (so-called anterior approach) is no longer the procedure of choice; it has been replaced by slow pathway ablation (so-called posterior approach) with a very high success rate and a very low risk of AV block. Among experienced centers, acute success rate approaches 99% with a 0.4% to 1% risk of AV block requiring pacemaker implant.

In slow pathway ablation, RF lesions are usually applied to right atrial posteroseptal sites that are close to the CS ostium. The safest and most effective approach appears to be a combined anatomic-electrogram approach in which RF lesions are applied at posteroseptal sites with slow pathway potentials (Fig. 2-9). Acute success of AVNRT ablation is predicated on noninducibility of the tachycardia. The goal in slow pathway ablation is to modify, but not necessarily eliminate, slow pathway conduction so that the arrhythmia is no longer inducible. Hence, the presence of residual dual antegrade AV nodal pathways and single AV nodal echoes may be acceptable therapeutic end points as long as AVNRT is noninducible. Effective delivery of RF energy to the slow pathway site is usually manifested as a junctional ectopic rhythm that is attributed to heating of the AV nodal cells with intrinsic pacemaker activity. While the duration of junctional ectopy is predictive of

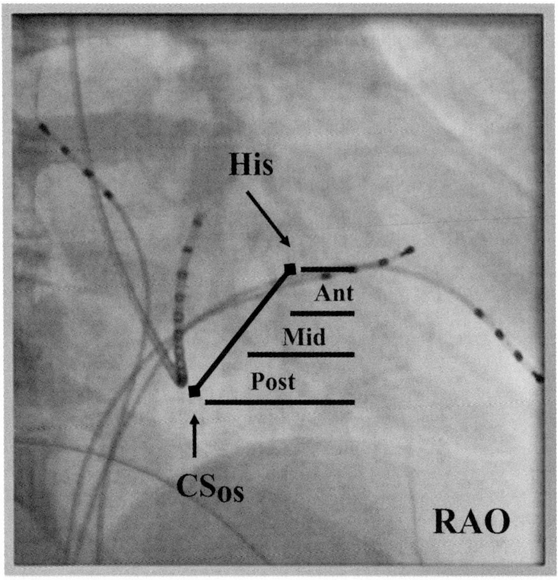

FIGURE 2-9. Anatomic approach to slow pathway ablation in AVNRT. The septal aspect of the tricuspid annulus from the CS ostium to the His bundle is divided in posterior (Post), mid (Mid), and anterior (Ant) sections (from the RAO view). The ablation catheter is initially placed in the posterior section and RF applications are started here. Successful ablation may require progressive advancement of the ablation catheter to the mid and then to the anterior sites with increased risk of AV block in the more superior and anterior sites. Coronary sinus, CS. (Reprinted from Lee KW, Badhwar N, Scheinman MM. Supraventricular tachycardia-I. *Curr Probl Cardiol.* Sep 2008;33(9):467–546, Copyright (2008).)

successful ablation, fast junctional ectopy has been implicated as a marker of AV nodal injury and impending AV block. A consistent increase in AV Wenckebach cycle length can also be taken as a reliable marker of elimination of slow pathway conduction and successful AVNRT ablation.

On rare occasions, despite apparently successful AV nodal modification for AVNRT, patients may report recurrent tachycardia symptoms. Sometimes these symptoms may initially be worse than the preablation ones. Although this may be due to a recurrence of AVNRT, in some cases, patients may actually have inappropriate sinus tachycardia. Ambulatory ECG monitoring can be used to confirm the diagnosis. Inappropriate sinus tachycardia has also been reported to occur after RF ablation of APs. This arrhythmia does not appear to be of major clinical significance and usually resolves spontaneously in 1 to 2 months. In rare cases, tachycardia symptoms may last much longer requiring treatment with beta-blockers.

While the risk of AV block from selective slow pathway modification of AVNRT in patients with normal baseline PR interval is very low, reports have suggested that the risk may be higher in patients with preexisting PR prolongation, especially in those with (i) a markedly prolonged PR interval (≥300 ms) at baseline, (ii) no demonstrable antegrade fast pathway at baseline, or (iii) who are older (>70 years old). Ablation of AVNRT in patients with prolonged AH interval at baseline has also been studied. In patients with prolonged AH interval at baseline, it appears that ablation of the slow pathway in patients with dual AV nodal physiology and ablation of the retrograde fast pathway in those without dual AV nodal physiology are effective and, for the most part, safe. Although rare, delayed onset of symptomatic AV block can develop and vigilant follow-up may be needed in those who are at risk. Long-term follow-up studies of patients who developed PR prolongation (3% to 4%) after the initial slow pathway ablation for AVNRT did not show further deterioration of PR interval.

Technological advances continue to improve safety for both the patient and the operator in AVNRT ablation. Besides significantly reducing fluoroscopic exposure to both the operator and the patient, the development of sophisticated, real-time, three-dimensional mapping systems has allowed precise localization ("tagging") of not only target ablation sites but also important peri-AV nodal sites (e.g., His bundle) so as to reduce the risk of inadvertent RF injury or mechanical trauma to these areas. Another advancement has been the development of cryomapping and cryoablation. The EP effects of cryomapping are completely reversible within minutes, thus allowing return of AV conduction in patients with inadvertent AV block during ablation. Another attractive feature of cryoablation is the adherence of the catheter tip to tissue during ablation. This enhances catheter stability and allows atrial pacing to assess slow pathway conduction during ablation. Junctional ectopy is not seen during cryoablation, but may be seen on rewarming. However, there is a higher recurrence rate with cryoablation as compared to RF ablation.

The development of magnetic guidance system has allowed operators to remotely navigate catheters to precise locations and effectively ablate SVTs. This has shown a trend toward shorter application of RF energy due to improved catheter stability. During the ablation procedure itself, the use of a remote navigation ablation system will also reduce orthopedic hazards associated with wearing protective lead apparel for a prolonged period of time.

WOLFF-PARKINSON-WHITE SYNDROME, ATRIOVENTRICULAR REENTRANT TACHYCARDIA

In 1930, Drs Wolff, Parkinson, and White reported on 11 young and healthy patients with peculiar ECG findings that included short PR interval and bundle branch block. These patients suffered from paroxysms of SVT. This eventually became known as the *Wolff-Parkinson-White (WPW) syndrome*. The wide QRS patterns seen in ventricular pre-excitation were initially thought to be related to a short PR and bundle branch block. Discrete extranodal AV connections accounting for ventricular pre-excitation were first proposed by Kent and later confirmed by Wood and Wolferth. Durrer and Wellens performed the first EP studies in these patients. They demonstrated that PACs or PVCs could initiate tachycardia (either orthodromic or antidromic), and furthermore, appropriately timed atrial or ventricular extrastimuli could be used to terminate the tachycardia.

EPIDEMIOLOGY

A major reason for the interest in the WPW syndrome and AVRTs over the years is their associated morbidity and mortality. There is a well-established relationship between the presence of symptoms and the risk of sudden death. In asymptomatic WPW patients, the sudden death rate is low and is estimated to be about 1 per 1,000 patient-years. In a symptomatic young patient with WPW syndrome, the lifetime incidence of sudden death has been estimated to be approximately 3% to 4%. In some patients, ventricular fibrillation was the first manifestation of this syndrome.

While EP study and pathway ablation is well established in symptomatic patients with WPW syndrome, the approach to asymptomatic patients is less clear. The improved safety of EP study and catheter-based ablation techniques provide an impetus for prophylactic pathway ablation. To support this, randomized studies have shown that in experienced arrhythmia centers, prophylactic pathway ablation in asymptomatic patients who are found to be at high risk for arrhythmias reduces the risk for life-threatening arrhythmias. Whether this proactive approach can be applied to all asymptomatic patients and to a broad electrophysiology community is not clear. Based on recommendations from the 2003 ACC/AHA/ESC Guidelines, asymptomatic pre-excitation is associated with a class IIa indication for catheter ablation.

The WPW syndrome is associated with numerous medical conditions, including various forms of congenital heart disease. Numerous reports delineate the association of Ebstein anomaly with the WPW syndrome with up to 5% affected with both conditions in some case series.

ELECTROPHYSIOLOGY

Patients with the *WPW pattern* have a short PR interval and a slurred upstroke of the QRS complex (*delta* wave) but may never have any arrhythmias. Those who have the *WPW syndrome* have both the WPW ECG pattern and paroxysmal tachyarrhythmias. Detailed clinicopathological studies have shown that APs are composed of microscopic strands of morphologically normal myocardium that are located along the cardiac annulus or septum (Fig. 2-10). More than 50% of APs are located at the left free wall, 20% to 30% at the posteroseptum, 10% to 20% at the right free wall, and 5% to 10% at the anteroseptum.

APs are classified into different types depending on their conduction properties. *Manifest* APs are those that conduct more rapidly in the antegrade direction than the AV node, resulting in a discernible delta wave on the surface ECG. *Concealed* APs only conduct in the retrograde direction. When the pathway is concealed, there is no delta wave on the ECG at baseline, in response to atrial decremental or extrastimuli pacing, or with vagal maneuvers. *Latent* APs are those that have the capability to conduct in the

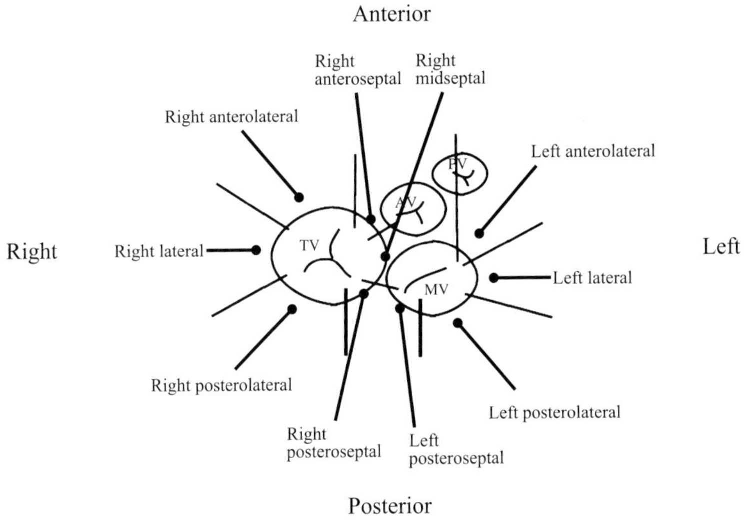

FIGURE 2-10. Diagram of AP locations at mitral and tricuspid annular sites. AV, aortic valve; PV, pulmonary valve; MV, mitral valve; TV, tricuspid valve. (Reprinted from Arruda MS, McClelland JH, Wang X, et al. Development and validation of an ECG algorithm for identifying accessory pathway ablation site in Wolff-Parkinson-White syndrome. *J Cardiovasc Electrophysiol.* Jan 1998;9(1):2–12, Copyright (2008).)

antegrade direction. Latent pathways are most often far left lateral pathways where the conduction time to the AV node is much shorter than to the pathway. Pacing closer to the pathway may elicit pre-excitation.

In some patients, the absence of overt retrograde conduction over APs may be due to a low resting sympathetic tone. Restoration of retrograde conduction with isoproterenol is not unusual and is most likely to be seen in those individuals with clinically documented SVT related to exercise. Adenosine can be a useful diagnostic tool. In patients with a minor degree of pre-excitation, adenosine can be used to unmask ventricular pre-excitation.

Numerous algorithms have been developed to localize APs from the surface ECG. Figure 2-11 shows an ECG algorithm for localizing AP based on delta wave polarity, as proposed by Arruda et al (1998). Figure 2-12 shows an ECG algorithm for localizing AP based on delta wave amplitude, sum of delta wave polarities, R/S wave ratio, and precordial QRS transition, as proposed by Fitzpatrick et al. (1994) Figure 2-13 shows 12-lead ECG from a patient with left posterolateral WPW.

In general, most ECG-based AP localization algorithms are based on delta wave polarity and/or R wave to S wave relationship. Any obscuring of these components will reduce the accuracy in pathway localization. Errors in pathway localization are usually due to (i) minimal pre-excitation on the surface ECG, (ii) multiple APs

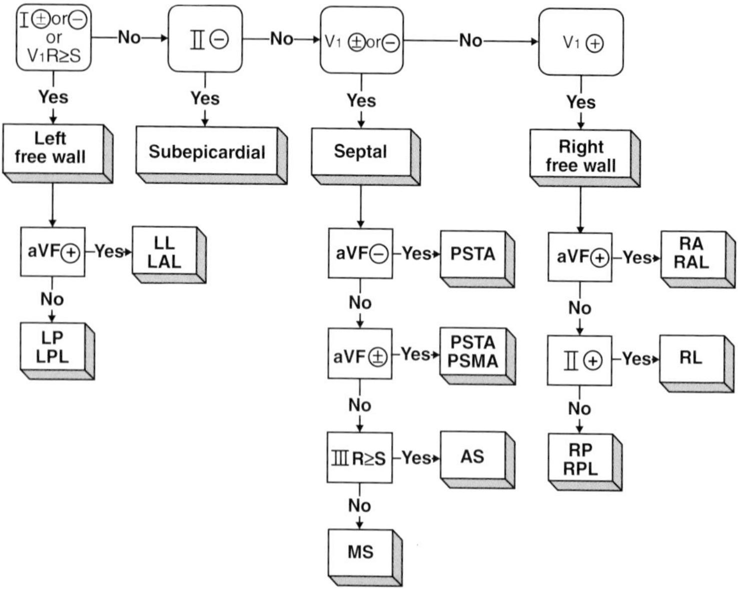

FIGURE 2-11. Stepwise ECG algorithm for localizing AP based on delta wave polarity. Delta wave polarity was determined by examining the initial 20 ms after the onset of the delta wave in the limb and precordial leads and was classified as +, −, or ±. LL, left lateral; LAL, left anterolateral; LP, left posterior; LPL, left posterolateral; RA, right anterior; RAL, right anterolateral; RL, right lateral; RP, right posterior; RPL, right posterolateral; PSTA, posteroseptal tricuspid annulus; PSMA, posteroseptal mitral annulus; AS, anteroseptal; MS, midseptal. (Reprinted from Arruda MS, McClelland JH, Wang X, et al. Development and validation of an ECG algorithm for identifying accessory pathway ablation site in Wolff-Parkinson-White syndrome. *J Cardiovasc Electrophysiol*. Jan 1998;9(1):2–12, Copyright (2008).)

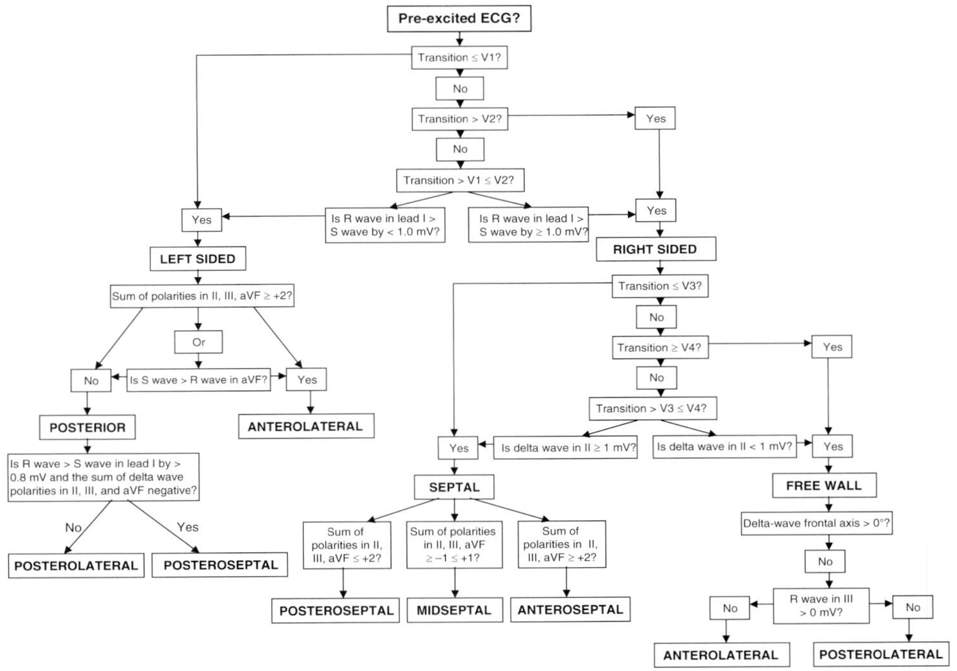

FIGURE 2-12. Stepwise ECG algorithm for localizing AP based on delta wave amplitude, sum of delta wave polarities, R/S wave ratio, and precordial QRS transition. Delta wave amplitude is calculated from the initial 40 ms of the pre-excited QRS complex in the limb and precordial leads and is classified as +, −, or 0. (Reprinted Fitzpatrick AP, Gonzales RP, Lesh MD, et al. New algorithm for the localization of accessory atrioventricular connections using a baseline electrocardiogram. *J Am Coll Cardiol*. Jan 1994;23(1):107–116, Copyright (1994).)

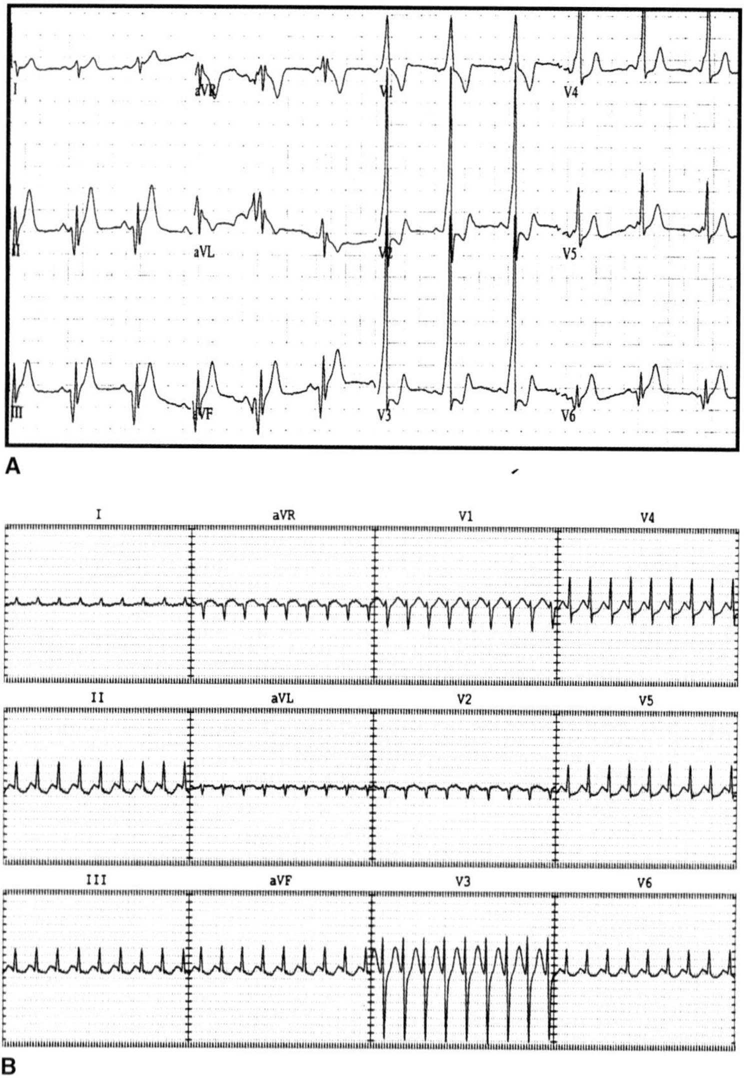

FIGURE 2-13. Twelve-lead ECG of a patient with a left posterolateral AP **(A)**. Delta waves may be subtle in this case due to the increased distance the sinus impulse has to travel to pre-excite the ventricle. **(B)** shows orthodromic AVRT using the AP as the retrograde limb of the circuit.

(seen in 2% to 20% of patients), and (iii) thoracic deformity or congenital cardiac disease. Localization algorithms are very useful in that they provide an excellent idea of the pathway insertion sites. Detailed intracardiac mapping is required for successful pathway ablation.

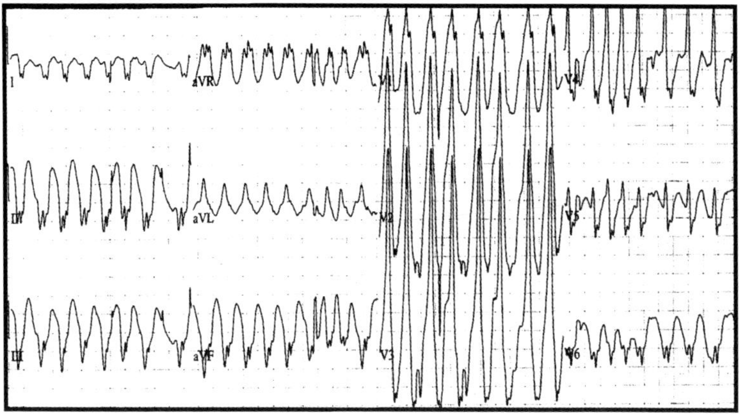

C

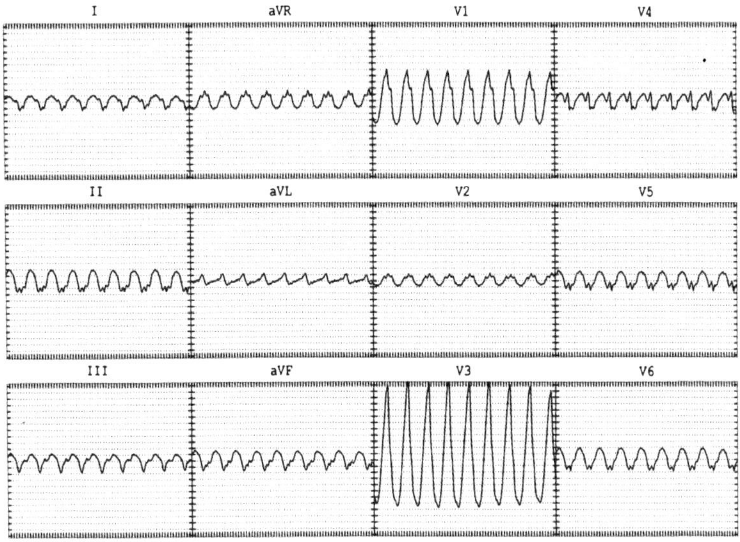

D

FIGURE 2-13. During atrial fibrillation, very rapid antegrade conduction over the pathway is evident **(C)**. **(D)** shows antidromic AVRT using the AP as the antegrade limb and AV node as the retrograde limb.

AVRT is a reentrant arrhythmia and is categorized into *orthodromic* and *antidromic* variants (Fig. 2-14). During orthodromic tachycardia, the antegrade limb is the AV node-His-Purkinje system and the retrograde limb is the AP. Fontaine first coined the term "antidromic" in describing the reentrant circuit whose antegrade limb is the AP and

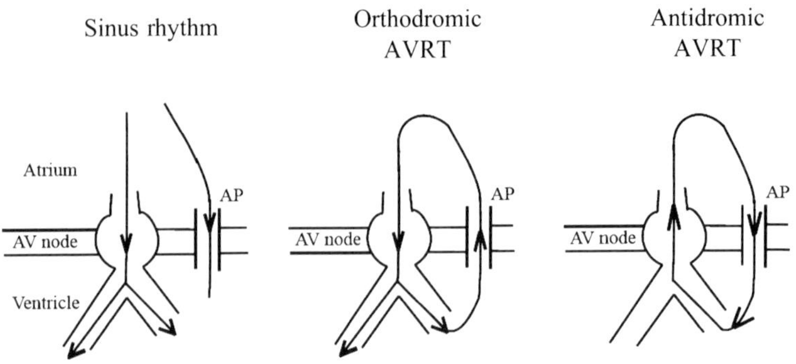

FIGURE 2-14. Schematic diagram of the AVRT reentrant circuit. During sinus rhythm **(left panel)**, the impulse conducts over the node and pathway. During orthodromic AVRT **(center panel)**, the impulse travels antegrade over the node and retrograde over the pathway. During antidromic AVRT **(right panel)**, the impulse travels antegrade over the pathway and retrograde over the node. (Reprinted from Lee KW, Badhwar N, Scheinman MM. Supraventricular tachycardia-I. *Curr Probl Cardiol.* Sep 2008;33(9):467–546, Copyright (2008).)

whose retrograde limb is the normal conduction system, i.e., the reverse of orthodromic. Since orthodromic AVRT uses the normal conduction system as its antegrade limb, it results in a narrow QRS complex tachycardia (Fig. 2-13B) (unless aberrant conduction is present). By contrast, antidromic AVRT results in a fully pre-excited tachycardia with wide QRS complexes (Figs. 2-13D and 2-15B).

Orthodromic AVRT constitutes approximately 95% of spontaneous and laboratory-induced AVRTs. For tachycardia initiation, a PAC, either spontaneous or induced by pacing in the EP laboratory, blocks at the AP and travels down the AV node-His-Purkinje system (Fig. 2-14). The conducted impulse reaches the ventricle and travels back up to the atrium over the AP, which has now recovered its excitability. The impulse then reenters the AV node-His-Purkinje system, perpetuating the tachycardia. Orthodromic tachycardia can also be initiated by a PVC. In this case, the PVC blocks the His-Purkinje system (or node) but travels over the AP up to the atrium. If the AV node-His-Purkinje system has recovered excitability, the impulse then travels down the node and reenters the ventricle and orthodromic tachycardia is started. The closer the PVC or PAC is to the site of insertion of the AP, the higher the likelihood of initiating orthodromic tachycardia.

P wave polarity during tachycardia may help in localizing the pathway: a negative P wave in lead I suggests that the atrial insertion of the pathway is in the left free wall, while negative P waves in the inferior leads suggest that it is in the posteroseptum or over an inferior right or left atrial insertion site.

Differentiating septal from free wall AP sites is important in helping to guide ablation. Spontaneous or induced bundle branch block during orthodromic AVRT can also provide important diagnostic clues. Lengthening of the tachycardia cycle length is seen in cases of AVRT when bundle branch block occurs *ipsilateral* to the free wall pathway. In this case, the impulse has to travel a greater distance from the ventricular insertion of the His-Purkinje system to the ventricular insertion of the AP, resulting in an increase in the VA interval by at least 35 ms. RBBB during orthodromic AVRT produces a smaller change in VA interval (15 to 20 ms) in those with anteroseptal AP while left bundle branch block (LBBB) produces a similar change in VA interval (15 to 20 ms) in those with posteroseptal AP.

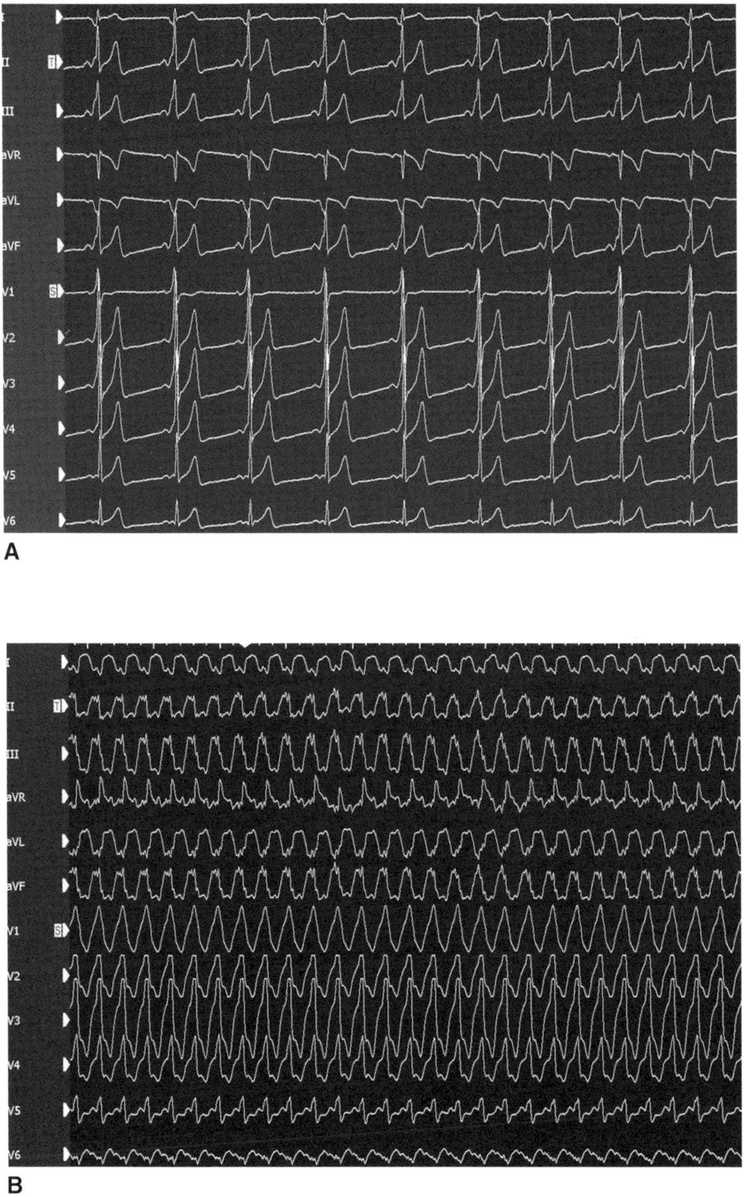

FIGURE 2-15. Patient with a left lateral AP. **(A)** shows the baseline pre-excited ECG; **(B)** shows 12-lead ECG during antidromic AVRT.

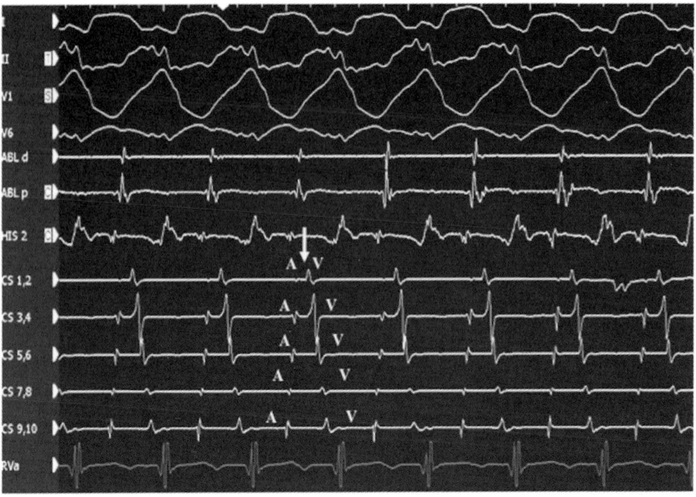

C

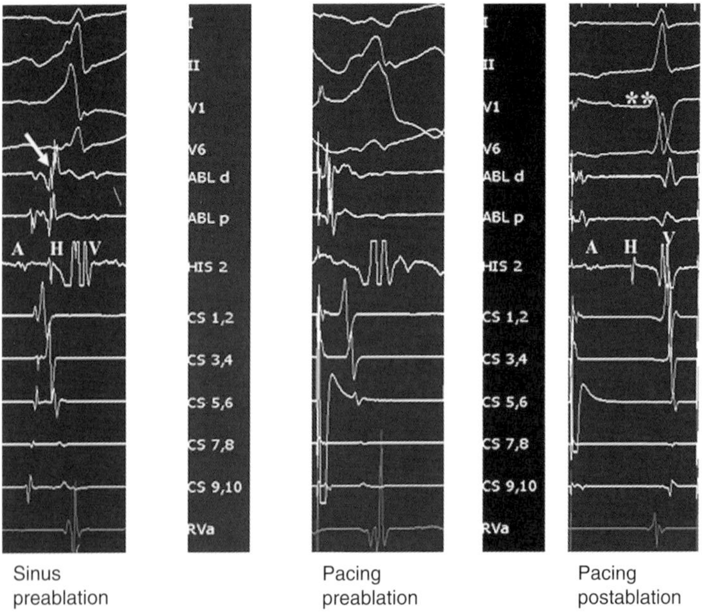

D

FIGURE 2-15. **(C)** shows surface and intracardiac tracings during antidromic AVRT, earliest antegrade ventricular activation is seen at the distal CS bipole (*arrow*); **(D)** shows successful RF ablation site at the lateral mitral annulus with elimination of pre-excitation and normalization of HV interval (**) (*arrow* denotes fused A and V electrograms). ABLp, proximal bipole of ablation catheter; ABLd, distal bipole of ablation catheter.

Other methods used to identify an AVRT include delivering a critically timed PVC late in the diastolic interval of the SVT, when the His bundle is depolarized, which results in an atrial activation with the *same* retrograde atrial activation sequence as during the tachycardia. If the tachycardia is reset or terminated, an AP exists and is likely required for the tachycardia circuit. In this case, retrograde conduction can occur only via an AP as the His bundle is refractory. In most cases, spontaneous termination of AVRT occurs in the AV node, as indicated by an atrial electrogram (or retrograde P wave) not followed by a His bundle potential.

Antidromic AVRT is much less common and constitutes approximately 3% to 6% of spontaneous and laboratory-induced AVRTs. Initiation and termination are the reverse of what is expected for its orthodromic counterpart (Fig. 2-14). Figure 2-15 shows a case of a patient with a left lateral AP capable of antegrade conduction only. The AP is capable of malignant potential since the shortest RR interval was less than 250 ms during atrial fibrillation.

Bystander APs conduct antegradely or retrogradely but are not active participants in AVRTs. Patients with the WPW syndrome have a higher incidence of dual AV nodal pathways and active participation by the AP in the tachycardia should be confirmed in the EP laboratory. It is important to note that bystander APs can still have a short antegrade refractory period and can cause rapid ventricular rates in the setting of atrial fibrillation.

Spontaneous and laboratory-induced atrial fibrillation (to a lesser extent atrial flutter) has been reported to occur in up to 32% to 58% of patients with the WPW syndrome. Several mechanisms have been documented or proposed, and they include (i) PAC-induced degeneration of AVRT to atrial fibrillation, (ii) PVC-induced atrial depolarization during the atrial vulnerable period leading to atrial fibrillation, and (iii) a reentrant circuit within the atrial branching insertion sites of the AP fibers. In patients without structural heart disease, susceptibility to subsequent atrial fibrillation is low (6% to 10%) after successful AP ablation. However, despite successful pathway ablation, some patients still have recurrence of their atrial fibrillation. The characteristics of these patients include (i) older age (>50 years old), (ii) a history of paroxysmal atrial fibrillation and presence of structural heart disease, (iii) no antegrade conduction in the AP, (iv) slow ventricular response during atrial fibrillation, and (v) inducible atrial fibrillation after AP ablation.

RISK STRATIFICATION

Criteria predictive of lower risk in patients with the WPW syndrome have also been reported. Individuals who lose antegrade AP conduction over time have lower mortality risk. Noninvasive techniques have been used to assess the duration of the antegrade refractory period of the AP. Intermittent loss of the pre-excitation is due to precarious conduction over the AP (long refractory period) and may portend a benign prognosis in the presence of atrial fibrillation. However, patients with intermittent loss of the pre-excitation may still have disabling symptoms due to AVRT, especially in the setting of high adrenaline states.

Treadmill exercise testing has been used to assess the robustness, or malignant potential, of an AP's antegrade conduction. The working hypothesis here is that in patients with APs whose effective refractory period (ERP) is longer than that of the normal AV conduction, the delta wave should disappear with exercise, while in patients with APs whose ERP is shorter than that of the normal AV conduction, the delta wave should persist. Some studies have shown that loss of delta waves on the surface ECG during exercise stress may suggest a less malignant AP. Whether this finding is predictive of lower long-term risk of sudden death is unclear and has not been systematically studied in a large patient population. Loss of delta wave during exercise is due to a balance between the relative effects of sympathetic stimulation on refractoriness of AP and AV node, and may neither be reflective of the robustness of an AP's antegrade conduction per se nor prognosticate the brevity of its ERP during rapid atrial fibrillation. Specifically, heightened sympathetic tone can accelerate conduction via the AV node-His-Purkinje system thereby masking antegrade conduction by the pathway and yielding a false sense of security in terms of pathway conduction.

IV medications can be used to assess the antegrade refractoriness of the AP. Lack of complete block in the AP with either IV procainamide or ajmaline suggests that the AP has a short antegrade ERP (<270 ms). However, the effects of IV procainamide have not been validated in other studies. In summary, none of the noninvasive techniques apart from spontaneous Mobitz type II block in the AP is a reliable indicator of low-risk malignancy potential.

The mechanism of sudden death for WPW patients is usually ventricular fibrillation due to atrial fibrillation conducting rapidly over the AP. EP testing methods via intracardiac or transesophageal routes have been used to identify asymptomatic patients who may be at risk for sudden death. Criteria predictive of increased risk include (i) presence of multiple pathways, (ii) short AP ERP (<270 ms), (iii) shortest RR intervals during inducible atrial fibrillation (<250 ms), (iv) inducibility of AVRT or atrial fibrillation, and (iv) septal AP location. In recent studies of asymptomatic WPW in children, inducibility of AVRT or atrial fibrillation or the demonstration of multiple pathways were predictive of a worse prognosis.

Syncope in patients with WPW syndrome as a potential harbinger of sudden death has been studied. The presence of syncope does not necessarily increase the chance of uncovering a particularly dangerous AP in some patient populations. In some adults, the prognostic value of syncope was less accurate and predictive than the shortest RR interval during atrial fibrillation and the antegrade ERP of the AP for the development of aborted sudden death. However, in young patients (<25 years old), the occurrence of AF with a rapid ventricular response during EP study correlated well with a history of syncope.

In general, symptomatic WPW patients should undergo ablation of the pathway. Indications for an invasive EP study to assess prognosis in asymptomatic patients with WPW pattern are controversial and may be warranted in certain patient populations (high responsibility professions, athletes, and family history of sudden death). Furthermore, although the complication rate of catheter ablation in experienced centers is extremely low, this does not lessen the controversy in regard to the issue of pathway ablation in asymptomatic patients since the risk of sudden death as the sentinel event is very low.

PHARMACOLOGIC TREATMENT

Drug treatment of AVRT is aimed at (i) reducing factors that precipitate the tachycardia (e.g., ectopy and atrial fibrillation) and (ii) targeting the weak link of the AVRT circuit (i.e., AV node or AP). In orthodromic AVRT circuit, the AV node is the weak link and drugs that prolong AV nodal refractoriness or depress its conduction can lead to block in the node resulting in tachycardia termination. Vagal maneuvers terminate tachycardia by causing block in the node. First-line drugs that are effective in acute termination of orthodromic AVRT include IV administration of adenosine, verapamil or diltiazem, or beta-blockers. IV digoxin is less effective due to its delayed onset of action. IV procainamide depresses conduction and prolongs refractoriness in most cardiac tissues (i.e., atrium, ventricle, and His-Purkinje system) and is a viable alternative. Procainamide also works by blocking conduction in the AP.

Oral class Ic drugs are more efficacious than class Ia drugs in blocking AP conduction; however, they should be avoided in patients with structural heart disease. Amiodarone has various EP effects but is not more effective than class Ic drugs used alone or in combination with beta-blockers. In general, amiodarone should be reserved for those who are drug-refractory, elderly, and not suitable candidates for ablative therapy. Sotalol can be effective in preventing tachycardia, although it is associated with a 4% risk of torsades de pointes, especially in those with significant structural heart disease and congestive heart failure. Oral digoxin is not effective as a monotherapy for orthodromic AVRT and most importantly, by its direct effects on the AP, this drug may actually accelerate conduction over the AP during atrial fibrillation. Therefore, digoxin should never be used for the treatment of patients with pre-excitation.

In antidromic AVRT, retrograde AV nodal conduction may be the weak link. IV calcium- channel blockers, beta-blockers, and adenosine can be used for acute termination of tachycardia if it is known to be antidromic AVRT. However, the role of the AP and its short antegrade refractory period permitting rapid ventricular response in the setting of atrial fibrillation must also be kept in mind. In some patients with pre-excited tachycardia, antegrade conduction may occur over one pathway and retrograde conduction over another pathway (not the AV node). IV adenosine should be used with caution since its can result in degeneration of the tachycardia into atrial fibrillation, and ventricular fibrillation may result if the AP has a short antegrade refractory period. IV procainamide is the drug of choice in the acute treatment of antidromic AVRT. Even if this drug does not terminate the tachycardia, it may slow the tachycardia rate. In the absence of contraindications, class Ic drugs are the drugs of choice for long-term oral treatment of antidromic tachycardia.

CATHETER ABLATION

Catheter-based ablation is the procedure of choice for patients with symptomatic WPW syndrome and for those who respond poorly to medical therapy. In most experienced centers, the success rate is 95% to 97% with a recurrence rate of 6%.

Successful ablation is critically dependent on accurate localization of the AP. Preliminary pathway localization can be obtained from delta wave and QRS morphologies. When pre-excitation is not maximal, rapid atrial pacing or IV adenosine can be used to obtain full pre-excitation so as to improve localization accuracy. This is especially useful in left lateral APs in which pre-excitation may be enhanced with left atrial pacing (from the CS catheter). A successful outcome requires detailed analysis of atrial and ventricular electrograms. Intracardiac electrogram criteria have been used to identify appropriate target sites for ablation of manifest pathways and include (i) presence of an AP potential (Fig. 2-15D), (ii) early onset of local ventricular activation relative to the delta wave onset, (iii) electrogram stability, and (iv) antegrade continuous electrical activity (i.e., fused atrial and ventricular electrograms). Electrogram criteria have also been used to identify appropriate target sites for ablation of concealed pathway and include (i) retrograde AP potential, (ii) retrograde continuous electrical activity with ventricular pacing or during tachycardia, and (iii) electrogram stability.

Left free wall pathways constitute the majority of APs and successful ablation requires detailed mapping of the lateral mitral annulus. Ablation can be guided by the CS catheter that is used to bracket the pathway's location. Left free wall pathways can be ablated via either a transseptal or a retrograde transaortic approach depending on the operator's experience and preference. Catheter ablation is associated with a very high success rate. Successful ablation of right free wall pathways requires detailed mapping of the lateral tricuspid annulus. The overall success rate for right free wall pathway ablation is the lowest of any of the APs with an average of 90% and a recurrence rate of 14%. Reasons for reduced success rates include catheter instability and lack of a right-sided CS structure that parallel the tricuspid annulus to aid in mapping. This can be improved with the use of deflectable sheaths for stability and a multielectrode mapping microcatheter placed in the right coronary artery for AP localization.

Ablation of anteroseptal and mid-septal pathways can be challenging due to their proximity to the AV node and His bundle. The location of the ablation catheter relative to the His catheter should be constantly monitored, preferably with a three-dimensional mapping system that can track these catheters continuously. Analogous to slow pathway modification in AVNRT ablation, RF ablation of anteroseptal and mid-septal pathways warrants high vigilance for any surface ECG or intracardiac electrogram clues of impending AV block. Cryoablation allows cryomapping and cryoadherence, and in difficult cases, it may be preferable to RF ablation. In some cases, RF ablation of anteroseptal pathways can be safely performed from the noncoronary aortic sinus when conventional approaches fail or are associated with a high risk of AV block. Anteroseptal and mid-septal pathways are more susceptible to catheter trauma during detailed mapping. This results in longer procedure times and lower success rates. A mapping system can be used to "tag" the sites of interest and can be invaluable. Ablation of anteroseptal and mid-septal pathways is associated with an overall success rate of 95% to 98% and a 1% to 3% risk of permanent AV block.

Ablation of posteroseptal pathways can be challenging due to the complex anatomy at the posteroseptum. Most posteroseptal pathways can be ablated from the right side, although in up to 20% of cases a left-sided approach is needed. ECG and EP clues that suggest a left-sided approach may be needed include (i) a positive delta wave or a positive QRS complex in V1, (ii) earliest retrograde atrial activation at the CS ostium, and (iii) increase in VA interval with LBBB during orthodromic tachycardia. Between 5% to 17% of posteroseptal and left posterior APs are located epicardially and ablation in the CS (most commonly the middle cardiac vein) is needed. A manifest AP that may require ablation within the CS is suggested by a negative delta wave in lead II. There also have been numerous case reports that suggest that the CS diverticulum may tend to harbor concealed posteroseptal pathways with the pathway actually making up part of the "neck" of the diverticulum. RF ablation in the CS should be done with caution, starting with low power, to minimize the risk of perforation and damage to the adjacent coronary arteries. Cooled (Chilli) ablation may be needed if conventional RF ablation at low power is unsuccessful. Cryoablation is a safe and efficacious ablation strategy in the CS. Ablation of posteroseptal APs is associated with an overall success rate of about 93% to 98%, a recurrence rate of 3% to 6% and a 1% risk of permanent AV block.

It appears that a small percentage of APs are epicardial. This is suggested by the finding of small or no pathway potentials during endocardial mapping and large pathway potentials in the CS. Left-sided pathways can be successfully ablated within the CS at sites with large AP potentials. However, successful ablation of APs at other epicardial sites may require a percutaneous epicardial approach, as an alternative to cardiac surgery. In specialized arrhythmia centers, up to 18% of patients referred for previously failed AP ablation may require a percutaneous epicardial approach for successful ablation.

Overall, ablation of AP is associated with a complication rate of 1% to 4% and a procedure-related death rate of approximately 0.2%. The complication of complete AV block occurs in about 1% of patients and is seen most frequently in patients undergoing ablation of septal pathways. Autonomic dysfunction and inappropriate sinus tachycardia are rare complications of RF ablation of AP and are less frequent than that seen in slow pathway ablation for AVNRT.

SUMMARY

SVTs remain a source of significant morbidity. Advances in the understanding of their mechanisms and anatomical locations have led to highly effective pharmacologic and nonpharmacologic treatment strategies. Catheter ablation has provided actual cure for thousands of patients with debilitating symptoms from paroxysmal SVTs; it also reduces risk of mortality in patients with WPW. Today, advances in catheter design, energy delivery systems, mapping systems, and remote navigation systems have made catheter ablation the therapy of choice for a majority of SVTs.

KEY POINTS

1. AVNRT and AVRT are the most common forms of PSVT commonly seen in patients without structural heart disease. AVNRT is more common in females while AVRT is more commonly seen in males.
2. Their mechanism is reentry that requires two distinct pathways with different speeds of conduction (fast and slow) and varying recovery times.
3. Typical AVNRT uses the slow pathway as the antegrade limb and the fast pathway as the retrograde limb and vice versa for atypical AVNRT.
4. Orthodromic AVRT is the most common tachycardia seen in patients with WPW. The AV node serves as the antegrade limb and an accessory pathway is the retrograde limb.
5. 12-lead ECG during AVNRT usually manifests as regular narrow complex tachycardia with pseudo R′ in V1 and pseudo S wave in the inferior leads. 12-lead ECG during AVRT usually manifests as short RP tachycardia.
6. The polarity of the delta wave and the R/S relationship on a 12-lead ECG can accurately localize the accessory pathway.
7. Catheter ablation is very effective and should be offered as the first line of treatment for patients with AVNRT and AVRT.

SELECTED REFERENCES

Anderson RH, Ho SY. The architecture of the sinus node, the atrioventricular conduction axis, and the internodal atrial myocardium. *J Cardiovasc Electrophysiol.* Nov 1998;9(11):1233–1248.

Arruda MS, McClelland JH, Wang X, et al. Development and validation of an ECG algorithm for identifying accessory pathway ablation site in Wolff-Parkinson-White syndrome. *J Cardiovasc Electrophysiol.* Jan 1998;9(1):2–12.

Blomstrom-Lundqvist C, Scheinman MM, Aliot EM, et al. ACC/AHA/ESC guidelines for the management of patients with supraventricular arrhythmias—executive summary. A report of the American college of cardiology/American heart association task force on practice guidelines and the European society of cardiology committee for practice guidelines (writing committee to develop guidelines for the management of patients with supraventricular arrhythmias) developed in collaboration with NASPE-Heart Rhythm Society. *J Am Coll Cardiol.* Oct 15, 2003;42(8):1493–1531.

Calkins H, Kim YN, Schmaltz S, et al. Electrogram criteria for identification of appropriate target sites for radiofrequency catheter ablation of accessory atrioventricular connections. *Circulation.* Feb 1992;85(2): 565–573.

Fitzpatrick AP, Gonzales RP, Lesh MD, et al. New algorithm for the localization of accessory atrioventricular connections using a baseline electrocardiogram. *J Am Coll Cardiol.* Jan 1994;23(1):107–116.

Friedman PL, Dubuc M, Green MS, et al. Catheter cryoablation of supraventricular tachycardia: Results of the multicenter prospective "frosty" trial. *Heart Rhythm.* July 2004;1(2):129–138.

Jackman WM, Beckman KJ, McCleland JH, et al. Treatment of supraventricular tachycardia due to atrioventricular nodal reentry by radiofrequency catheter ablation of slow-pathway. *N Engl J Med.* July 1992;327(5):313–318.

Jackman WM, Wang XZ, Friday KJ, et al. Catheter ablation of accessory atrioventricular pathways (Wolff-Parkinson-White syndrome) by radiofrequency current. *N Engl J Med.* June 6, 1991;324(23):1605–1611.

Lee KW, Badhwar N, Scheinman MM. Supraventricular tachycardia-I. *Curr Probl Cardiol.* Sep 2008;33(9): 467–546.

Lee KW, Badhwar N, Scheinman MM. Supraventricular tachycardia-II. *Curr Probl Cardiol.* Oct 2008;33 (10):557–622.

Lee MA, Morady F, Kadish A, et al. Catheter modification of the atrioventricular junction with radiofrequency energy for control of atrioventricular nodal reentry tachycardia. *Circulation.* Mar 1991;83(3):827–835.

Lockwood D, Otomo K, Wang Z, et al. Electrophysiologic characteristics of atrioventricular nodal reentrant tachycardia: Implications for the reentrant circuits. In: Zipes DP, Jalife J, eds. *Cardiac Electrophysiology: From Cell to Bedside*. 3rd Ed. Philadelphia, PA: W. B. Saunders; 2004:537–557.
Orejarena LA, Vidaillet H Jr, DeStefano F, et al. Paroxysmal supraventricular tachycardia in the general population. *J Am Coll Cardiol*. Jan 1998;31(1):150–157.
Rosen KM, Mehta A, Miller RA. Demonstration of dual atrioventricular nodal pathways in man. *Am J Cardiol*. Feb 1974;33(2):291–294.
Scheinman MM, Huang S. The 1998 NASPE prospective catheter ablation registry. *Pacing Clin Electrophysiol*. June 2000;23(6):1020–1028.
Scheinman MM, Morady F, Hess DS, et al. Catheter-induced ablation of the atrioventricular junction to control refractory supraventricular arrhythmias. *JAMA*. Aug 20, 1982;248(7):851–855.
Sun Y, Arruda M, Otomo K, et al. Coronary sinus-ventricular accessory connections producing posteroseptal and left posterior accessory pathways: Incidence and electrophysiological identification. *Circulation*. Sep 10, 2002;106(11):1362–1367.
Wellens HJJ. The electrophysiologic properties of the accessory pathway in the Wolff-Parkinson-White syndrome. In: Wellens HJJ, Kie KI, Janse MJ, eds. *The Conduction System of the Heart*. Leiden, The Netherlands: HE Stenfert Kroese B.V.; 1976:567–588.
Wood KA, Drew BJ, Scheinman MM. Frequency of disabling symptoms in supraventricular tachycardia. *Am J Cardiol*. Jan 1997;79(2):145–149.
Wu D, Denes P, Amat YLF, et al. An unusual variety of atrioventricular nodal re-entry due to retrograde dual atrioventricular nodal pathways. *Circulation*. July 1977;56(1):50–59.

CHAPTER 3

Atrial Arrhythmias

Jonathan S. Steinberg, Aysha Arshad, and Tina Sichrovsky

ATRIAL FIBRILLATION

DIAGNOSIS AND EPIDEMIOLOGY

Atrial fibrillation (AF) is the most commonly sustained arrhythmia observed in clinical practice, encountered in a variety of clinical settings including the ambulatory clinic, the emergency room, and inpatient units. It may occur in isolation, be precipitated by an acute and reversible cause, or complicate a chronic cardiovascular or noncardiovascular condition. The current prevalence in the US is believed to be close to 2.5 million.

The ECG diagnosis of AF is made based on an undulating or oscillating pattern of atrial activity that is inconstant and disorganized and conducted with an irregularly irregular ventricular response. There is a distinct absence of regular, consistent and organized atrial activity. The inferior leads of the ECG are often helpful in distinguishing AF from other atrial arrhythmias that may have irregular ventricular rates such as atrial flutters (AFLs) and tachycardias. The hallmark of AF is the absence of regular and organized atrial activity.

AF is strongly age related. It infrequently presents below the age of 50 or 60 but is extremely common when patients reach the age of 80 and above (about one in ten). Population studies confirm the relationship of age in AF, independent of cardiovascular conditions (Fig. 3-1). It is likely that age-dependent atrial pathophysiologic processes are responsible for the increasing prevalence of AF relative to age. In addition, the success in treating chronic cardiovascular conditions such as hypertension and coronary heart disease makes AF more likely to occur in the elderly. In addition, population studies consistently observe that men are more likely to experience AF than women, with an increased prevalence of approximately twofold.

The development of AF in population-based studies was associated with an increased risk of death. This appeared to be independent of other known predictors of mortality but the specific underlying mechanism of death was unclear. Possible contributing factors may include the increased risk of stroke and heart failure associated with AF. Additional possibilities include coronary ischemia, systemic thromboembolic state, toxic drug therapy, and associated cardiovascular diseases.

Although most patients with AF have an associated cardiovascular condition, some patients have no known precipitating cause or associated cardiovascular disease, and in these patients, AF is termed "lone" AF or idiopathic AF. Anywhere from 5% to 30% of patients with AF may fall into this category, depending on the setting. It is thought that these patients may face a lower long-term risk of cardiovascular complications because of the absence of associated cardiovascular disease, although age-related risks are still important, especially that of age-related stroke risk.

The most common associated cardiovascular cause of AF in the Western world is hypertension, responsible for approximately 40% of cases of AF in most studies. Additional causes (Table 3-1) include coronary heart disease and acute myocardial infarction (MI), valvular heart disease, heart failure and cardiomyopathy, cardiac and valvular surgery, and pericardial diseases. Additionally, some noncardiovascular causes may precipitate AF including hyperthyroidism, acute and chronic pulmonary diseases, and toxic exposure, particularly excess alcohol intake.

Although rheumatic heart disease is seen much less frequently in contemporary medicine, the presence of mitral valvular disease is a potent risk factor for AF. The strongest association is found with mitral stenosis, and a less potent association is seen with mitral regurgitation. Although the risk of developing AF long-term is relatively small with

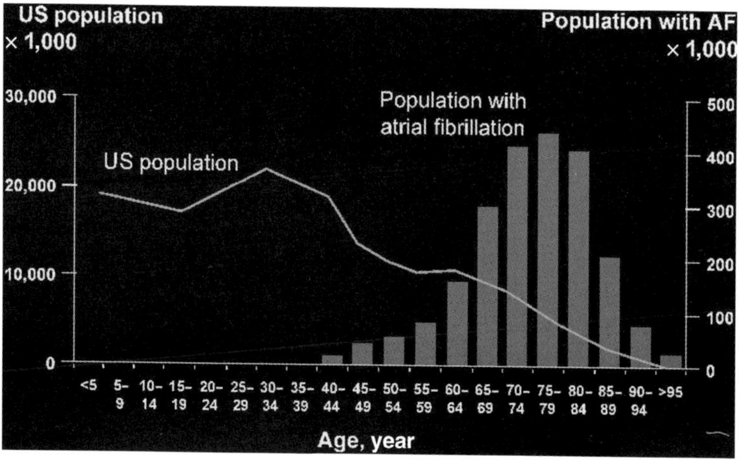

FIGURE 3-1. The age-related prevalence of AF relative to the US population. (Reprinted from Feinberg WM, Blackshear JL, Laupacis A, et al. Prevalence, age distribution, and gender of patients with atrial fibrillation. *Arch Intern Med.* 1995;155:469–473, with permission.)

TABLE 3-1 Conditions Associated with AF

Cardiovascular	Noncardiovascular
Hypertension	Pulmonary
Valvular heart disease	Sepsis
Coronary heart disease and MI	Central nervous system
Pericardial disease	Autonomic (vagal, adrenergic)
Congenital heart disease	Hyperthyroidism
Cardiomyopathy and heart failure	Post-noncardiac surgery
Electrical conditions (sick sinus syndrome, WPW, familial)	Toxin exposure (alcohol)
Postcardiac surgery	Idiopathic

MI, myocardial infarction.

coronary heart disease, its prevalence makes this an important risk factor for AF in the general population. In addition, AF may be seen in approximately 10% of patients in the early period after acute MI, usually in unstable patients with extensive myocardial damage when atrial injury has also occurred. AF in this setting is often short-lived.

AF is an extremely common postoperative finding in patients who have undergone all forms of cardiac surgery. Following coronary artery bypass surgery, AF may occur in approximately 20% to 25% of patients, but in valvular surgery, it may be seen in up to 40% of patients. Risk factors for the development of AF in this setting include age, left ventricular (LV) hypertrophy, right coronary artery bypass, intra-atrial conduction delay detected on signal-averaged ECG, and absence of beta-blocker therapy. AF lengthens hospital stay and may be associated with thromboembolic events. However, AF in this setting is generally transient, resolving within the hospital stay or shortly thereafter. The peak incidence occurs on postoperative days 2 to 3.

AF may be seen in patients who have overt or subclinical (occult) hyperthyroidism. The latter is particularly important to identify in the elderly patient. AF is associated with the significant risk of thromboembolic events in this clinical setting and rapid ventricular rates are often observed. AF is often difficult to control until the patient is rendered euthyroid.

AF may occur when patients have consumed large amounts of alcohol, i.e., binge drinking, giving rise to a "holiday heart syndrome." There may be no underlying cardiac disease and the AF may be a transient phenomenon.

PATHOPHYSIOLOGY

The electrophysiologic (EP) mechanism(s) underlying AF are likely varied and dependent upon atrial substrate and underlying cardiovascular conditions. Well-established AF, such as that of persistent or permanent AF, is likely due to multiple wave reentry. Multiple wave reentry is defined as the simultaneous presence of multiple reentrant circuits, which vary in size, number, and position during ongoing atria fibrillation. A critical mass of atrial tissue is required to maintain multiple wave reentry, likely requiring at least five or six simultaneous reentrant circuits. Alternatively, a smaller number of reentrant circuits, perhaps one or two, termed rotors, can anchor in a stable or variable position, usually in the left atrium (LA), and have a short cycle length (CL). Activation spreading from this reentrant circuit source may be so rapid that atrial tissue cannot keep up with this rapid rate and becomes disorganized, so-called fibrillatory conduction. Finally, many episodes of AF may be generated by a focal source, most commonly emanating from the pulmonary veins, or perhaps other large thoracic veins, firing at a very rapid CL but also associated with fibrillatory conduction. Combinations of these mechanisms are likely to exist as well, most commonly a focal trigger emanating from the pulmonary veins precipitating multiple wave reentry in atrial tissue (Fig. 3-2).

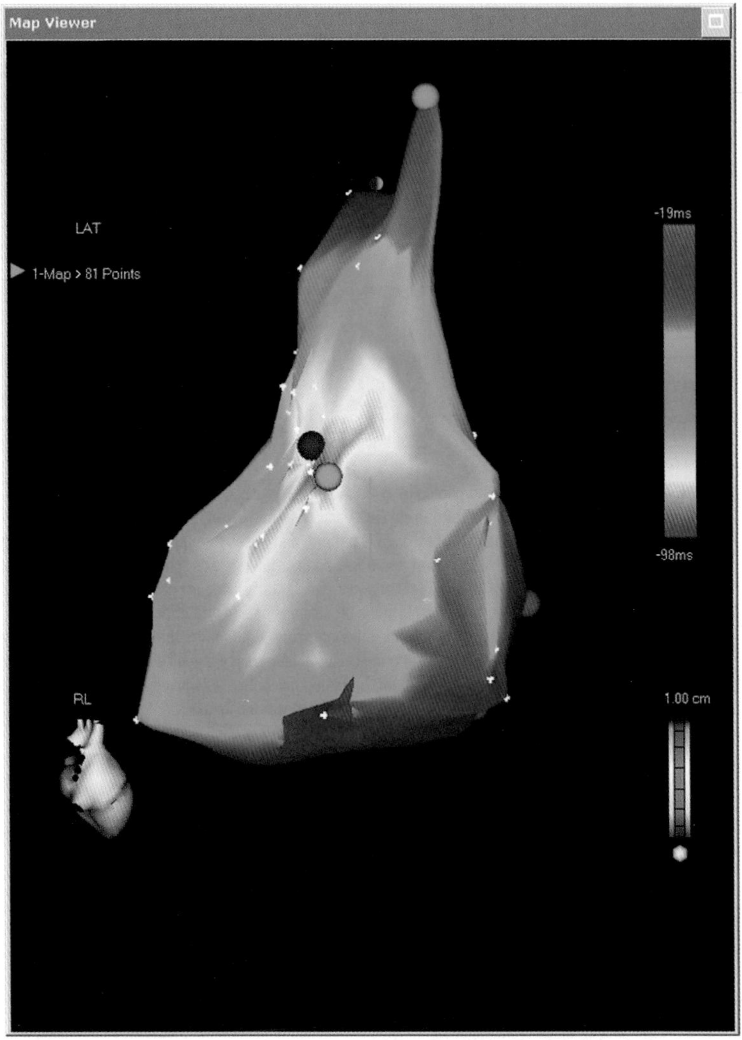

FIGURE 3-13. Endocardial activation mapping showing earliest activation at upper portion of crista terminalis in patient with focal origin.

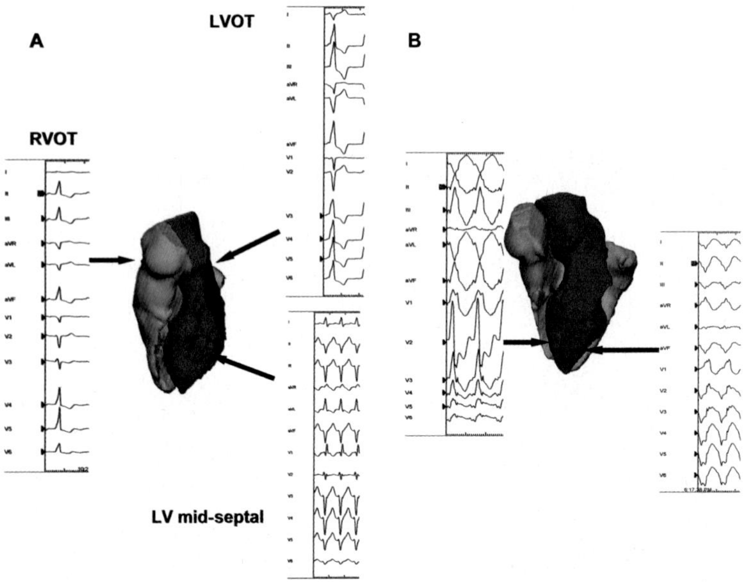

FIGURE 4-2. Representative ECG morphologies during VT and corresponding sites of origin. A cast of the RV (*blue*) and LV (*red*) is shown in the left lateral **(left)** and posterior **(right)** projections. **A:** Idiopathic VT patterns. RVOT VT has a left bundle, inferior axis ECG pattern, and arises from just beneath the pulmonary valve. LVOT VT (from the sinuses of Valsalva) has a left bundle, inferior axis, but the precordial R wave transition is earlier because the LV is more posterior. LV mid-septal VT has a right bundle, superior axis. **B:** Two examples of right bundle morphology VTs in the presence of healed infarction. Both of these VT morphologies are RBBB, signifying origin away from the intraventricular septum. VTs that arise from the septum have a left bundle configuration. VT in the setting of structural heart disease typically arises from areas of scarring, either in healed infarction or in the setting of dilated myopathy, perivalvular fibrosis. In the latter setting, epicardial involvement may be more extensive than endocardial involvement.

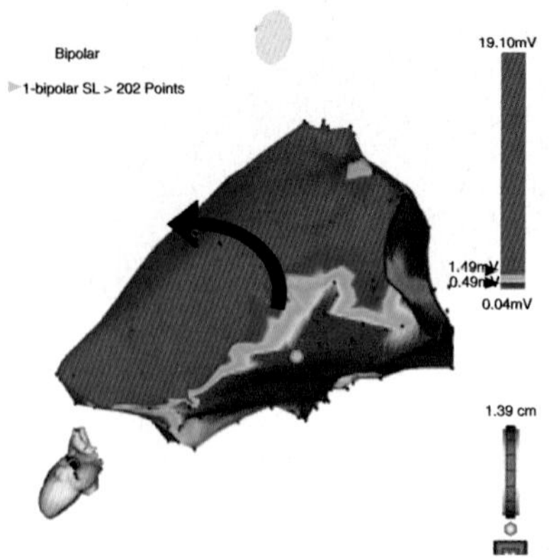

FIGURE 4-4B. Sinus voltage map of a patient with a large inferior scar extending to the lateral wall. VT exits from the lateral wall based on the QRS morohology during VT.

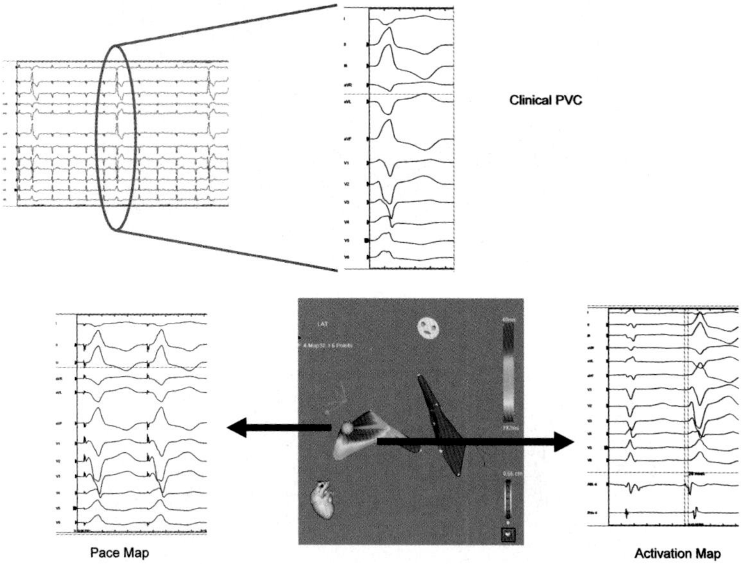

FIGURE 4-5. Idiopathic VT arising from the left coronary cusp. The surface ECG, electroanatomic map of the RVOT and left cusp (color patterns signify activation time during the PVC: red is early, purple is late), pacemapping and activation mapping at the site of origin are shown. Complementary techniques used for focal VT/PVC ablation. Activation mapping is used to locate the area of earliest activity, typically 15 to 45 ms pre-QRS. Pace mapping is used to locate the area of focal exit. Typically, both areas overlap allowing the frequency of PVC/VT to dictate which approach is selected.

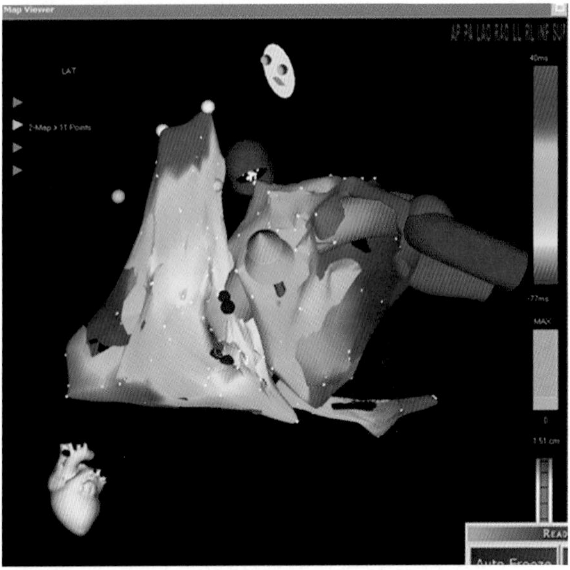

FIGURE 7-3. Electroanatomic activation maps of the right and left atria in a patient with a focal left atrial tachycardia tachycardia.

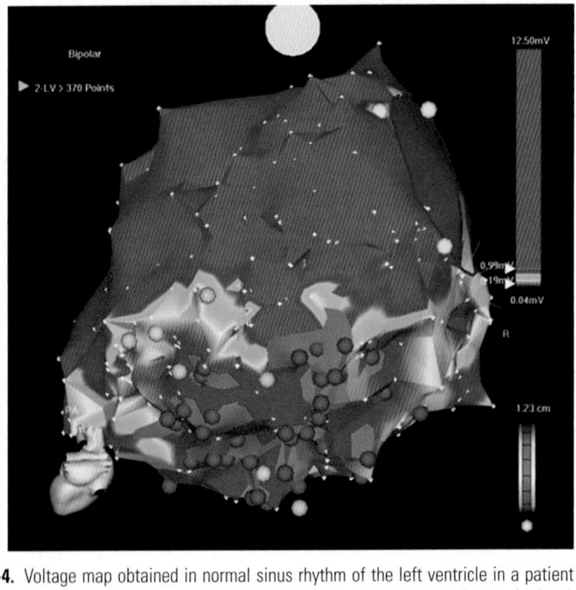

FIGURE 7-4. Voltage map obtained in normal sinus rhythm of the left ventricle in a patient with extensive scar and ventricular tachycardia. Areas displayed in purple are healthy tissue with local electrogram voltages >1.5 mV. Whereas areas displayed in red demonstrate voltages <0.5 mV. Areas displayed in gray demonstrate no appreciable electrograms and are electrically unexcitable.

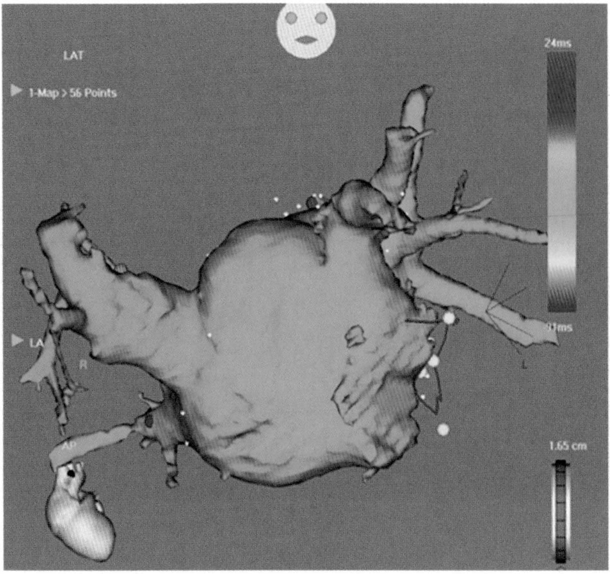

A

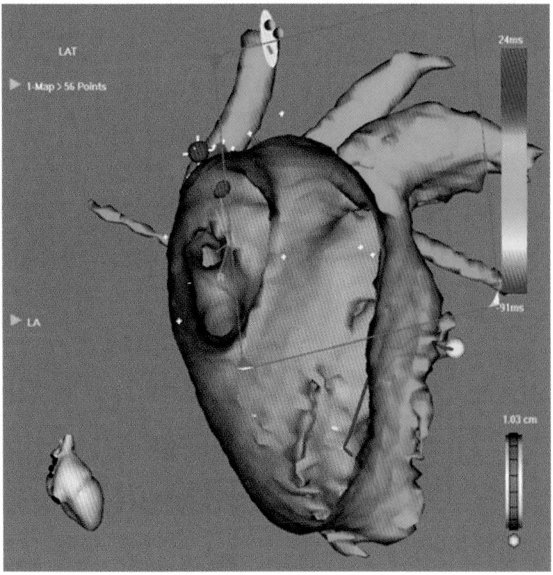

B

FIGURE 7-5. A: Three-dimensional image of the left atrium registered to the electroanatomic map of the left atrium and used to demonstrate the left atrial anatomy and guide catheter positioning during ablation of atrial fibrillation. **B:** Open "clipped" view demonstrating the pulmonary vein ostia around which RF lesions will be placed.

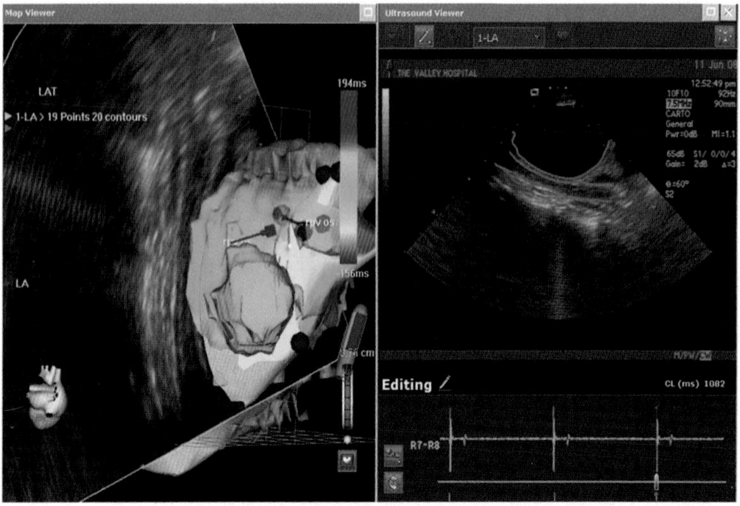

FIGURE 7-7. Three-dimensional imaging of the left atrium during an ablation procedure for atrial fibrillation. The left panel shows the three-dimensional shell created with ultrasound imaging in gray, the color represents points obtained with the mapping catheter and displayed on the shell and registered to a three-dimensional CT image in blue. The two-dimensional ultrasound fan demonstrates the real time position of the esophagus behind the posterior wall of the right atrium near the right sided pulmonary veins. The right panel shows the two-dimensional echocardographic image with the left atrium and esophagus outlined in green.

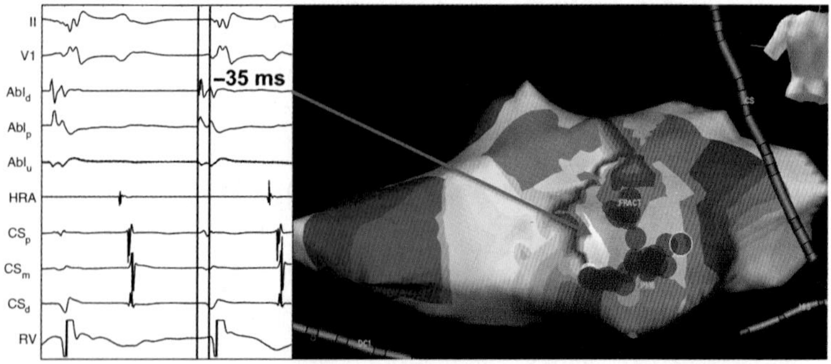

FIGURE 9-3. Activation map of ventricular tachycardia. Local activation time at hundreds of individual sites are recorded and displayed on an electroanatomic map, with colors to indicate timing as compared to a constant reference. The earliest local activation is at the white area, latest at the purple area. Local electrogram recorded from the site indicated by the *arrow* showed local activation 35 ms before onset of QRS complex in a beat of ventricular tachycardia. After ablation lesions at early sites (*brown circles*) with abnormal electrograms, the tachycardia was not inducible. Abl end, endocardial ablation catheter; HRA, high right atrial catheter; CS, coronary sinus catheter (p, proximal; m, middle; d, distal); RV, right ventricular catheter; HIS, His bundle catheter; FRACT, fractionated local EGM; PM5; pace map 5.

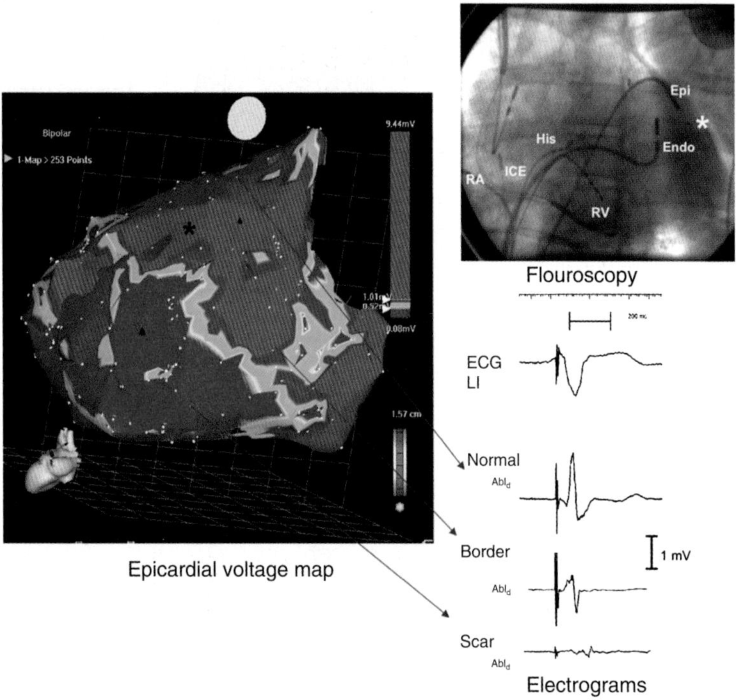

FIGURE 9-6. Electroanatomic map of epicardial surface in a patient with nonischemic cardiomyopathy and a large epicardial scar. Also shown are fluoroscopy of catheter positions, and representative local electrograms from normal tissue, border zone, and dense scar regions. RA, right atrial catheter; ICE, intracardiac echocardiogram catheter; RV, right ventricular catheter; Endo, endocardial left ventricular mapping catheter; Epi, epicardial left ventricular mapping catheter; ECG LI, electrocardiogram lead I; Abl d, ablation distal bipole. (Courtesy of David Cesario, MD, PhD, University of Southern California.)

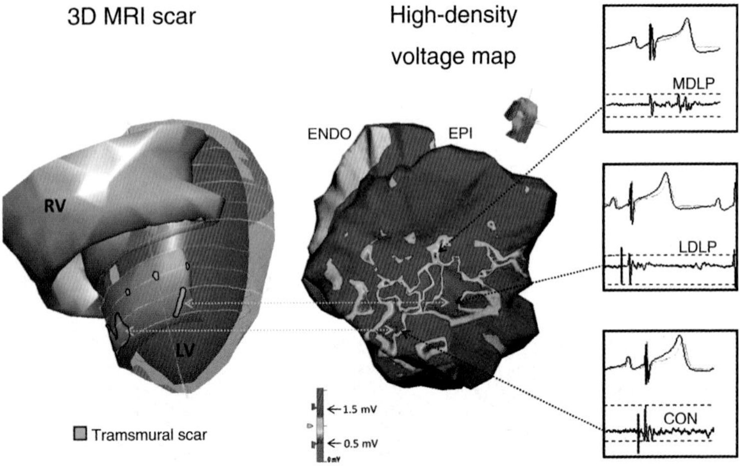

FIGURE 9-7. Substrate mapping correlating magnetic resonance imaging (MRI) with electroanatomic voltage map. Areas of scar on MRI correlate with low-voltage areas on electroanatomic map. Late potentials are recorded within scar and in scar border zones. RV, right ventricle; LV, left ventricle; ENDO, endocardial surface; EPI, epicardial surface; MDLP, mid-diastolic late potential; LDLP, late-diastolic late potential; CON, continuous electrical activity. (Courtesy of Shiro Nakahara, MD, PhD, UCLA.)

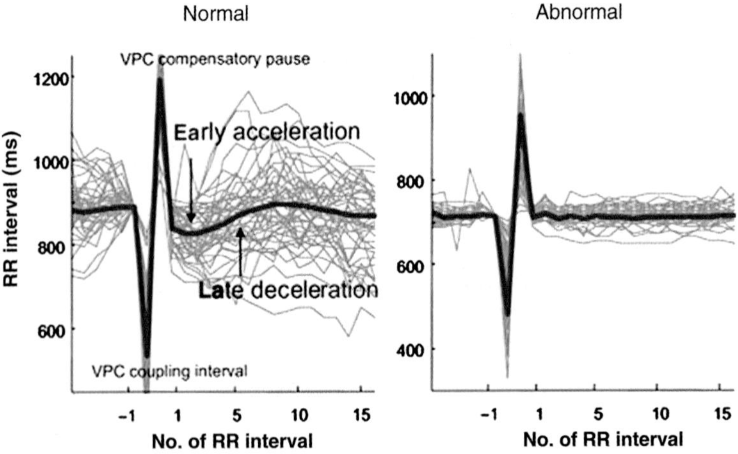

FIGURE 11-4. Heart rate turbulence. VPC tachograms showing normal **(left)** and abnormal **(right)** HRT. HRT is composed of the transient acceleration phase of heart rate (RR interval shortening) immediately after the compensatory pause followed by a subsequent and gradual deceleration phase (RR interval prolongation). *Orange curves* show single VPC tachograms. *Bold brown curves* show the averaged VPC tachogram over 24 h. (Reproduced from Bauer A, Malik M, Schmidt G, et al. Heart rate turbulence: Standards of measurement, physiological interpretation, and clinical use-International society for Holter and noninvasive electrophysiology consensus. *J Am Coll Cardiol.* 2008;52:1353–1365, with permission.)

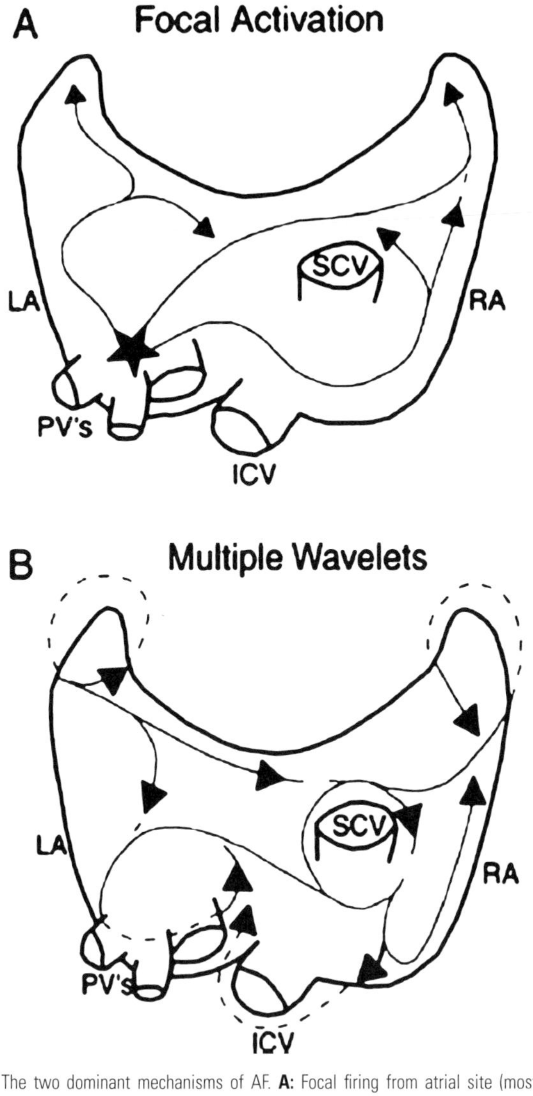

FIGURE 3-2. The two dominant mechanisms of AF. **A:** Focal firing from atrial site (most often pulmonary vein) with fibrillatory conduction. **B:** Multiple wavelets or unstable reentrant circuits throughout atria. (Reprinted from Fuster V, et al. ACC/AHA/ESC 2006 Guidelines for the management of patients with atrial fibrillation—Executive Summary: A Report of the American College of Cardiology/American Heart Association Task Force on Practice Guidelines and the European Society of Cardiology. *J Am Coll Cardiol* 2006;e149–e246, with permission from Elsevier.)

On a cellular level, AF is associated with a variety of abnormal functional properties. Patients may exhibit abnormal shortened action potential duration, changes in calcium handling, and alterations in a variety of potassium and other channel functions. On a larger scale, cellular tissue may have disorders of gap junctions which will interfere with propagation of the atrial impulse. Autonomic modulation may also play a role, with parasympathetic and sympathetic effects both resulting in shortened action potential duration, which facilitates the development of reentry.

Very importantly, perpetuation of AF generates enhanced abnormal atrial EP properties resulting in perpetuation and prolongation of AF episodes. This process, known as atrial remodeling, contributes to recurrences of AF, inability to terminate AF effectively, or ultimately, in the continuous presence of AF. Restoration of sinus rhythm may normalize or restore electrical function, a process termed reverse remodeling. Ultimately, however, prolonged AF may result in structural or permanent abnormalities, including pathologic development of atrial fibrosis. The sum total of these EP consequences is abnormal atrial conduction, shortened atrial repolarization, heterogeneous atrial refractory periods, and abnormal atrial dynamic repolarization properties.

Those patients with AF and underlying cardiovascular conditions often have abnormal atrial chamber size, function, and pathology. Enlargement of the atrial chambers or thickening of atrial muscle is associated with abnormal atrial electrical function. Many patients with AF have atrial fibrosis, fatty or amyloid tissue deposition, or inflammation. All of these will contribute to the abnormal functional properties associated with AF, and the continuing pathologic evolution will likely contribute to incremental functional changes and worsening of atrial substrate.

Some patients have patterns of AF that strongly suggest influence of the autonomic nervous system. A vagal form of AF is suspected when patients describe onset exclusively after meals or while lying down or sleeping. Less commonly, exercise-induced AF suggests the influence of the adrenergic nervous system.

CLASSIFICATION

AF may occur episodically with spontaneous termination or prolonged and continuous requiring pharmacologic or electrical therapy for termination. The former is termed paroxysmal AF and generally self-terminates within 24 to 48 h. On other occasions, the AF may spontaneously terminate after a more prolonged period, often when the patient is on an antiarrhythmic drug program. AF that continues without spontaneous termination is categorized based on the duration of AF or the intentions of therapy. When AF has been present continuously for more than 7 days and up to 1 year, it is termed persistent AF. When AF has continued for longer than 1 year, when there has been failed efforts to restore and maintain sinus rhythm, and/or when sinus rhythm is no longer sought, this form of AF is termed permanent. A more recently developed category, long-lasting persistent AF, is reserved for a group of patients whose AF has lasted from 1 to 3 years but in whom efforts are being made to restore sinus rhythm usually by catheter ablation.

These categories are useful for clinical management because AF is a progressive condition, with patients often passing from one phase to another. Hence, AF patients can be further classified based on the first occurrence of AF or when a pattern is recurrent. Most, but not all, patients present with paroxysmal AF. The frequency and duration of AF is quite variable but often the AF burden increases over time and the patient will pass into a phase of persistent AF.

Because of underlying atrial pathophysiology (defined above) the overall pattern of AF opens a window into the likely progression of atrial remodeling, i.e., the longer the AF has been present or the greater the burden, the more likely there has been progression of pathophysiologic substrate. The pace of progression of AF is highly variable, even among similar clinical conditions or even in the absence of underlying cardiovascular disease. However, paroxysmal AF will progress to more long-lived or permanent forms at a rate that may be in the range of about 5% per year.

SYMPTOMS AND CLINICAL PRESENTATION

AF may complicate the course of patients with a number of serious medical illnesses especially pneumonia, MI, viral pericarditis, and sepsis. The clinical presentation is dominated by these underlying conditions.

Much more frequently, patients present with AF as the primary event. They may be seen in the emergency room, an ambulatory care clinic, or be hospitalized. The most common symptoms include a sense of irregular or rapid heart beating, fatigue or weakness, dyspnea especially with exertion, anginalike chest discomfort, and light-headedness. Less frequently, patients describe polyuria and near syncope, and very rarely, syncope. Syncope may result from tachyarrhythmia but also from associated bradyarrhythmia, especially sinus bradycardia and pauses posttermination ("tachy-brady syndrome").

Symptoms of AF are due to the underlying arrhythmic condition, namely irregular ventricular activation, rapid ventricular rate, and loss of atrioventricular (AV) synchrony. Any one or a combination of these three underlying mechanisms may play a role. In other words, some patients may not be tachycardic yet experience severe symptoms due to loss of atrial kick.

In particular, patients with severe cardiac conditions may have a more profound presentation. Irregular ventricular rates can compromise ventricular function. Rapid ventricular rates shorten diastole and thus interfere with ventricular filling and coronary perfusion. Loss of AV synchrony, and thus, the atrial kick can decrease stroke volume by up to 40% in patients who are dependent upon atrial systole for ventricular filling, such as patients with hypertrophic cardiomyopathy and congestive heart failure. Patients with hypertrophic cardiomyopathy sometimes present with extremely serious and life-threatening findings including hypotension and shock.

Many patients can describe the onset of symptoms, and thus with reasonable accuracy, clinicians can gauge the duration of the AF. Other patients have a more vague recollection of when symptoms had started and it is difficult to determine how long AF has been present. In these situations, concerns are increased regarding the development of atrial thrombus. Very importantly, up to one third of patients with AF have no symptoms whatsoever. In these patients, it is impossible to know how long they have had AF and in fact they may have had a varying pattern and long history of AF without diagnosis. In these patients, it is helpful to determine if they have had medical examinations and ECGs in the past so a window of AF duration can be calculated. This is an important issue because the longevity of AF, especially if present for more than 1 year, will greatly influence the likelihood for successful restoration and maintenance of sinus rhythm. Finally, even patients who have clear-cut symptoms will have asymptomatic episodes intermixed with symptomatic ones; indwelling pacing devices have made this scenario abundantly clear.

INITIAL EVALUATION

The key to diagnosis is of course the electrocardiogram. Ideally, a 12-lead ECG should be obtained during symptomatic and asymptomatic arrhythmias. Multiple recordings are useful as many patients can experience more than one type of arrhythmia, for example, AF, AFL, atrial tachycardia (AT), and atrial ectopic beats. In some patients, ambulatory monitoring including transtelephonic ECG is useful to diagnose paroxysmal arrhythmias that occur in the outpatient setting. Prolonged monitoring is also useful to document the patterns of AF including whether AF, and the ventricular rates, is persistent, especially during activities of daily living. Single-lead ECG recordings are less useful because at times they can be misleading and the underlying fibrillatory wave pattern may not be apparent or in other circumstances an organized atrial arrhythmia may be difficult to discern. Thus multilead recordings or 12-lead ECGs are most useful.

Historical variables are critical to review including the symptoms described in the previous section and the AF frequency, duration, and initial onset. Classification of AF as described in a preceding section is critical for planning management. It should be recognized that even patients with symptomatic episodes will frequently have asymptomatic events as well. Additional historical variables that should be sought include the presence of cardiovascular conditions that can promote AF as well as noncardiovascular conditions that are associated with AF. The potential complications of AF, including neurologic incidents, should be elicited.

Besides historical variables, it is important to determine whether the patient has underlying heart disease, which at times may be occult or a secondary phenomenon related to the AF (e.g., tachycardia-induced cardiomyopathy). Thus, it is typically useful to perform an echocardiogram to evaluate ventricular function, valvular heart disease, and LA dimension. The latter will give insight into the mechanism of AF or may be indicative of the duration of AF as patients with prolonged AF often have progressive atrial dilatation. The LA has been shown to enlarge by about 5 mm in diameter over a 1-year observation period. LA enlargement (especially greater than 55 to 60 mm) has been associated with failure to maintain sinus rhythm after successful cardioversion.

Transesophageal echocardiography may be required to exclude the presence of atrial thrombus, specifically LA appendage thrombus, when a cardioversion is required and a patient has not yet had the requisite 3 consecutive weeks of therapeutic anticoagulation. The transesophageal echo is particularly useful to detect the presence of thrombus and more frequently the presence of spontaneous echo contrast or "smoke" which is a marker of stasis in the atrial chamber. The presence of thrombus is a contraindication for cardioversion but the presence of smoke is not. Nonetheless, stroke risk is increased in the presence of smoke and also in the presence of reduced LA appendage emptying velocity. Up to approximately 25% of patients with AF of more than a few days duration may have LA appendage thrombus if they have not been inadequately anticoagulated.

Additional cardiac tests can be individualized and include exercise testing, cardiac catheterization, cardiac MRI, etc. EP study is generally not required for most patients with AF unless another primary arrhythmia is suspected (e.g., supraventricular tachycardia [SVT], Wolff-Parkinson-White [WPW] syndrome, AFL, or tachycardia) or if catheter ablation of AF or associated arrhythmias is planned (see below).

PROGNOSIS AND COMPLICATIONS

AF can have adverse consequences but the nature and frequency of complications vary, primarily related to underlying heart disease and age. Population studies such as the Framingham cohort have determined that patients with AF have an increased rate of death compared to counterparts in the population without AF. For men, the death rate is increased 1.5-fold and for women, 1.9-fold (Fig. 3-3). The cause-specific mortality composition is uncertain but may be related to an increased risk of stroke and its consequences, aggravation or precipitation of heart failure, worsening of coronary ischemia, development of a hypercoagulable state, ventricular electrical instability, complications and proarrhythmia from drug therapy, and other causes.

AF by virtue of rapid and/or irregular ventricular rates can contribute to LV dysfunction. A pure form of tachycardia-induced cardiomyopathy can exist when patients' heart rates are excessive for much or all of the 24 h period. However, the proportion of time and the degree of tachycardia that is required to precipitate LV dysfunction in a clinical environment is uncertain. Indeed, the diagnosis of tachycardia-induced cardiomyopathy must be made in retrospect, i.e., when rate or rhythm control is achieved, there is improvement of the LV dysfunction and/or resolution of cardiomyopathy. A high index of suspicion should be maintained in all patients. An even more difficult scenario unfolds when patients

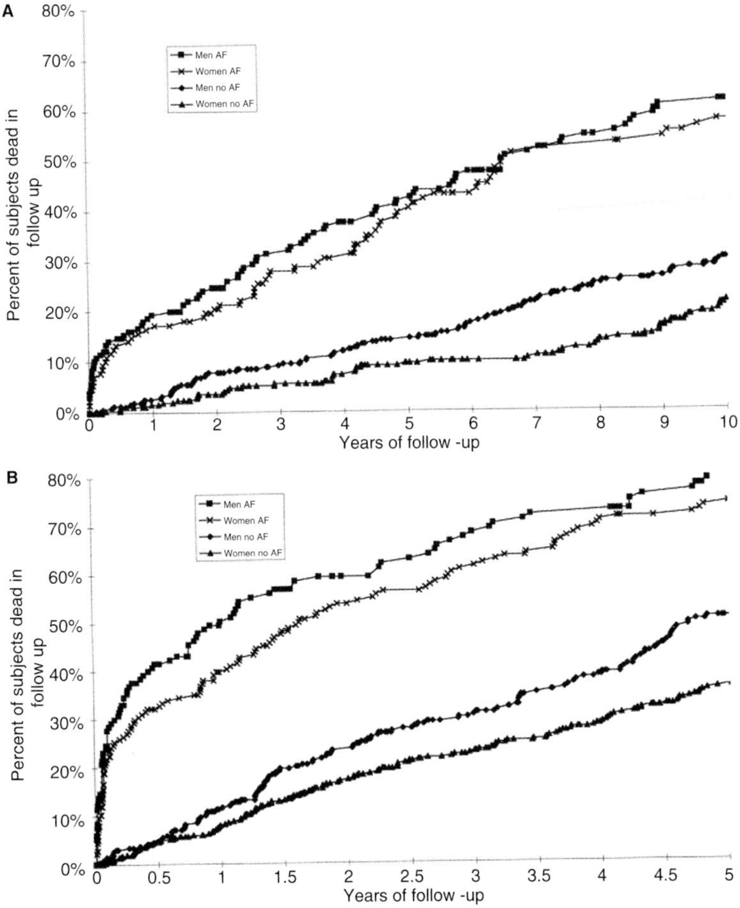

FIGURE 3-3. The risk of death is increased for all patients with AF versus those without for patients identified in the age group of 55 to 74 years **(A)** or in the age group of 75 to 94 years **(B)** in the Framingham cohort. (Reprinted from Benjamin EJ, Wolf PA, D'Agostino RB, et al. Impact of atrial fibrillation on the risk of death: The Framingham Heart Study. *Circulation.* 1998;98:946–952, with permission.)

have preexisting heart disease and superimposed AF, which can aggravate rather than create a cardiomyopathic process. This "impure" form of tachycardia-induced cardiomyopathy is even more difficult to recognize but should be considered possible in all such patients with a high index of suspicion. Thus, patients should not be allowed to have excessive ventricular rates without adequate control.

Patients with AF may have a risk of stroke and systemic thromboemboli. Cardioemboli resulting from AF are usually cerebrovascular rather than systemic (peripheral, spenic, etc). The risk of stroke is extremely variable and relates in large part to the presence of cardiovascular diseases and the patient's age. In its most benign context, AF in the absence of cardiovascular disease and in a young patient, particularly when paroxysmal without atrial remodeling, is not associated with an increased risk of stroke relative to the general population (Fig. 3-4). Thus these patients with lone AF do not necessarily require chronic anticoagulation. However, in the setting of cardiovascular disease and advanced age (variably defined as age 65 or 75 and above), there is a measurably increased risk of stroke. The projected stroke risk is related to a number of risk factors (see below), and guidelines have been published based on a vast literature confirming the importance of chronic anticoagulation in these patients. AF is the most important cardiac cause for stroke and may account for approximately 15% of all strokes. The annual stroke rate in high risk patients is estimated to be 5% to 8% per year. Strokes that complicate AF are often dense, large, and permanent. Once a patient has experienced a stroke, the long-term prognosis is compromised. A stroke that occurs despite anticoagulation is often smaller than anticipated and more reversible, and these patients will have an improved prognosis relative to those who are unanticoagulated.

Because oxygen demand is governed in large part by heart rate, patients with underlying coronary artery disease may have aggravation of ischemia in the presence of AF. Patients who have AF have activation of the coagulation cascade, and it is conceivable that this hypercoagulable state may contribute to coronary thrombosis as well.

Antiarrhythmic drug therapy which is sometimes used for patients with AF may have a distinct long-term risk as well. Many antiarrhythmic drugs possess potent channel blocking properties and may be associated with pro-arrhythmia in specific contexts. For example, class Ic antiarrhythmic drugs have a potent negative effect on outcome in patients with underlying coronary heart disease and LV dysfunction, but this concern should probably be extended to patients with LV dysfunction from any cause, coronary artery disease without LV dysfunction, and perhaps any patient with structural heart disease. Drugs that block the potassium channels may have a risk of torsade de pointes which can be life-threatening. Finally, the AFFIRM trial has indicated that a rhythm control strategy that employs antiarrhythmic drugs may be associated with an increased risk of noncardiovascular death over time in older patients treated for AF.

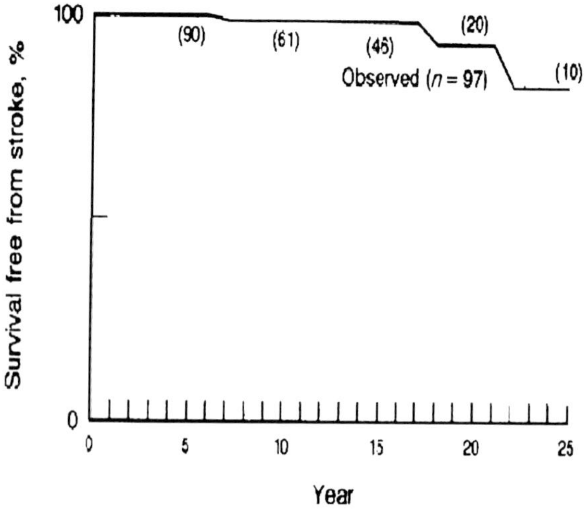

FIGURE 3-4. Risk of stroke in patients with lone AF. (Reprinted from Kopecky SL, Gersh BJ, McGoon MD, et al. The natural history of lone atrial fibrillation. A population-based study over three decades. *New Eng J Med.* 1987;317:669–674, with permission. Copyright © 1987 Massachusetts Medical Society. All rights reserved.)

ANTITHROMBOTIC THERAPY

In most patients identified as having an increased risk of stroke and systemic thromboemboli, chronic anticoagulation is the cornerstone of therapy. An initial assessment of stroke risk is mandatory when the diagnosis of AF is made, repeatedly during follow-up as underlying cardiovascular conditions may change or as the patients age. Multiple risk stratification schemes (Table 3-2) have been created, generally based on data accumulated in large multicenter trials of anticoagulation, and should be applied in clinical practice. One of the most popular schema is the $CHADS_2$ risk index. Using risk factors of congestive heart failure, hypertension, age above 75 years, diabetes and prior stroke, or other thromboembolism, patients can have risk scores calculated between 0 and 6 points (Table 3-3, Fig. 3-5). One point is awarded for each one of these risk factors except for the presence of prior stroke/TIA which is counted as two points. Current guidelines suggest that a risk score of 2 or greater necessitates long-term anticoagulation unless there is a specific and validated contraindication. A risk score of 1 is considered an optional indication for chronic anticoagulation.

Contraindications to chronic therapy are generally few or temporary. Multiple surveys have determined that physicians are overly cautious in administering anticoagulant therapy to patients at risk of stroke due to AF and may overestimate the risk of potential bleeding complications. This is especially true in the elderly who, although often at slightly greater risk of bleeding complications, also have a much greater risk of stroke due to their age and associated cardiovascular conditions. Contraindications to chronic

TABLE 3-2 AHA/ACC/ESC Guidelines for Antithrombotic Therapy for Patients with AF

Risk Category	Recommended Therapy
No risk factors	Aspirin 81 or 325 mg daily
1 moderate risk factor	Aspirin or warfarin (target INR 2.0–3.0)
1 high-risk factor or >1 moderate risk factor	Warfarin

Less Validated or Weaker Risk Factors	Moderate Risk Factors	High-Risk Factors
Female gender	Age >75 years	Prior stroke, TIA or systemic embolism
Age 65–74 years	Hypertension	Mitral stenosis
Coronary artery disease	Heart failure	Prosthetic heart valve (target INR 2.5–3.5 if mechanical)
Thyrotoxicosis	LVEF < 35%	
	Diabetes mellitus	

TABLE 3-3 Stroke Risk According to the $CHADS_2$ Index

$CHADS_2$ Risk Criteria	Score
Prior stroke or TIA	2
Age >75 years	1
Hypertension	1
Diabetes mellitus	1
Heart failure	1

warfarin therapy include rare hypersensitivity reactions, active bleeding or recent surgical procedures, bleeding diatheses, or serious hemorrhagic complication during therapeutic anticoagulation with warfarin.

On the basis of the results of multiple randomized clinical trials (Fig. 3-6), chronic warfarin therapy is the antithrombotic therapy of choice in patients at risk of stroke. It has been determined that the INR is ideally maintained in a range of 2.0 to 3.0 to maximize therapeutic efficacy and limit bleeding risk. In general, these clinical trials have indicated an approximate two-third risk reduction of stroke if patients are treated with

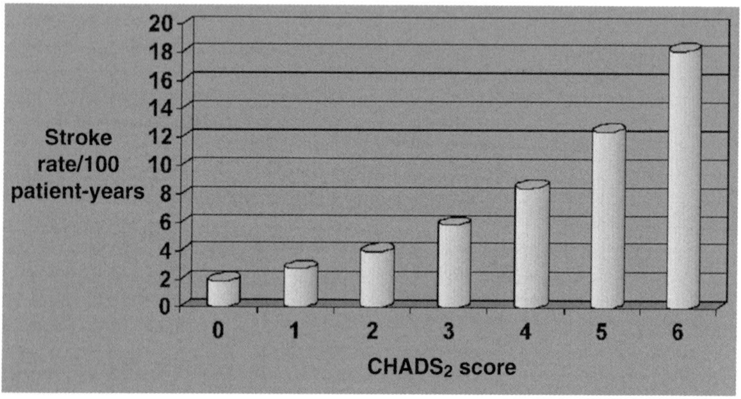

FIGURE 3-5. Adjusted annual stroke risk relative to the $CHADS_2$ risk score. (Adapted from Gage BF, et al. Validation of clinical classification schemes for predicting stroke: Results from the National Registry of Atrial Fibrillation. *JAMA.* 2001;285:2864–2870.)

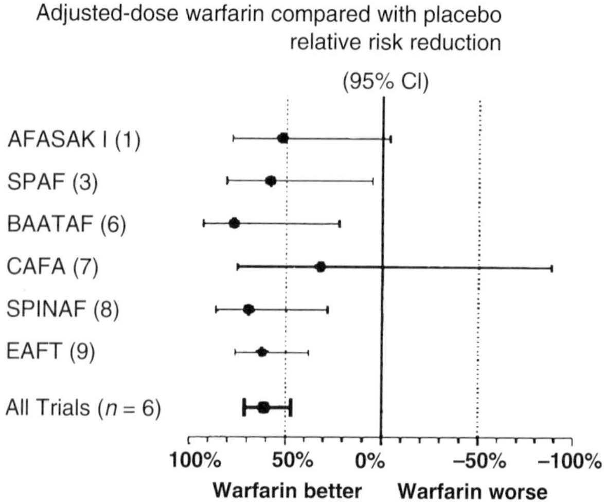

FIGURE 3-6. Risk of all strokes in patients with nonvalvular atrial fribrillation treated with warfarin versus placebo. (Adapted from Hart RG and Halperin JL. Atrial fibrillation and thromboembolism: A decade of progress in stroke prevention. *Ann Int Med.* 1999;131:688–695.)

warfarin. If patients can be maintained on the therapeutic dose of warfarin on a consistent basis, the risk reduction may range as high as 80%. The risk of major bleeding is in the range of approximately 1% per year, most notably including intracerebral hemorrhage. Thus, clearly, the use of warfarin in patients must include a stroke risk that significantly outweighs this potential bleeding risk, and thus the use of the risk stratification schemes. The flip side of this argument is that patients who have little or no risk, such as those with lone AF at a younger age, are generally not candidates for anticoagulation except preceding (for 3 weeks) and following cardioversion (for 4 weeks).

Echocardiographic risk factors were not consistently obtained in large scale clinical trials but may be of additional value as well. LA enlargement and LV dysfunction have been identified as risk factors. The former may develop in patients with long standing AF who have no other risk factors, and some would consider this an indication that the LA is becoming structurally abnormal and may become a potential nidus for atrial thrombus.

Several clinical trials also tested the value of aspirin alone as an antithrombotic regimen and in general these trials found that aspirin did not provide statistically significant risk reduction although one large-scale trial found otherwise. A metaanalysis of all published data suggests modest benefit from aspirin and thus aspirin is considered only a second-line therapy in patients who have a bona fide contraindication to warfarin or in patients who are at low risk and do not require warfarin therapy. More recent clinical trial data have tested other potent antiplatelet regimens, specifically combining clopidogrel with aspirin therapy. In the ACTIVE studies, this combination was shown to provide inferior protection against stroke versus targeted warfarin therapy, and the trial was prematurely terminated.

It is important to recognize that challenges exist to warfarin usage including multiple drug interactions, food interactions, inconstant INR results, and a narrow therapeutic window. Frequent INR testing is required to ensure a consistent therapeutic action. In the early phases of warfarin initiation, INR values will need to be determined approximately twice weekly. As the therapeutic level is maintained on a stable warfarin dose regimen, this can be initially decreased to once weekly and later, once monthly. This of course is subject to change should new medications be introduced that have the potential to alter the INR, notably amiodarone which potentiates the therapeutic effect of warfarin. It is crucial to maintain the INR value within the targeted range because values consistently below 2.0 are associated with an increased stroke risk, and as values rise above 3.0, there is no additional benefit of stroke protection but there is much greater risk of bleeding.

There is at present no indicated alternative to warfarin with similar efficacy. Direct thrombin inhibitors have been tested in randomized clinical trials and were found to be equivalent but had significant hepatotoxicity and have thus not been approved for clinical use. New direct oral thrombin inhibitors are currently undergoing randomized clinical trials. Factor Xa inhibitors have also been tested but were associated with excessive bleeding relative to warfarin. Mechanical devices have been developed that can be placed transvenously via transeptal puncture into the LA appendage in an effort to exclude this primary source of atrial thromboemboli. Small studies have shown feasibility albeit with a significant complication rate, and a large multicenter trial is ongoing. Surgical excision of the LA appendage is commonly employed in some cardiac surgical procedures, especially mitral valve repair or replacement. Nonrandomized surgical series have suggested a significant reduction in stroke rate but the results are not definitive. An ongoing randomized multicenter trial of high risk patients undergoing coronary artery bypass graft surgery will test the value of routine prophylactic LA appendage excision. Finally, catheter or surgical ablation to eliminate the presence of AF and thus potentially stroke risk has not undergone rigorous randomized examination to test the potential to mitigate stroke risk. Nonetheless, current guidelines suggest there are certain subsets of patients who may safely come off anticoagulant therapy after successful ablation procedures (see below).

PHARMACOLOGIC THERAPY FOR RHYTHM AND RATE CONTROL; CARDIOVERSION

Because most patients with AF have recurrent, progressive or chronic arrhythmia burden, it is reasonable to consider whether patients should undergo pharmacologic or electrical cardioversion to restore sinus rhythm and consider antiarrhythmic drug therapy for maintenance of sinus rhythm.

Certainly, for patients with acute hemodynamic or other serious complications when presenting with AF, electrical cardioversion via external transthoracic shock is appropriate. In order to prevent the progressive remodeling that occurs with prolonged AF, interruption of a prolonged event with cardioversion is also reasonable. Pharmacologic conversion can be accomplished by intravenous ibutilide and by some oral agents (for details regarding antiarrhythmic drug therapy, see Chapter 14). Oral dofetilide seems to be particularly advantageous as an oral agent for pharmacologic conversion, in that approximately two thirds of patients will convert during the initiation phase. Amiodarone, commonly employed agent, has a lower incidence of conversion, approximately 25%.

Clearly, restoration and maintenance of sinus rhythm will relieve the pantheon of consequences of AF. The challenges that confront physicians caring for patients with AF are that the antiarrhythmic drug therapies that are currently available are inherently limited. In general, most agents can be expected to be beneficial for maintenance of sinus rhythm in approximately half of the patients who receive an individual drug. Amiodarone may have a slightly higher rate of success, perhaps around 60%. Randomized use of antiarrhythmic drug therapy in AFFIRM and other studies support the superiority of amiodarone, but of course noncardiac adverse effects limit its long-term usage. Drug therapy is useful not only to fully suppress AF, but also to delay the next event or shorten its duration. In some patients this may be an acceptable end point.

Whether all patients with AF should have a routine effort made to maintain sinus rhythm using antiarrhythmic drugs was a matter of controversy until recent clinical trial data became available. The largest and most important of these trials, AFFIRM, enrolled over 4,000 patients over the age of 65 with risk factors for stroke and mortality. Patients were randomly assigned to either undergo a strategy designed to control rhythm or to control rate. Rhythm control was generally achieved by cardioversion when needed and long-term antiarrhythmic drug therapy, most commonly amiodarone. Rate control was achieved by AV nodal blockers including beta-blockers and calcium channel blockers, and if needed, AV junctional ablation. Although almost twice as many patients in the rhythm control arm remained in sinus rhythm, the long-term outcome during 5 years of follow-up demonstrated that the primary end point, all-cause mortality, was equivalent between the two groups. Indeed, there was a slightly higher all-cause mortality in the rhythm control arm. Subsequently, analyses of the AFFIRM data indicated that the rhythm control patients had a substantially higher rate of noncardiovascular mortality; the reasons underlying this observation are uncertain but may be related to the long-term effects of antiarrhythmic drugs outside the cardiovascular system.

Secondary end points including quality of life, cardiac arrest, disabling stroke, and so on were also no different between the two groups. In addition, because patients in the rhythm control were more frequently in sinus rhythm, there was a tendency to reduce the intensity of anticoagulation or eliminate it entirely. A greater than expected risk of stroke was thus observed in the rhythm control arm, providing powerful evidence that even when there is apparent rhythm control, a risk of stroke remains, likely due to asymptomatic AF, and these patients should continue chronic warafin therapy.

This important randomized clinical data lead one to the inevitable conclusion that routine or first-line administration of antiarrhythmic drug, at least in the older population or those with cardiovascular conditions, should be avoided. Instead, selective administration of antiarrhythmic drugs for relief of symptoms related to AF, for prevention or elimination of tachycardia-induced cardiomyopathy, or to improve exercise capacity and hemodynamic function, should be judiciously employed and individualized to patient care. Administration of chronic antiarrhythmic drugs should be undertaken with careful analysis of the risk-benefit ratio. Whether antiarrhythmic drug therapy has a similar lack of benefit in other patient populations, such as the young, is uncertain.

A post hoc analysis of the AFFIRM data tested the hypothesis that consistent maintenance of sinus rhythm conferred a favorable survival advantage. In a complex multivariate analysis, the presence of sinus rhythm was associated with reduction in the risk of death by approximately 50%. Counterbalancing this benefit was the increased risk of death by approximately 50% related to the use of antiarrhythmic drugs. Hence there was a neutral outcome of the trial. However, a theoretical benefit of consistent sinus rhythm was suggested by this analysis, further raising the question of whether alternative pharmacologic or nonpharmacologic therapy may be advantageous in the future.

The AFFIRM trial largely did not enroll patients with congestive heart failure. A subsequent study, the *AF-CHF trial*, specifically targeted patients with NYHA classes II to IV heart failure and an LVEF≤35%. Similar to AFFIRM, patients were randomly assigned to a rhythm or rate control strategy. At the end of follow-up, this trial also failed to demonstrate any advantage to the routine use of a rhythm-control strategy. The primary end point, cardiovascular death, was virtually identical, as were all major secondary end points, between the two arms.

Should antiarrhythmic drug therapy be undertaken, specific drugs should be used in specific clinical contexts. For young patients with no or minimal heart disease, a class Ic drug such as flecainide or propafenone may be useful. In the presence of heart failure, first-line agents are amiodarone and dofetilide. In the presence of coronary artery disease, with or without LV dysfunction, class Ic drugs should be avoided and instead patients may consider dofetalide or sotalol. Patients with hypertension and significant LV hypertrophy may have a greater risk of torsade de pointes so class III agents should be avoided. Instead, amiodarone may be considered. In the absence of LV hypertrophy, class Ic or III antiarrhythmic drugs may be used.

Selecting strategies for selection of the various competing therapeutic modalities are a complex process. In general, symptom status is the most important criterion to guide the clinical choice of therapy. In the setting of recurrent paroxysmal AF but with no or minor symptoms, a simple rate control regimen is reasonable. Anticoagulation is based on the risk of stroke as described in the preceding section. If symptoms are disabling, antiarrhythmic drug therapy can be considered, with catheter ablation as an alternative when drugs fail. It is important to recognize that drug therapy need not be undertaken after the initial episode of AF until a pattern has been established.

For persistent AF, the initial goal is restoration of sinus rhythm. If recurrent, symptom burden again will dictate the need for antiarrhythmic drugs. Recurrent cardioversion may be required as well. Catheter ablation is available should drug therapy fail. In addition, some patients may benefit from episodic antiarrhythmic drug therapy designed to convert an acute event rather than to chronically suppress recurrences. This so-called pill in the pocket therapy has been shown in a randomized trial to provide more rapid restoration of sinus rhythm than conventional means. Typically, propaphenone and flecainide in higher than usual doses can be employed for this purpose in the outpatient setting when there is no severe structural heart disease. When the patient has evolved to permanent AF and no efforts are undertaken to restore sinus rhythm, rate control is appropriate.

The definition of rate control is important to emphasize. Resting rate should be maintained below 80. In addition, rates during a variety of usual activities should be sampled as well, usually by ambulatory ECG recording. The peak ventricular rate should be assessed throughout the day and generally maintained below approximately 110 to 120 beats/min. Scrupulous attention to rate control will avoid the potential risk of tachycardia-induced cardiomyopathy. Rate control can be achieved in the vast majority of patients with medical therapy using calcium channel blockers such as diltiazem and verapamil and/or beta-blockers such as metoprolol, propranolol, carvedilol, atenalol, etc. Careful dose titration needs to balance rate control, bradyarrhythmias, and adverse affects is often required. When pharmacologic therapy fails, in selected patients, an AV junctional ablation can be considered (see below).

Nonantiarrhythmic drugs, such as inhibitors of the renin angiotensin system, polyunsaturated fatty acids and fish oils, and statins, might modify the underlying atrial substrate or improve the underlying cardiovascular condition and thus limit the potential for AF. Retrospective analyses of large multicenter trials that employed statins and angiotensin converting enzyme inhibitors/angiotensin receptor blockers have suggested that there is a lesser likelihood of developing AF. However, there is no prospective clinical trial data that provides evidence that would advocate the routine use of these medications to prevent AF. However, many patients with AF have associated cardiovascular conditions that necessitate the use of one or more of these medications, and thus, these patients may benefit from their long-term use for a variety of reasons. Prospective clinical trials are anticipated to clarify the use of statins and fish oils. Finally, atrial pacing in the setting of sick sinus syndrome may lower the likelihood for the development of AF but is not advocated as a stand alone treatment for AF in the absence of symptomatic bradycardia due to sick sinus syndrome necessitating permanent pacemaker placement. Although sleep apnea is a common concomitant condition that may provoke AF, treatment of obstructive sleep apnea with CPAP does not eliminate the AF.

CATHETER AND SURGICAL ABLATIVE THERAPY

The seminal surgical ablation technique pioneered by Cox et al., was based on the concept of a sufficient critical mass of atrial muscle required to maintain AF. The "Maze" procedure divided the atria into smaller subsegments and clinical observational series provided proof of concept that this intervention was capable of eliminating AF in up to 90% of treated patients. Because the procedure was very invasive and had a small but important morbidity and mortality, as a stand alone approach, it was not highly popular. Initial catheter attempts to mimic the Maze procedure were successful in very small series but were associated with significant morbidity.

In the mid-1990s based on the pioneering work of Haissaguerre et al., it became clear that a powerful new strategy could be developed based on the predictability of trigger sites of AF from one or more of the pulmonary veins. This facilitated the development of catheter ablation strategies, i.e., in some manner, isolating the pulmonary veins from the LA and preventing the initiation of AF. Over the first decade of catheter ablation therapy for AF, a consensus has developed that isolation of all major pulmonary veins is the cornerstone of catheter ablation therapy. In many published clinical series, the 6 to 12 month success rate is in the range of 67% to 80%. Although the end point has been measured in a variety of different ways, generally speaking, it should reflect symptomatic elimination of AF and as much as possible, confirmation by long-term monitoring, and the ability to discontinue antiarrhythmic therapy. The complication rate from this procedure is greater than other ablation procedures and in the range of 2% to 4%. Most prominently, adverse consequences may include complications related to venous access, embolic events including stroke and MI, cardiac perforation and tamponade requiring pericardiocentesis, pulmonary vein stenosis, and LA-esophageal fistula. Some of these complications can be limited with careful selection of patients, targeted energy delivery and adjustments of energy power and duration, online intraprocedure monitoring with intracardiac ultrasound, accurate delineation of important anatomic sites such as the ostia of the pulmonary veins and the esophagus, etc. Nonetheless, these procedures are generally longer and more complex than other ablation procedures and thus have an inherently increased risk.

Ideal candidates for catheter ablation are those who remain highly symptomatic despite medical therapy (Table 3-4). Medical therapy generally involves AV nodal blockers

TABLE 3-4 Indications for Catheter Ablation of AF
• Symptomatic AF refractory to or intolerant of ≥1 class I or III antiarrhythmic drug
• Paroxysmal, persistent, or long-lived persistent AF
• In rare circumstances, first-line therapy
• Selected symptomatic patients with heart failure or LV dysfunction

and often at least one class I or III antiarrhythmic drug. Patients with paroxysmal AF are generally treated with a simple pulmonary vein isolation procedure. A redo procedure is required in a minority of patients and often involves simple reisolation.

The ideal treatment strategy for patients with persistent or longstanding persistent AF is unresolved at this point. Various alternative or adjunctive techniques to pulmonary vein isolation are employed to improve the success rate in persistent AF. These may include conversion of the persistent AF patient to a paroxysmal pattern by aggressive medical therapy in advance to the procedure to effect reverse remodeling; the addition of "substrate" ablation targeting important areas of the LA that are thought necessary to maintain AF including the LA roof between the two upper pulmonary veins, the mitral isthmus between the left lower pulmonary vein and the mitral annulus, or other important sites determined by mapping of triggers or atrial electrogram characteristics (e.g., "complex fractionated atrial electrograms"), targeting of the vagal ganglia, and mapping and ablation of other identified more organized atrial tachyarrhythmias. A general rule is that the more longlasting the AF has been, the more likely the procedure will require additional ablation strategies and/or additional procedures.

Prior to an ablation procedure, patients are therapeutically anticoagulated and a TEE or intracardiac ultrasound is needed to exclude intra-atrial thrombus. All patients, regardless of generic stroke risk, must be anticoagulated after the procedure for about 2 months. Generally speaking, most patients are monitored with ambulatory ECG recordings of some type that supplement symptom status to evaluate response to the procedure. It should be noted that in some patients who have had a long-lived response to an ablation procedure, AF may recur months or even years after apparent success.

There are some patients who continue to have AF despite best efforts to maintain sinus rhythm and who continue to be highly symptomatic. Some of these patients may best be managed with an AV nodal ablation which will eliminate the rapid and irregular rates of AF, although not the AF itself. These patients will require permanent pacing and the use of right ventricular or biventricular pacemakers will be determined based on the presence of heart failure or LV dysfunction. If patients have LVEF less than 35% or advanced heart failure or both, a biventricular device may be preferred. However, it should be noted that some patients with chronic right ventricular pacing may go on to develop new or worsening heart failure and may need upgrade to a biventricular device. These patients will all require chronic anticoagulation as the AF has not been eliminated.

Surgical procedures have been designed to isolate the pulmonary veins and mimic the linear atrial lesions described above. Surgical series that are largely observational have suggested a significant response rate. These procedures are generally employed as an adjunct to another surgical need such as bypass surgery and mitral valve repair/replacement but can in selected patients be used as a primary treatment approach.

ATRIAL FLUTTER

DEFINITION

AFL is a common reentrant tachycardia originating in the atrium with a variable, often 2:1 AV conduction.

EPIDEMIOLOGY

Incidence

Incidence rates range from 5/100,000 in patients less than 50 years to 587/100,000 in patients less than 80 years. There are about 200,000 new cases of AFL diagnosed in the US annually. AFL is diagnosed for the first time more than twice as often as paroxysmal supraventricular tachycardia (PSVT) and is approximately 2.5 times more common in men than women.

Risk Factors

Typical AFL frequently occurs in the absence of structural heart disease, so-called lone atrial flutter. The risk of developing AFL increases 3.5 times in individuals with heart failure and 1.9 times in individuals with chronic obstructive pulmonary disease (COPD). Prior instrumentation of the atria resulting in scar, including open-heart surgery and prior ablation with extensive radiofrequency (RF) delivery, increases the risk of developing *atypical* AFL. Class Ic antiarrhythmic drugs given for AF can organize the atrial rhythm and transform AF to AFL.

CLINICAL PRESENTATION

Symptoms

Many patients present with palpitations as the only symptom. Prolonged episodes, especially in patients with reduced cardiopulmonary reserve, can lead to heart failure symptoms or exacerbation.

Electrocardiogram

AFL is a macroreentrant atrial tachyarrhythmia and is organized in contradistinction to AF. The ECG is characterized by a regular and consistent pattern of atrial activation called flutter (F) waves. F waves are usually visible in leads II, III, and aVF, without

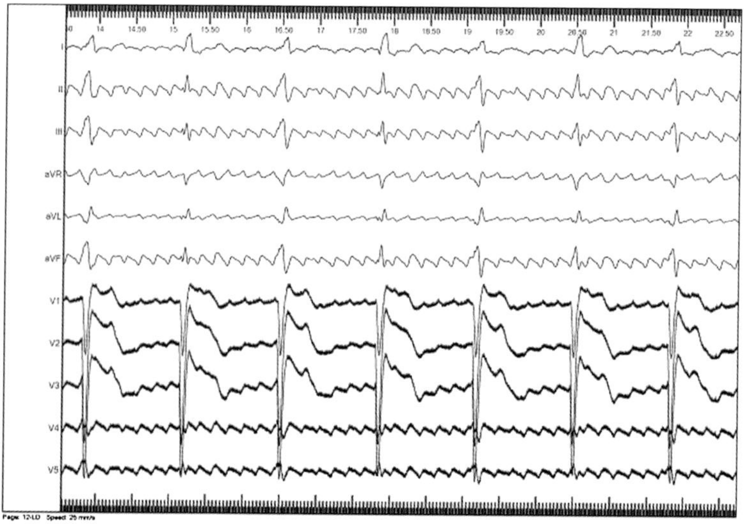

FIGURE 3-7. Typical counterclockwise AFL.

an isoelectric baseline between deflections (in contrast to AT). In case of typical AFL, F waves are negative in ECG leads II, III, and aVF, often in a "sawtooth" pattern, and positive in lead V1 (Fig. 3-7). The atrial rate typically ranges from 240 to 320 beats/min. If untreated, there is often 2:1 AV conduction resulting in a ventricular rate of approximately 150 beats/min, but 1:1 conduction as well as higher degree of AV nodal block are possible, especially if treated with AV blocking agents. One-to-one AV conduction can result in aberrant ventricular conduction, which can make the distinction form ventricular tachycardia (VT) difficult. Lead V1 can sometimes be misleading, demonstrating more organization than other leads, which can lead to misdiagnosis of AF as AFL, and should therefore not be used as sole lead to make the diagnosis (Fig. 3-8).

In untreated subjects with lone AFL, the F wave polarity can often give reliable clues to the origin and direction of AFL:

(1) *Right-sided AFL*:
   (a) Typical (counterclockwise) AFL: negative in II, III, and aVF, positive in V1.
   (b) Reverse typical (clockwise) AFL: positive in II, III, and aVF, negative in V1.
(2) *Left-sided AFL*: Often negative in I and aVL, flat or positive in V1, often positive in II, III, and aVF. Patients who underwent prior open heart surgery (OHS) or ablation can have typical AFL but present with atypical ECG features.

Complications

Similar to AF, AFL predisposes to intracardiac thrombus formation, which can lead to embolic events including stroke. The same risk factors, which govern the risk of stroke during AF, are applicable to AFL.

Persistent AFL with rapid ventricular conduction can lead to a tachycardia-induced cardiomyopathy, which is usually reversible within several weeks to months once the ventricular rate is controlled or sinus rhythm is restored. Thromboembolic events and heart failure from tachycardia-induced cardiomyopathy can sometimes be the initial presentation.

PATHOPHYSIOLOGY

Mechanism

AFL is a macroreentrant rhythm. As such, it occurs when typical requirements for reentry are met: (i) two anatomically or functionally distinct pathways (often separated by a central obstacle), (ii) slow conduction in one limb, and (iii) unidirectional block.

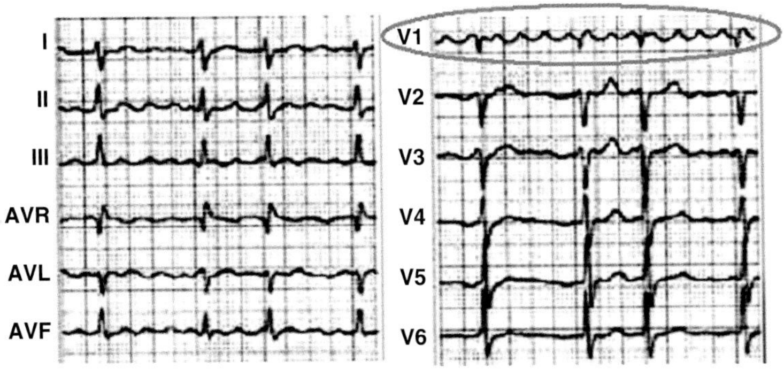

FIGURE 3-8. Coarse AF. (With permission of Ashish Nabar, MD, PhD; Department of Cardiology, Academic Hospital Maastricht.)

Origin

AFL can originate within the right atrium (RA) or LA. Obstacles in AFL can consist of natural barriers (in the RA: tricuspid valve, superior vena cava, inferior vena cava, coronary sinus (CS), and crista terminalis; in the LA: mitral valve and pulmonary veins) or scar.

Categorization

AFL can be isthmus dependent or nonisthmus dependent (Fig. 3-9). In right-sided AFL the impulse travels along the tricuspid annulus, passing through an electrically isolated isthmus. This isthmus is bordered anteriorly by the tricuspid valve, inferiorly by the inferior vena cava, and posteriorly by the ostium of CS. The impulse can travel in a counterclockwise (ccw) (Fig. 3-10) or clockwise (cw) fashion. The former is much more common, representing about 90% of isthmus-dependent cases.

Left-sided AFL: Predisposing factors are prior instrumentation of the LA resulting in a scar, like prior open-heart surgery, including Maze procedure which carries a risk of the development of AFL in the future of up to 30%, and prior LA ablation, especially for AF:

(1) After a segmental pulmonary vein isolation, in approximately 8% of patients, focal previously ablated pulmonary vein-LA connections can recover and fire rapidly. This can result in a regular AT. This mechanism is not macroreentry but focal—automatic, triggered, or microreentrant.

(2) After extensive linear ablation, similar to AFL post-Maze, gaps or recovering sites within ablation lines can lead to macroreentrant AFL in about 20% of patients.

DIAGNOSIS

Pharmacologic Maneuvers

During AFL, the AV node and the ventricles are activated passively and are not required to maintain the tachycardia. Thus, AV nodal blockade does not terminate AFL but merely exposes the F waves.

Giving intravenous adenosine can sometimes help distinguish AFL with 2:1 or 1:1 conduction from SVT or VT, respectively.

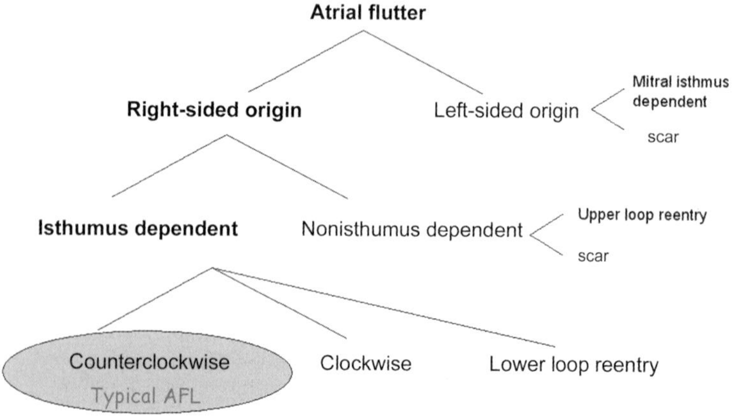

FIGURE 3-9. Categorization of AFL.

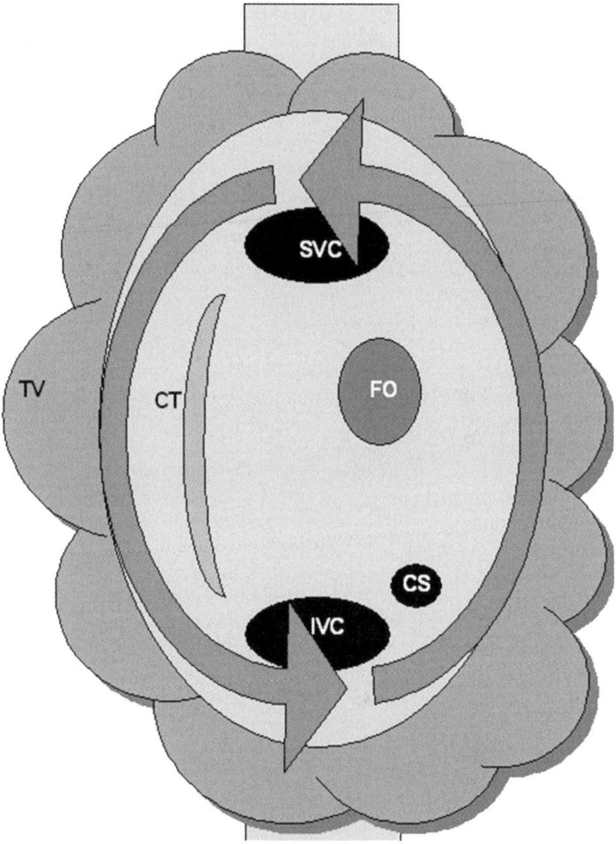

FIGURE 3-10. Typical counterclockwise AFL. TV, tricuspid valve; CT, crista terminalis; SVC, superior vena cava; IVC, inferior vena cava; CS, coronary sinus; FO, fossa ovalis.

Electrophysiologic Maneuvers

In the EP lab, the mechanism, origin, and direction of AFL can be determined by (i) Intracardiac activation sequence, (ii) Entrainment mapping, and (iii) Electroanatomic mapping. If the patient presents in sinus rhythm, pacing maneuvers (atrial extrastimuli and especially burst pacing) can often induce AFL, but not as reliably as SVT. Sometimes administration of isoproterenol is helpful.

(1) Intracardiac activation sequence: Once AFL is present, the atrial activation sequence can be determined using a multipolar catheter which can be deflected to a circular shape, to record from sites around the tricuspid annulus.

In the case of typical counterclockwise AFL, the catheter is activated in a continuous fashion from proximal to distal, with a caudo-cranial pattern on the septal wall and a cranio-caudal pattern on the lateral wall.

(2) Entrainment mapping: Entrainment is a diagnostic pacing maneuver that

(a) confirms reentry as mechanism, (b) localizes tachycardia circuit, and

(c) diagnoses presence of a protected isthmus.

During pacing at a CL slightly below (approx. 20 ms faster) than tachycardia CL, the tachycardia should speed up to the pacing CL to confirm capture of atrial tissue and entrainment of the tachycardia.

Atrial activation (intracardiac activation sequence and F wave morphology on surface electrogram) during entrainment can be identical (concealed entrainment) or different (manifest entrainment) compared to tachycardia.

Upon cessation of pacing, the first postpacing interval (PPI) is measured: if within approximately 30 ms of tachycardia CL, the pacing site is within tachycardia circuit.

The longer the PPI compared to tachycardia CL, the further away the pacing site is from the circuit.

In the case of isthmus depended AFL, entrainment from the isthmus should demonstrate concealed entrainment with a PPI of ≤30 ms.

Concealed entrainment means that a myocardial site lies within an electrically protected site (isthmus) and stimulating this area will always lead to activation of the surrounding myocardium in the same sequence, regardless of activation through pacing or the tachycardia itself.

Origin of AFL: There are several ways to distinguish left- from right-sided AFL:

In left-sided AFL, entrainment mapping shows that during RA stimulation the PPI is long and that the shortest return interval is found in the CS. CS activation is often inverse and proceeds from the distal or mid part of the CS to the proximal part.

(3) Electroanatomic mapping: Electroanatomic mapping uses computer software that creates a three-dimensional map of the chamber of interest.

This can be done via catheter contact, using coordinates from every area of the endocardium, which is touched by the ablation catheter during tachycardia, to determine the timing within tachycardia cycle and voltage of that site. Adding all points together, either an activation map or a voltage map can be created. Another software uses a balloon inflated in the chamber of interest. No catheter contact or sustaining of tachycardia is necessary for activation mapping.

An activation map can demonstrate if the tachycardia mechanism is focal versus macroreentrant. A focal tachycardia would have a central earliest site from which subsequent activation spreads centrifugally. A macroreentrant mechanism would demonstrate that earliest site meets late sites of the circuit and at least 90% of the circuit CL can be recorded within the chamber of interest. A voltage map can differentiate areas of scar from viable areas. This is especially important for atypical flutter related to scar, to find critical isthmuses amenable for ablation.

THERAPY

Acute Treatment

(1) Rate control: Achieving sufficient AV block to control ventricular conduction can be difficult in AFL, so much more for AF. Beta-blockers, calcium channel blockers (nondihydropyridines), and digoxin can be tried.

(2) Rhythm control

(a) Pharmacologic: The overall efficacy of antiarrhythmic drugs in acutely converting AFL is approximately 30% to 90%, class III drugs are more effective than class I, and ibutilide may be useful for this purpose.

(b) Electrical cardioversion is highly effective for acute conversion and safe.

(c) Ablation: see below.

(d) Anticoagulation: see below.

Long-term Treatment

(1) Pharmacologic: Overall long-term maintenance of sinus rhythm with antiarrhythmic drugs is successful in less than 50% of cases and decreases as time progresses. More than 60% of patients will have recurrence after 2 years.
(2) Ablation: see below.
(3) Anticoagulation: see below.

Catheter Ablation

In the case of typical AFL, a line of ablation points is created from the tricuspid annulus to the inferior vena cava across the subeustachian isthmus (Fig. 3-11). This can be done while the patient is in AFL, terminating AFL abruptly once the line is completed, or in sinus rhythm. In either case, pacing maneuvers can confirm if isthmus block was achieved. Catheter ablation has a long-term success rate of more than 95% with a periprocedural

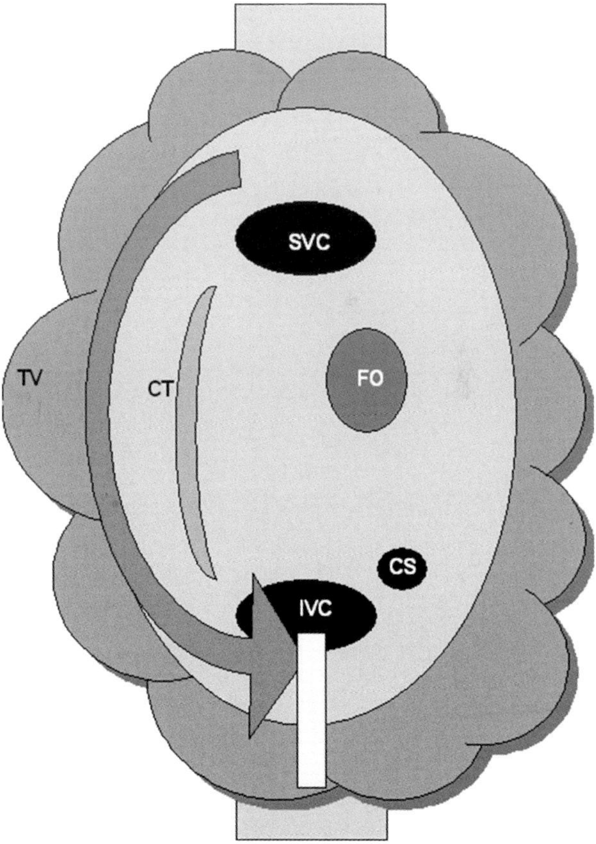

FIGURE 3-11. RA after isthmus ablation. TV, tricuspid valve; CT, crista terminalis; SVC, superior vena cava; IVC, inferior vena cava; CS, coronary sinus; FO, fossa ovalis.

risk of approximately 1%. Long-term recurrence rates after ablation performed in experienced centers are less than 5%, compared to 60% at 2 years if treated medically. This justifies proceeding with ablation as first-line therapy.

Anticoagulation

Patients with AFL carry a stroke risk similar to those with AF and a higher risk for subsequent development of AF than the general population.

Anticoagulation with warfarin should be considered for all patients with a $CHADS_2$ score ≥1. Even if AFL is apparently suppressed with antiarrhythmic drug therapy, anticoagulation should be continued for the likely occurrence of asymptomatic and therefore undetected episodes of AFL. If AFL has been present for ≥24 to 48 h, intracardiac thrombi need to be ruled out by transesophageal echocardiogram prior to ablation or cardioversion—electrical or pharmacologic.

If ablation terminates AFL, which has been present more than 24 to 48 h prior procedure, anticoagulation should be continued for at least 1 month. Unfractionated or low molecular weight heparin needs to be used for bridging until warfarin is therapeutic. Due to the low recurrence rates of typical AFL after initial successful ablation, anticoagulation can be discontinued after about 1 to 3 months postprocedure, if no concomitant AF is present.

ATRIAL TACHYCARDIA

AT is an uncommon arrhythmia. The term AT encompasses several types of tachycardia that originate in the atria and do not require the participation of the AV node for maintenance of the arrhythmia. These tachycardias have differing arrhythmia mechanisms and are often related to anatomical structures. Mechanisms include abnormal automaticity, triggered activity, and reentry (Fig. 3-12).

DEFINITIONS AND CLASSIFICATIONS

Previous classifications of regular ATs were based exclusively on the ECG. Differentiation between AFL and AT depends on a rate cutoff less than 240 to 250/min and the presence of isoelectric baseline between atrial deflections in AT, but not in AFL. However, AT mechanisms, defined by EP studies and RF catheter ablation, do not always correlate with these ECG patterns, and a certain amount of confusion is evident in the literature at the time of assigning appropriate terms to specific arrhythmias.

With the advent of curative RF ablation targeted to the anatomic or EP substrate, it has become necessary to clarify the relations between the AT and the underlying mechanism of arrhythmia, including its anatomic bases. Recently, a statement from the professional societies has sought to redefine the classification of AT.

From their classification, two types of AT are relatively well-known and can be defined clearly based on their EP mechanisms (Table 3-5):

(1) Focal AT (due to an automatic, triggered, or microreentrant mechanism)
(2) Macroreentrant AT (including typical AFL and other well-characterized macroreentrant circuits in the RA and LA.

EPIDEMIOLOGY

Sustained AT is relatively rare. In asymptomatic young individuals, the prevalence of AT has been calculated to be 0.34%, with a prevalence of 0.46% in symptomatic patients. AT accounts for 5% to 15% of adults undergoing EP studies, with higher rates in children. Automatic AT tends to be a condition that affects the young, whereas AT due to microreentry/macroreentry is more common in older patients. In contrast to AV nodal reentry and AV reentrant tachycardia, there appears to be no gender difference in AT incidence.

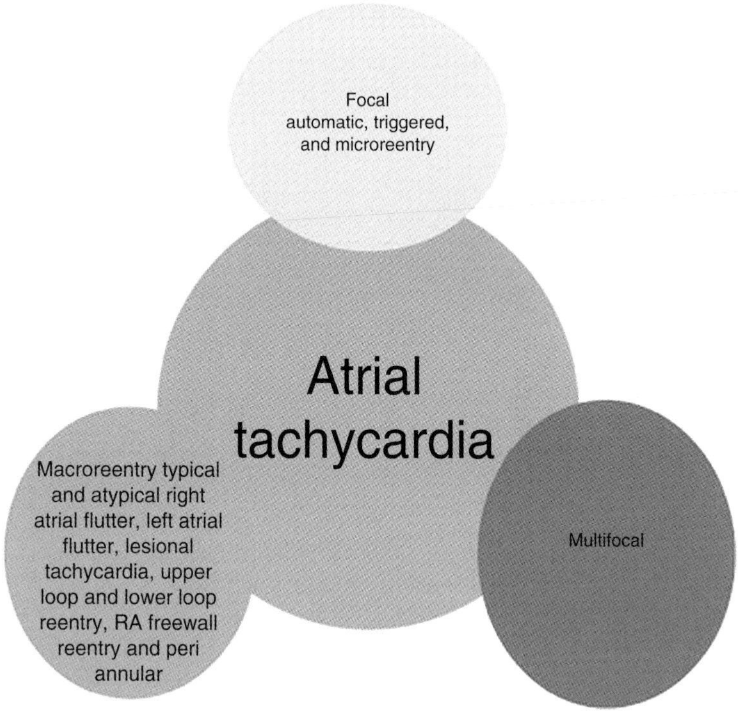

FIGURE 3-12. Atrial tachyarrhythmias are commonly classified as either focal, macroreentrant, or multifocal.

PROGNOSIS

The outlook of patients with AT is usually benign, with the exception of patients with incessant forms, which may lead to tachycardia-induced cardiomyopathy. Chen et al. reported that 63% of patients with focal AT had LV dysfunction. Of these, 73% had tachycardia-induced cardiomyopathy, and often the AT was a result of abnormal automaticity. Patients with faster heart rates seem more likely to develop cardiomyopathy; however,

TABLE 3-5 Classification of ATs and Common Characteristics

AT	PES Induction	PES Termination	Catecholamine Facilitation	Ca Blocker Sensitivity
Focal				
Automatic	No	No	Yes	No
Triggered	Yes	Yes	Yes	Yes
Microreentry	Yes	Yes	±	No
Macroreentry				
Typical (RA)	Yes	Yes	±	No
Atypical right and left AFL	Yes	Yes	±	No

it remains unclear why some patients develop cardiomyopathy and others maintain normal LV function. The cardiomyopathy usually reverses spontaneously following correction of the tachycardia, with the majority of patients achieving normal or near-normal LV function. Thus, a high index of suspicion should be routine in patients with incessant AT and LV dysfunction. Embolic events and stroke have rarely been reported in patients with AT.

MANAGEMENT

The management of AT has changed in recent times due to advances in RF ablation techniques and mapping tools. Previously, the use of antiarrhythmic medication was the mainstay of therapy, but there remains a paucity of trials comparing the efficacy of different treatment regimens. The efficacy of various therapies is also difficult to assess because the clinical definition of AT is challenging to rigorously apply, and focal AT may spontaneously regress.

ACUTE THERAPY

Vagal maneuvers, such as carotid sinus massage, are normally unsuccessful in terminating focal AT but may produce AV block allowing a clear view of the P wave and a definitive diagnosis. Adenosine also has utility in distinguishing the mechanism underlying an AT. Adenosine has antiadrenergic effects on myocardial tissue by decreasing intracellular cAMP, which results in inhibition of inward calcium currents. Triggered rhythms usually terminate with adenosine, while automatic rhythms are transiently suppressed, both of which are felt to be cAMP mediated. Adenosine response has a high sensitivity and specificity for identifying focal ATs, as macroreentrant ATs are usually insensitive to adenosine. However, a minority of focal ATs are insensitive to adenosine as well. Recent evidence has demonstrated that these adenosine insensitive focal ATs are often due to microreentry.

The effectiveness of DC cardioversion is limited for automatic AT. Similarly, overdrive pacing transiently suppresses automatic AT but does not result in termination, whereas it is often successful in terminating AT due to microreentry and triggered activity.

AV-nodal blocking agents are useful in controlling the ventricular rate. Nonautomatic AT is frequently terminated by verapamil. Intravenous beta-blockers may also terminate AT due to abnormal automaticity and triggered activity. Class Ic drugs have been shown to be efficacious in terminating some focal AT via suppression of automaticity.

LONG-TERM PHARMACOLOGIC THERAPY

There are no long-term, randomized, placebo-controlled studies on the use of antiarrhythmic therapy in AT. The available studies regarding long-term medical therapy are observational, with small numbers. The majority focus on automatic AT in children and infants, with only a few studies in adults. There is widespread agreement that antiarrhythmic agents have low efficacy in the treatment of focal AT. Calcium channel blockers and beta-blockers are recommended as first-line agents due to their low side-effect profile. These medications, along with digoxin, have a role in controlling the ventricular rate. The ACC/AHA/ESC Guidelines for the Management of supraventricular arrhythmias regard classes Ia, Ic, and III agents as second-line agents. In view of the limited long-term efficacy of pharmacologic therapy, RF ablation may be considered as a first-line therapeutic modality for patients with significant symptoms or an incessant pattern.

Focal AT is characterized by atrial activation starting rhythmically at a small area (focus) from which it spreads centrifugally. Frequent locations of focal ATs include RA structures (67%), such as the crista terminalis and tricuspid annulus, and LA structures (37%), such as the pulmonary veins and mitral annulus. The CS, atrial appendages, and intra-atrial septum are involved to a lesser degree. When a focus is located high in the crista terminalis, atrial activation sequence will not be very different from that during sinus rhythm or inappropriate sinus tachycardia (Fig. 3-13). Only sharp changes in the rate with minor, but significant, changes in origin of activation detected by endocardial mapping permit diagnosis. Multiple AT foci have been described and can be the cause of recurrences after surgical or RF ablation.

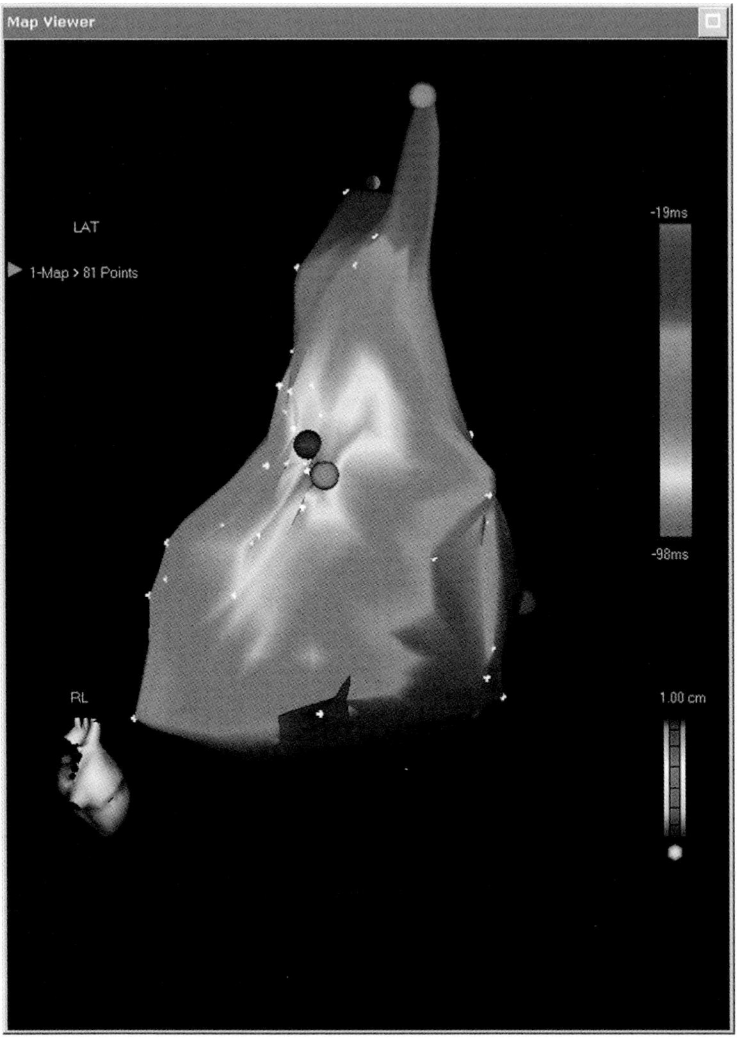

FIGURE 3-13. Endocardial activation mapping showing earliest activation at upper portion of crista terminalis in patient with focal origin (see color insert).

Over a prolonged period of observation, focal AT CL can exhibit important variations. Progressive rate increase at tachycardia onset (warm up) and/or progressive decrease in CL before termination (cool down) are suggestive of an automatic mechanism. Exercise and adrenergic stimulation also may have this effect. Relatively small reentrant circuits may resemble focal AT especially if a limited number of endocardial recordings are collected. EP mechanisms of focal ATs include enhanced automaticity, triggered activity, or microreentry. Automatic tachycardias result from cells with enhanced diastolic phase 4 depolarization and thus an increased firing rate compared with normal pacemaker cells. Triggered activity is probably responsible for the majority of focal ATs. It refers to tachycardia as a consequence of afterdepolarizations, which result in new triggered action potentials. Afterdepolarizations occur either during the phase 2 or 3 (early) or phase 4 (late) of the action potential. Microreentry refers to a small reentrant loop that is below the resolution of current three-dimensional mapping systems.

MULTIFOCAL ATRIAL TACHYCARDIA

Multifocal AT (MAT) also known as chaotic atrial rhythm is a poorly understood but not uncommon atrial tachyarrhythmia. It is usually seen as a complicating feature in a variety of acute cardiorespiratory illnesses, especially respiratory insufficiency associated with COPD. The condition is characterized by the electrocardiographic finding of (i) multiple (at least three) distinct P wave morphologies; (ii) irregular PP intervals; (iii) isoelectric baseline between P waves; and (iv) ventricular rate of more than 100 beats/min.

Patients presenting with MAT have been reported to have a high in-hospital mortality rate. The mainstay of therapy has been the correction of underlying acute pulmonary disease, thus to limit the utilization of inhaled beta-agonists and IV methylxanthines because of possible arrhythmogenic effects. Although attempts to control the heart rate and rhythm disturbance have employed direct-current cardioversion, digitalis, and antiarrhythmic agents, such efforts are often ineffective. Amiodarone has been reported to be effective in limited studies, but the concern over pulmonary toxicity limits its utility. While beta-blocking agents have been reported to be effective, they are often contraindicated due to concomitant heart and lung disease. Verapamil may also be used to decrease the ventricular rate, but its utility may be limited by its tendency to worsen hypoxemia by negating hypoxic pulmonary vasoconstriction in underventilated alveoli. IV magnesium has been reported to have some limited clinical utility. In small series, AV junction modification has been shown to be an effective therapy for controlling ventricular rate in medically refractory MAT.

Ultimately, long-term cardiovascular outcome depends principally on treating the underlying condition.

Macroreentrant AT is largely represented by AFL and is discussed in further detail earlier in this chapter.

MAPPING AND ABLATION STRATEGY FOR ATRIAL TACHYCARDIA

Endocardial mapping can trace the origin of activation to a specific area, from which it spreads centrifugally to both atria. Unipolar recordings will be helpful by showing negative ("QS") patterns with sharp initial deflections at the location of the focus. Spread of activation from the focus or origin may or may not be uniformly radial, as conduction can be directed by anatomic or functional pathways and barriers. There is generally an electrically silent period in atrial CL that is reflected on the ECG by an isoelectric line between atrial deflections. Intracardiac mapping will show significant portions of the CL without recorded activity, even when recording from the whole RA, LA, and/or CS.

The mechanism of macroreentrant AT is reentrant activation around a "large" central obstacle, generally several centimeters in diameter, at least in one of its dimensions. The central obstacle may consist of normal or abnormal structures. The obstacle can be fixed, functional, or a combination of the two. There is no single point of origin of activation, and atrial tissues outside the circuit are activated from various parts of the circuit. Description of macroreentrant AT mechanisms must be made in relation to atrial anatomy, including a detailed description of the obstacles or boundaries of the circuit and the critical isthmuses that may be targets for therapeutic action.

Currently with three-dimensional mapping technology, AT ablation series have reported acute success rates between 69% and 100%. Recurrence rates are generally low, varying between 0% and 33%. In an analysis of 16 studies, the recurrence rate was 7%. In that study, the authors analyzed predictors of success of RF ablation. A RA location was the only independent predictor of successful RF ablation. In contrast, another study noted that patients who were male had multiple foci and had repetitive forms of AT had lower acute success rates. Similarly, older patients, patients with other cardiac diseases, and those with multiple foci had a higher risk of recurrence. Prior to the advent of RF ablation, surgery was the treatment of choice for AT refractory to medical therapy. However, as ablation techniques have become more advanced, surgical treatment for focal AT is unusual.

KEY POINTS

ATRIAL FIBRILLATION

1. AF is the most common sustained arrhythmia, and its prevalence is strongly related to age.
2. The most commonly associated cardiovascular condition is hypertension, and a substantial minority have lone AF.
3. There is an increased risk of stroke and death in population studies of patients with AF.
4. All patients should be profiled regarding stroke risk, and chronic warfarin should be used when risk is elevated.
5. It is useful to classify AF as first or recurrent, and as paroxysmal, persistent, long-lasting persistent, and permanent.
6. Symptoms are variable, ranging from asymptomatic to disabling. Symptoms are caused by rapid and/or irregular ventricular patterns and loss of AV synchrony.
7. Rhythm control by antiarrhythmic drugs or catheter ablation should be judiciously employed in select patients.

ATRIAL FLUTTER

1. AFL is macroreentrant arrhythmia typically originating in RA.
2. The ECG hallmark of typical AFL is negative sawtooth flutter waves in the inferior leads.
3. AFL carries a similar risk of stroke as AF.
4. A high recurrence rate of AFL when treated with cardioversion and/or antiarrhythmic drugs justifies ablation as first-line strategy.

ATRIAL TACHYCARDIA

1. AT is defined as a SVT in which an atrial source drives the tachycardia with an atrial rate generally less than 250 bpm and more than 100 bpm.

(*Continued*)

2. The mechanism of AT may be automatic, triggered, or less commonly reentrant, and ECG criteria are insensitive for delineating the mechanism.
3. Diagnostic maneuvers such as adenosine administration and EP study are useful to clarify the underlying mechanism.
4. For patients who do not respond to drug therapy or who have incessant or poorly tolerated ATs, catheter ablation is often an effective and low-risk strategy.
5. Entrainment, activation and electroanatomic mapping are all techniques used to localize and then ablate ATs and hence a cure may be achieved in a high proportion of patients.

SUGGESTED READINGS

Alessie M, Ausma J, Schotten U. Electrical, contractile and structural remodeling during atrial fibrillation. *Cardiovasc Res.* 2002;54:230–246.

Chen SA, Tai CT, Chiang CE, Ding YA, Chang MS. Focal atrial tachycardia: Reanalysis of the clinical and electrophysiologic characteristics and prediction of successful radiofrequency ablation. *J Cardiovasc Electrophysiol.* 1998;9:355–365.

Cox JL, Schuessler RB, Boineau JP. The surgical treatment of atrial fibrillation. *J Thorac Cardiovasc Surg.* 1991;101:402–405.

Da Costa A, Thevenin J, Roche F, et al. Results from the Loire-Ardeche-Drome-Isere-Puy-de-Dome (LADIP) trial on atrial flutter: A multicentric, prospective, randomized study comparing amiodarone and radiofrequency ablation after the first episode of symptomatic atrial flutter. *Circulation.* 2006;114:1676–1681.

Fuster V, Ryden LE, Cannom DS, et al. ACC/AHA/ESC 2006 Guidelines for the management of patients with atrial fibrillation. *J Am Coll Cardiol.* 2006;e149–e246.

Haissaguerre M, Jais P, Shah DC, et al. Spontaneous initiation of atrial fibrillation by ectopic beats originating in the pulmonary veins. *N Engl J Med.* 1998;339:659–666.

Hart RG, Halperin JL. Atrial fibrillation and thromboembolism: A decade of progress in stroke prevention. *Ann Intern Med.* 1999;131:688–695.

Kamath G, Steinberg JS. Cardiac resynchronization therapy and atrial fibrillation. *Cardiol J.* 2009;6:295–301.

Marchilinski F, Callans D, Gottlieb C, et al. Magnetic electroanatomical mapping for ablation of focal atrial tachycardias. *PACE.* 1998;21:1621–1635.

Markowitz SM, Nemirovksy D, Stein KM, et al. Adenosine insensitive focal atrial tachycardia. *J Am Coll Cardiol.* 2007;49:1324–1333.

Manning WJ, Silverman DI, Keighley CS, et al. Transesophageal echocardiographically facilitated early cardioversion from atrial fibrillation using short-term anticoagulation: Final results of a prospective 4.5 year study. *J Am Coll Cardiol.* 1995;25:1354–1361.

Steinberg JS, Sadaniantz A, Kron J, et al. Analysis of cause-specific mortality of the atrial fibrillation investigation follow-up investigation of rhythm management trial. *Circulation.* 2004;109:1973–1980.

Roberts KC, Kistler, PM, Kalman JM. Focal atrial tachycardia 1. *PACE.* 2006;29:643–652.

Roberts KC, Kistler, PM, Kalman JM. Focal atrial tachycardia 2. *PACE.* 2006;29:769–778.

Wilbur DJ, Packer DL, Stevenson WG. *Catheter Ablation of Cardiac Arrhythmias: Basic Concepts and Clinical Applications.* 3rd Ed. Malden, MA: Blackwell Futura; 2008.

Wood MA, Brown-Mahoney C, Kay GN, et al. Clinical outcomes after ablation and pacing therapy for atrial fibrillation: A meta-analysis. *Circulation.* 2000;101:1138–1144.

Wyse DG, Waldo AL, DiMarco JP, et al. A comparison of rate control and rhythm control in patients with atrial fibrillation. *N Eng J Med.* 2002;347:1825–1833.

CHAPTER 4

Ventricular Tachycardia

Shuaib Latif and David J. Callans

Sustained ventricular tachycardia (VT) is a cause of significant morbidity and mortality in patients with cardiac pathology. In addition, idiopathic VT can occur in patients with structurally normal hearts. Antiarrhythmic medications reduce the risk of recurrent ventricular tachyarrhythmias with variable efficacy and with significant side effects. While implantable cardiac defibrillators (ICD) reduce the mortality associated with ventricular arrhythmias, recurrent ICD discharges result in reduced quality of life. Catheter-based ablation reduces the incidence of ventricular arrhythmias and improves quality of life. The approach to VT in the electrophysiology (EP) laboratory is determined by the myocardial substrate and the mechanism of the arrhythmia. Prior to arrival in the EP lab, an adequate assessment of the myocardium must be undertaken. While sustained monomorphic ventricular tachycardia (MMVT) is often related to structural heart disease, 10% of all sustained MMVT occurs in the setting of a structurally normal heart (idiopathic VT). These VTs typically occur in specific locations and have specific VT morphologies. The overall approach to VT ablation involves inducing tachyarrhythmia, creating ablation lesions in the area of interest, and attempting to re-induce tachyarrhythmia.

PREABLATION ASSESSMENT

Prior to an EP procedure, the presence or absence of structural heart disease should be adequately defined. Specifically, the presence and location of wall motion abnormalities, the presence of thrombus, the severity of valvular disease, and the severity of coronary artery disease are all important in helping to assess not only the approach taken but also the risk of the procedure as well. Electrocardiograms of the clinical VTs or premature ventricular contractions (PVCs) should be obtained if possible. In addition, EGM morphologies from implanted devices should be obtained as well as these may provide a useful comparison of the targeted clinical VT during the procedure. Left ventricular (LV) access is required for VTs originating from this chamber; as such, determination of the degree of peripheral vascular disease and aortic valve disease is important as some patients may require a transseptal approach. In patients with an epicardial origin of VT, which is fairly common in patients with nonischemic cardiomyopathy and some patients with idiopathic VT, access to the pericardial space is required; patients with prior cardiac surgery or prior pericardial inflammation may have significant adhesions limiting such access.

Attempts at induction of VT are often done in the EP lab in order to assess its mechanism and the effect of ablation. In patients with structural heart disease, VT is often poorly tolerated and leads to hemodynamic collapse requiring rapid restoration of sinus rhythm. Prior to the procedure, patients should be managed with this in mind. Volume status should be optimized. A recent coronary evaluation is necessary as tachycardia and hypotension can worsen ischemia. If possible, antiarrhythmic medications should be discontinued.

MECHANISMS OF VT

Determining the mechanism of VT is important in planning an ablation strategy. The two basic mechanisms of tachycardia are enhanced impulse formation and abnormalities of conduction leading to reentry (Fig. 4-1). Enhanced impulse formation is due to either enhanced automaticity (enhanced phase 4 activity) or to triggered rhythms (early or delayed after depolarizations). While it may be challenging to determine the mechanism of MMVT, generalizations may be made depending on the presence of structural heart disease and the response to programmed stimulation.

Ventricular tachyarrhythmias due to an automatic focus are rare and not well-characterized. They are more often seen in younger patients (usually <50 years old). Automatic VT may arise from anywhere within the right ventricle (RV) or LV although typical areas do exist (mitral annulus, para-hisian region, and RV inflow tract). It is thought to result from adrenergically mediated automaticity as it is often precipitated by exercise and is sensitive to beta-blockers. Automatic VTs cannot be initiated or terminated with programmed stimulation.

Triggered activity refers to ventricular complexes that result from abnormal afterdepolarizations occurring during a prior ventricular beat. Early afterdepolarizations (EADs) occur in late phase 2 or early phase 3 of the action potential while delayed afterdepolarizations (DADs) occur during late phase 3 or phase 4 of the action potential. In both cases, a net inward current causes premature depolarization of the myocardium. EADs occur more often during bradycardia or during pauses and can initiate torsade de pointes. DADs develop in the setting of increased intracellular calcium concentrations; adrenergic stimulation increases intracellular cAMP levels, which triggers release of calcium from the sarcoplasmic reticulum. This leads to an increased inward sodium current with a resultant depolarization (DAD).

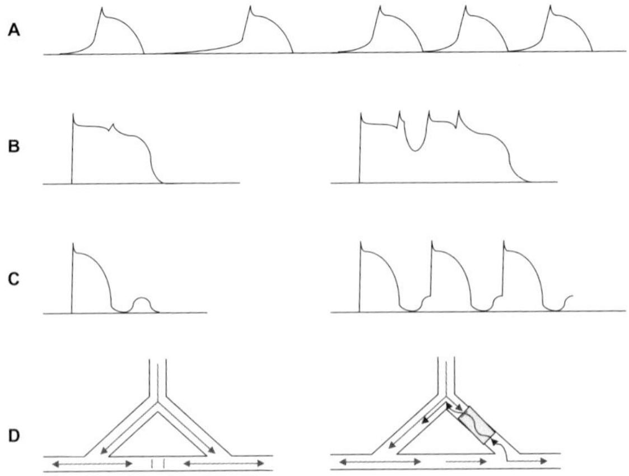

FIGURE 4-1. Mechanisms of VT. **A:** Increased automaticity is a rare cause of VT but is typically induced by exercise and catecholamines and is not induced by programmed stimulation. In addition, cell damage may increase automaticity leading to VT. **B:** Early afterdepolarizations (EADs) occur before repolarization is complete and are associated with abnormalities that prolong the action potential. EADs can trigger polymorphic VT such as torsade de pointes. **C:** Delayed afterdepolarizations (DADs) occur after repolarization is complete and are due to increased cellular calcium release. If threshold is reached, the cell will depolarize again. DADs are thought to be the mechanism behind triggered VTs such as outflow tract VTs. **D:** Reentry relies on areas of nonhomogenous conduction through tissue and is most commonly the mechanism of scar based VT. Differential conduction through a zone of tissue with dissimilar refractory periods is needed to sustain reentry.

In the EP lab, triggered rhythms, can be initiated by programmed stimulation in about 60% of cases, typically rapid atrial or ventricular pacing. Adrenergic stimulation (e.g., isoproterenol and epinephrine) facilitates initiation of these tachyarrhythmias. Adenosine terminates cAMP-mediated triggered arrhythmias through antiadrenergic effects.

In patient with structural heart disease, the bulk of evidence suggests that the mechanism of sustained MMVT is reentry. Reentry requires two pathways with unidirectional block in one while the other sustains slow conduction (allowing the blocked pathway to recover excitability). More specifically, the refractory period of the blocked pathway must be shorter than the conduction time down the unblocked pathway. Patients with structural heart disease typically have areas of slow conduction allowing for reentry. In contrast to focal rhythms, reentrant rhythms are able to be reproducibly initiated and terminated by timed extrastimuli in the EP lab.

ECG LOCALIZATION

An ECG of the clinical VT should be obtained if possible as it helps direct one to the area of interest (Fig. 4-2). The majority of VT associated with structural heart disease arises from the area of scar. While several factors affect the QRS, including amount and

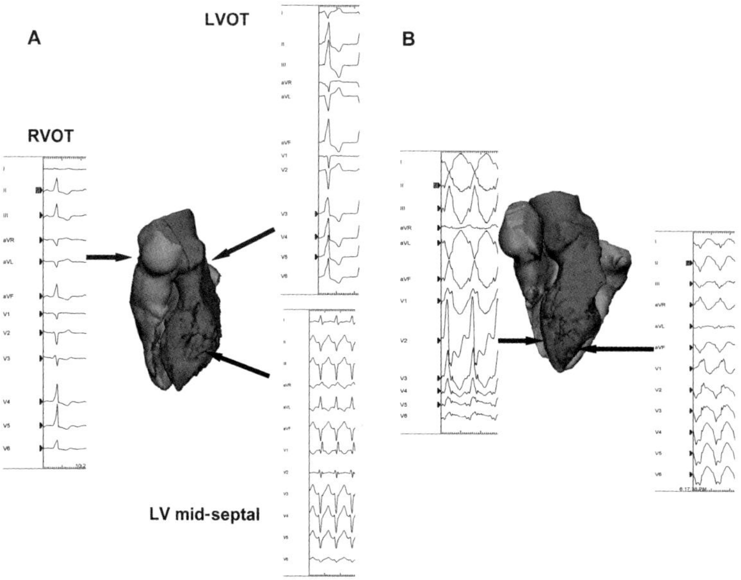

FIGURE 4-2. Representative ECG morphologies during VT and corresponding sites of origin. A cast of the RV (*blue*) and LV (*red*) is shown in the left lateral **(left)** and posterior **(right)** projections. **A:** Idiopathic VT patterns. RVOT VT has a left bundle, inferior axis ECG pattern, and arises from just beneath the pulmonary valve. LVOT VT (from the sinuses of Valsalva) has a left bundle, inferior axis, but the precordial R wave transition is earlier because the LV is more posterior. LV mid-septal VT has a right bundle, superior axis. **B:** Two examples of right bundle morphology VTs in the presence of healed infarction. Both of these VT morphologies are RBBB, signifying origin away from the intraventricular septum. VTs that arise from the septum have a left bundle configuration. VT in the setting of structural heart disease typically arises from areas of scarring, either in healed infarction or in the setting of dilated myopathy, perivalvular fibrosis. In the latter setting, epicardial involvement may be more extensive than endocardial involvement (see color insert).

distribution of the scar, orientation of the heart in the chest, antiarrhythmic medications, the morphology, axis, and precordial transition indicate the area of exit of VT. VT with a left bundle branch block (LBBB) morphology typically arises from the RV or the interventricular septum, while VT with a right bundle branch block (RBBB) morphology arises from the LV. The precordial transition indicates the exit location between the base and apex. Dominant R waves suggest a basal exit while dominant S waves suggest an apical exit. The frontal plane axis localizes the exit to either the anterior wall, producing an inferiorly directed axis, or the inferior wall, producing a superiorly directed axis. A broad QRS morphology with slurred initial activation may indicate a subepicardial origin.

Common patterns exist for patients with VT and no structural heart disease. Typically, these are focal in nature and originate in the outflow tracts and near the fascicles. Outflow tract tachycardias typically exhibit a left bundle inferior axis morphology. The transition in the precordial leads helps to localize the focus to either the right ventricular outflow tract (RVOT), the left ventricular outflow tract (LVOT), or the aorto-mitral continuity. Idiopathic left VT often exhibits a right bundle left axis morphology.

ABLATION OF VT IN STRUCTURAL HEART DISEASE

SCAR-RELATED SUSTAINED MONOMORPHIC TACHYCARDIA

In patients with structural heart disease, reentry in the area of scar is the most common mechanism of sustained VT. Myocardial scar is typically nonhomogenous with variable areas of fibrosis causing conduction block interspersed with surviving damaged myocytes with limited intercellular coupling creating areas of slow conduction and a suitable environment to sustain reentry.

Reentrant VT is typically viewed as a wave front that traverses through a protected channel (the isthmus) not seen on surface ECG. Rather, the surface ECG reflects the point of exit from the isthmus; after exiting, the wave front then activates the ventricles. The wave front then continues around the circuit back to the entrance point of the isthmus. Different VT morphologies can often be induced and may be due to different circuits in different areas of scar or different exits within the same area of scar.

ENTRAINMENT MAPPING

VT that is hemodynamically tolerated offers the opportunity to map during tachycardia. The wave front is mapped as it progresses through the isthmus to the exit. Mid-diastolic potentials identify the wave front as they travel through the isthmus while presystolic potentials identify the wave front at the exit site.

Electrogram mapping alone is not reliable in defining a circuit as scars can sustain multiple conduction paths. Entrainment mapping can be used to verify the importance of a site of interest (Fig. 4-3). Reentrant circuits have an excitable gap at each point in the circuit, defined as the time of recovery from the last depolarization to the arrival of the next wave front. Pacing at an appropriate time interval during tachycardia produces a wave front that propagates to the reentrant circuit and depolarizes an area of the circuit during the excitable gap. The wave front then propagates in two directions: the orthodromic wave front propagates in the direction of the reentrant circuit resetting the circuit, while the antidromic wave front propagates in the reverse direction of the reentrant circuit until it collides with a previous orthodromic wave front. The response to a single stimulus is termed resetting, while continuous resetting is termed entrainment.

Entrainment of a reentrant rhythm satisfies the Waldo criteria. Specifically, entrainment demonstrates fixed fusion (QRS morphology between the native tachycardia and pure ventricular pacing) during pacing with progressive fusion (QRS morphology more closely resembling the purely paced morphology) at faster pacing cycle lengths. The tachycardia resumes after pacing starts and the last paced beat is entrained but not

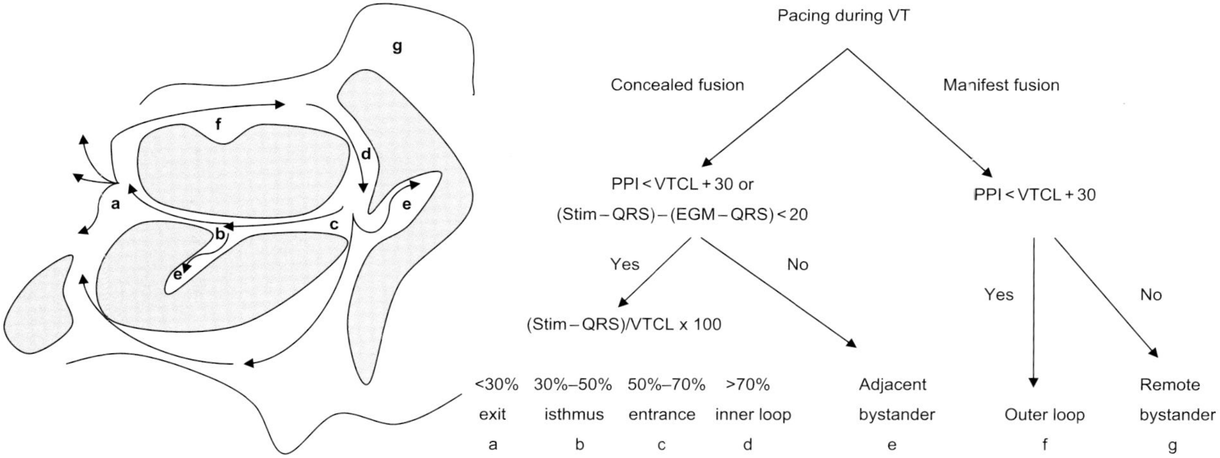

FIGURE 4-3. Entrainment mapping. If pacing entrains tachycardia, response to pacing can be used to assess the location of the pacing site within the circuit.

fused. The postpacing interval (PPI) indicates the proximity of the pacing site to the reentrant circuit. The PPI is measured from the last entrained stimulus to the next activation at the pacing site. The PPI reflects the time taken to travel to the circuit, around the circuit, and back to the site of pacing. At pacing sites within the reentrant circuit, the PPI is roughly equal to the tachycardia cycle length (TCL). As the pacing sites move progressively further away from the reentrant circuit, the PPI increases compared to the TCL. A PPI-TCL of 30 ms or less often indicates a pacing site within the circuit. However, it does not specify what portion of the circuit (i.e., outer loop, entrance, isthmus, exit, etc.).

When pacing is performed during tachycardia, the native wave front and the paced wave front collide and alter the QRS morphology on the surface ECG, indicating fusion. Typically, the PPI indicates these are outside of the circuit. Reentrant circuits often rotate around areas of scar with a protected isthmus area and a larger outer loop area. The outer loop area is a part of the circuit; pacing in this area produces a fused QRS complex but a PPI that demonstrates it is within the circuit. Ablation at these areas is unlikely to interrupt tachycardia. Pacing within an isthmus limits the propagation of the paced wave front to the orthodromic and the antidromic direction. At these sites, the antidromic wave front collides with the orthodromic wave front within or near the isthmus and is not evident in the surface ECG. As a result, the paced QRS morphology appears the same as the native tachycardia morphology and is referred to as concealed fusion. Concealed fusion with an acceptable PPI demonstrates a pacing site within an isthmus where ablation is likely to terminate tachycardia (Fig. 4-4). The relative location of the pacing site within the isthmus is then identified by the stimulus-QRS time. As the pacing site moves backwards through the isthmus from exit to entrance, the stimulus-QRS time increases. Typically, this time is expressed relative to the TCL; a ratio of less than 0.3 indicates a site that is likely at the exit, while a ratio of between 0.3 and 0.7 reflects a position within the isthmus. A ratio of greater than 0.7 is often at the entrance.

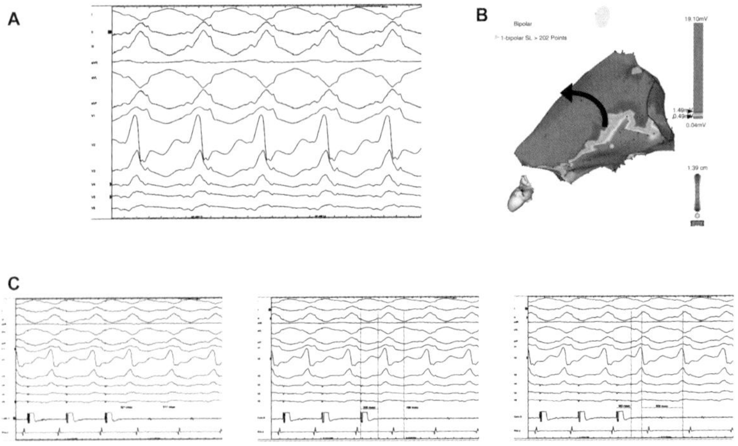

FIGURE 4-4. Entrainment mapping. **A:** Monomorphic VT with right bundle right inferior axis. **B:** Sinus voltage map of a patient from **(A)** demonstrating large inferior scar extending to the lateral wall. VT exits from lateral wall based on VT morphology (see color insert). **C:** Pacing from indicated site in **(B)** during VT satisfied entrainment criteria and demonstrated concealed fusion with pacing site at isthmus location by response to entrainment (ECG1: PPI-TCL = 10 ms ECG2: (Stim-QRS) – (Stim-EGM) = 10 ms ECG3: (Stim-QRS)/TCL × 100 = 36). VT terminated with ablation at this site and was subsequently noninducible.

Ablation at entrance and exit sites is less likely to affect tachycardias as these sites may be relatively broad compared to the protected isthmus. Ideally, ablation at the isthmus interrupts tachycardia.

Entrainment mapping of VT requires a stable VT circuit that is hemodynamically tolerated. It is not useful if pacing alters tachycardia or terminates it or if tachycardia leads to hemodynamic collapse. In such instances, substrate mapping can be helpful.

SUBSTRATE MAPPING

For multiple and unstable VTs, substrate mapping can be used to identify areas of scar which may support reentry. Voltage maps are created during sinus or a stable paced rhythm. Low-voltage regions (<1.5 mV in bipolar recordings) are identified as scar. In sinus rhythm, low-amplitude late potentials (potentials appearing after the end of the QRS) indicate areas of slow conduction, which may represent a potential isthmus. Pacing in the region of VT isthmus then replicates the VT morphology on surface ECG. However, the scar area is often significant in size and many areas may demonstrate slow conduction allowing pacing wave fronts to exit in a variety of paths. Portions of scar that are electrically unexcitable (i.e., cannot be paced from) represent areas of dense fibrosis and represent areas of block. Tagging such areas on 3D maps potentially allows the visualization of channels, which can be further explored. Often, substrate mapping can be used in sinus rhythm to help narrow the area of interest allowing the amount of time spent in VT to be minimized.

ABLATION OF VT IN IDIOPATHIC HEART DISEASE

Idiopathic monomorphic VT usually presents in younger individuals. Typical triggers include exertion or emotional stress. These arrhythmias often have a focal origin originating from the outflow tract. However, another relatively common variety of idiopathic VT results from reentry in the area of LV Purkinje fascicles. Structural heart disease must be excluded. The prognosis is generally good and the risk of sudden death is low in idiopathic VTs. However, closely coupled outflow tract PVCs can cause polymorphic VT or ventricular fibrillation (VF) in a patient with a structurally normal heart. In addition, heavy PVC burden or incessant VT can cause depressed LV function that improves after treatment. Medical therapy includes beta-blockers and calcium channel blockers but can prove ineffective in a significant number of cases.

OUTFLOW TRACT TACHYCARDIAS

The outflow tract encompasses the RV region between the pulmonary and tricuspid valves, the basal LV including the outflow tract, the aortic cusps, and the epicardial outflow tract area. RVOT tachycardias demonstrate a characteristic LBBB pattern with an inferior axis and a precordial transition after lead V3. A free wall origin is suggested by a QRS duration more than 140 ms and notching in the inferior leads. The RVOT is an angled structure that wraps around the right anterior portion of the aorta; the posterior portion of the RVOT extends slightly rightward while the anterior portion extends leftward. A Q wave in lead I indicates an anterior focus in the RVOT, while an R wave in lead I indicates a posterior focus in the RVOT. LVOT tachycardias manifest similar clinical features to RVOT tachycardias. As in RVOT tachycardias, they demonstrate a LBBB pattern on ECG. Typically, the transition in the precordial leads is earlier occurring at or before V2. VT from the aortic cusps occurs as well. These may demonstrate an early precordial transition (at or before VT) indicating a leftward focus with notching in V1 or V2. Most VTs from this area arise from the left coronary cusp. While ECG morphology is helpful in narrowing the area of interest, localization is ultimately achieved in the EP lab with pace mapping and activation mapping.

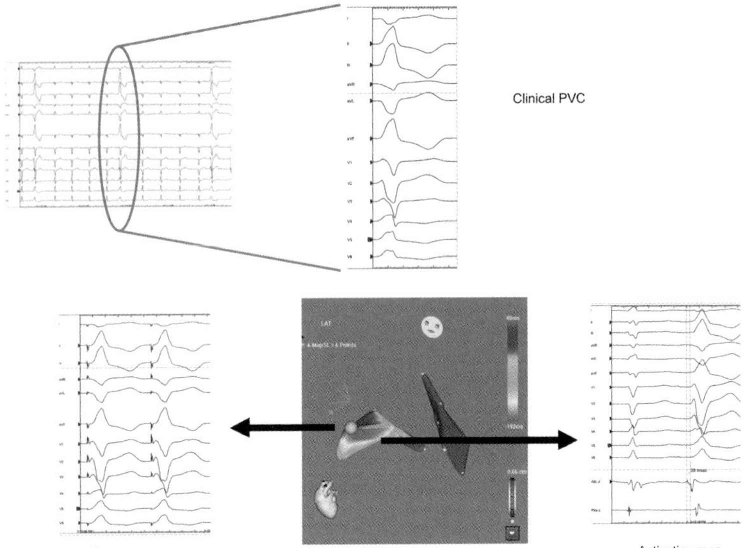

FIGURE 4-5. Idiopathic VT arising from the left coronary cusp. The surface ECG, electroanatomic map of the RVOT and left cusp (color patterns signify activation time during the PVC: red is early, purple is late), pacemapping and activation mapping at the site of origin are shown. Complementary techniques used for focal VT/PVC ablation. Activation mapping is used to locate the area of earliest activity, typically 15 to 45 ms pre-QRS. Pace mapping is used to locate the area of focal exit. Typically, both areas overlap allowing the frequency of PVC/VT to dictate which approach is selected (see color insert).

MAPPING

For tachycardias with a focal origin, pace mapping and activation mapping are used to locate the origin prior to ablation (Fig. 4-5). Pacemapping can be used to narrow down the area of interest or if VT or PVCs are not readily induced. Pacemaps should be identical to the QRS morphology of the VT or PVC in all 12 leads. Low-pacing outputs should be used with ablation catheters with small interelectrode distances. In addition, pacemapping should be carried out at a rate as close to that of the VT as possible to minimize the risk of aberrant conduction. Near-identical pacemaps may be obtained from multiple sites in the area of interest requiring additional lesions. Activation mapping can be used if the VT or PVC of interest is frequently present or easily inducible. The mapping catheter is moved around the area of interest in an attempt to locate the earliest myocardial activation. In the unipolar recording, a QS complex is present at the site of earliest activation. Earliest activation during VT or during PVCs typically precede the QRS by 15 to 45 ms. Ablation at such a site often induces VT with acceleration followed by termination of VT. Typically, VT or PVCs are no longer inducible.

LV FASCICULAR VT

Verapamil-sensitive idiopathic VT is seen most often in patients between 15 and 40 years old. It typically manifests a RBBB morphology with left axis deviation. Most evidence indicate localized reentry as the predominant mechanism. The tachycardia can be initiated with programmed atrial or ventricular stimulation. The majority of these VTs involve the posterior fascicle of the left bundle branch. During VT, Purkinje potentials or late diastolic potentials are targeted. In situations where the tachycardia cannot be induced in the EP lab, an empiric linear lesion set can be placed in the area of the posterior fascicle guided by Purkinje potentials.

SUMMARY

VT is an increasingly common arrhythmia that causes significant morbidity and mortality. Catheter ablation reduces symptoms and improves quality of life. Prior to catheter ablation, a comprehensive preablation assessment must be conducted. In the EP lab, understanding the mechanism of the tachycardia is important in planning an ablation strategy. Various techniques can be used to localize the area of interest. Overall success is generally good in experienced centers. As such, catheter ablation should be considered in the therapeutic armamentarium in treating these arrhythmias.

KEY POINTS

1. VT ablation can reduce symptoms.
2. Mechanisms of VT include reentry, triggered activity, and increased automaticity.
3. The ECG morphology of VT can localize the exit site.
4. Preablation assessment should include an evaluation of cardiac function.
5. VT in structural heart disease is often due to reentry within a scar.
6. In structural heart disease, VT can be mapped during tachycardia using entrainment while late potentials indicating areas of slow conduction can be targeted as well.
7. In idiopathic VT, activation mapping and pace mapping are complementary techniques that can be utilized during ablation.
8. Typical foci in idiopathic VT include the outflow tracts and the fascicular system.
9. The prognosis for patients with idiopathic VT is typically good.

SUGGESTED READINGS

Badhwar N, Scheinman MM. Idiopathic ventricular tachycardia: Diagnosis and management. *Curr Probl Cardiol.* 2007;32:7–43.

Huang SKS, Wood MA, ed. *Catheter Ablation of Cardiac Arrhythmias.* Philadelphia, PA: Elsevier Inc.; 2006.

Josephson ME. *Clinical Cardiac Electrophysiology.* Philadelphia, PA: Lippincott Williams & Wilkins; 2008.

Latif S, Dixit S, Callans DJ. Ventricular arrhythmias in normal hearts. In Miller JJ, ed. Ventricular arrhythmias. *Cardiol Clin.* 2008;26(3):367–380.

Lin D, Ilkhanoff L, Gerstenfeld E, et al. Twelve-lead electrocardiographic characteristics of the aortic cusp region guided by intracardiac echocardiography and electroanatomic mapping. *Heart Rhythm.* 2008;5(5):663–669.

Stevenson WG, Khan H, Sager P, et al. Identification of reentry circuit sites during catheter mapping and radiofrequency ablation of ventricular tachycardia late after myocardial infarction. *Circulation.* 1993;88:1647–1670.

Stevenson WG, Soejima K. Catheter ablation for ventricular tachycardia. *Circulation.* 2007;115:2750–2760.

Wilbur DJ, Packer DL, Stevenson WG, ed. *Catheter Ablation of Cardiac Arrhythmias.* Malden, MA: Blackwell Publishing; 2008.

CHAPTER 5

Syncope

Suneet Mittal

Syncope is defined as the sudden loss of consciousness associated with the absence of postural tone and is usually followed by a complete and rapid recovery. It is a very common clinical problem with an overall incidence of a first report of syncope being 6.2 per 1,000 person-years. The incidence rate increases with age, especially after age 70; the estimated 10-year cumulative incidence of syncope is 6% and up to 22% of patients experience recurrent syncope. The differential diagnosis of syncope is extensive (Fig. 5-1). The management of the patient who presents with syncope begins with the history and physical examination and almost always includes an electrocardiogram (ECG) and echocardiogram. The initial step in diagnosis involves distinguishing cardiac from noncardiac causes of syncope.

CARDIAC SYNCOPE

Cardiac causes of syncope include disorders of autonomic function such as neurally mediated syncope (e.g., vasovagal syncope and carotid sinus hypersensitivity), chronic orthostatic intolerance (i.e., postural orthostatic tachycardia syndrome [POTS]), and orthostatic hypotension (secondary to volume depletion, systemic illness, use of a vasoactive drug, or pure autonomic failure/multiple system atrophy), disorders related to obstruction to blood flow, and arrhythmias (brady and tachyarrhythmias). Patients in whom syncope results from obstruction to blood flow are readily identified by echocardiography (in conjunction with the clinical history and physical examination)

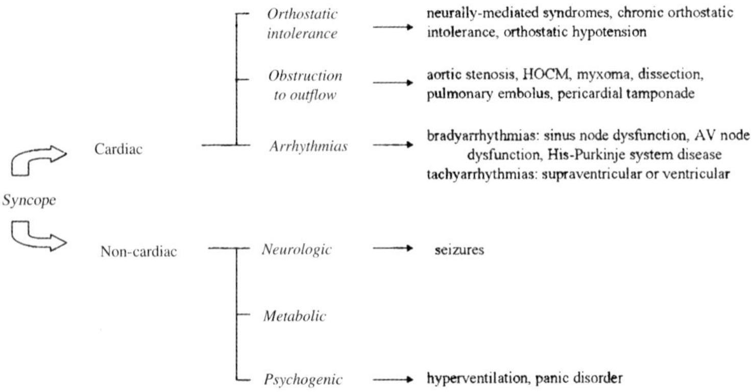

FIGURE 5-1. Differential diagnosis of syncope. HOCM, hypertrophic cardiomyopathy.

and pose less of a diagnostic or therapeutic dilemma. Therefore, the remainder of this chapter will focus on differentiating patients with syncope due to autonomic dysfunction from those with an arrhythmic etiology. This differentiation has prognostic implications since the mortality of patients with arrhythmic syncope is double that of patients without a history of syncope or those in whom syncope is vasovagal in etiology.

DISORDERS OF AUTONOMIC FUNCTION

These disorders are usually not associated with underlying structural heart disease. Therefore, in a patient (especially in a younger patient) with a normal ECG and no structural heart disease, one of the disorders of autonomic function should be strongly considered. The most common disorder of autonomic function is neurally mediated syncope, which includes vasovagal and carotid sinus syncope. Additionally, micturition, defecation, deglutition, and posttussive syncope are common "situational" forms of neurally mediated syncope. In these conditions, syncope results from bradycardia and/or hypotension. It is important to note that in many patients with carotid sinus hypersensitivity the hemodynamic alterations may be manifest only in the upright state and that in nearly a third of patients the major hemodynamic effect is a pure vasodepressor response. Therefore, in diagnosing carotid sinus hypersensitivity, patients should be evaluated while supine *and* upright with use of one of several commercially available devices capable of recording beat-to-beat blood pressure noninvasively.

Chronic orthostatic intolerance, formerly referred to as the postural orthostatic tachycardia syndrome, is characterized by pronounced orthostatic tachycardia without associated hypotension. By definition, the orthostatic symptoms are long-standing (≥6 months) and not attributable to an underlying cause such as a debilitating disease, substantial weight loss, prolonged bed rest, peripheral neuropathy, and/or medications. This is a disorder of the young (age 14 to 45 years) with a female predominance (4:1). The disorder may follow a viral illness in 30% to 40% of cases. The predominant symptoms include light-headedness, dizziness, palpitations, chest pain, and syncope. In some patients, this condition is related to a defect in the norepinephrine transporter, which results in an increase in the norepinephrine concentration. In the upright state, the heart rate increases by ≥30 bpm (usually to an absolute rate ≥120 bpm); upright norepinephrine levels characteristically exceed 600 pg/mL.

Although most commonly a result of volume depletion, orthostatic hypotension may represent a sign of generalized autonomic dysfunction. An identifiable cause is often present such as a systemic disease (e.g., diabetes mellitus), toxic agents (e.g., alcohol), or use of a vasoactive medication. Often a cause cannot be identified; in these instances, one must consider pure autonomic failure (when other neurologic features are absent) or multiple system atrophy (associated with other neurologic features).

Tilt table testing is useful in differentiating these syndromes. In neurally mediated syncope, in response to upright tilt, the heart rate and blood pressure initially remain stable. However, there is then an abrupt decline in the heart rate and/or blood pressure, which results in syncope. In contrast, patients with chronic orthostatic intolerance have an immediate increase in heart rate (≥30 bpm to ≥120 bpm) without a change in blood pressure, and patients with orthostatic hypotension due to autonomic dysfunction exhibit a progressive decline in blood pressure (≥20 mm Hg) without a change in heart rate.

Although tilt testing is widely used to evaluate patients with suspected neurally mediated syncope, there is no standardized tilt test protocol. Current protocols usually consist of an initial drug-free tilt phase followed by a phase using pharmacologic provocation, most commonly with isoproterenol, nitroglycerin, or adenosine (see Chapter 11). A major problem with tilt testing remains its poor sensitivity when using a protocol that maintains high specificity. In addition, the sensitivity of tilt testing worsens significantly as the patient population being evaluated becomes older. Furthermore, prospective studies have demonstrated that in patients without structural heart disease who present with syncope, the clinical outcome is similar irrespective of the tilt test response. As a result, the clinical role for tilt testing remains controversial. Figure 5-2 summarizes an approach to the clinical incorporation of tilt table testing when a disorder of autonomic function is suspected.

Another frustrating area relates to the treatment of patients with vasovagal syncope. For one, the natural history of vasovagal syncope is variable. Multiple events often occur over a relatively short period and are followed by longer, relatively symptom-free periods. Interestingly, the frequency of syncopal episodes decreases substantially following tilt testing, whether patients are treated on not. Therefore, it has been difficult to evaluate the therapeutic effect of any single intervention.

The need to initiate therapy needs to be highly individualized; in general, therapy is attempted in patients with recurrent episodes of syncope or in those in whom syncope is associated with trauma. An important cornerstone for therapy is encouraging patients to hydrate aggressively (until urine output is consistently clear), liberalize salt intake, and avoid behaviors/situations known to provoke vasovagal syncope. Isometric counter-pressure maneuvers involving the arms (hand grip and arm tensing) and legs (crossing of the legs) rapidly increase blood pressure and may abort syncope in some patients if initiated at the onset of symptoms. Some clinicians advocate "tilt training" (standing against a wall for 5 min and increasing gradually to 30 min daily) to "desensitize" patients to the effect of orthostatic stress; however, the long-term compliance is poor. Nonetheless, these nonpharmacological "physical" maneuvers are rapidly emerging as first-line treatments in patients suffering from recurrent vasovagal syncope.

A variety of additional therapies have been suggested for patients with vasovagal syncope. The most commonly used treatments include beta-blockers, selective serotonin reuptake inhibitors, alpha-agonists, anticholinergic agents, mineralocorticoids, and permanent pacemakers. Unfortunately, most of these therapies have been evaluated in only

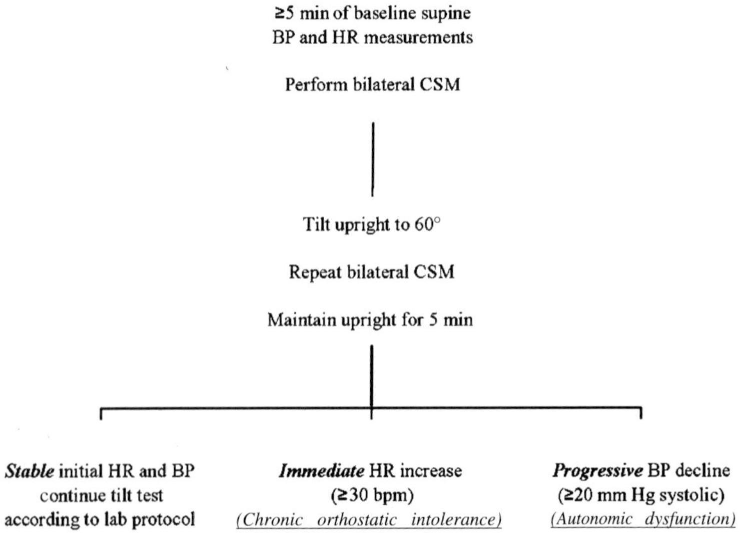

FIGURE 5-2. An approach to tilt table testing in patients with a suspected disorder of autonomic function. BP, blood pressure; CSM, carotid sinus massage; HR, heart rate.

small, short-term, uncontrolled, and unblinded studies. Of note, no pharmacologic therapy is approved by the Food and Drug Administration for the management of vasovagal syncope. To date, only the SSRI agent paroxetine has been shown in a double-blind, randomized, placebo-controlled clinical trial to significantly reduce the incidence of recurrent syncope. However, a confirmatory study is still needed. In general, convincing data for any pharmacotherapy in patients with vasovagal syncope are lacking; as a result, current practice guidelines on syncope management advocate *against* the routine institution of these medications. Given the relative futility of pharmacotherapy, there was great initial enthusiasm for using permanent pacemakers (with enhanced features such as rate-drop programming) in these patients. However, the negative results of North American Vasovagal Pacing Study II effectively eliminated the routine use of pacing in patients with vasovagal syncope.

ARRHYTHMIAS

An important arrhythmic cause for syncope is a bradyarrhythmia, such as sinus bradycardia resulting from sinus node dysfunction or atrioventricular (AV) block resulting from AV node or His-Purkinje system dysfunction. Electrophysiologic (EP) studies are most useful when the patient's baseline ECG demonstrates sinus bradycardia or conduction system disease (prolonged PR interval and/or bundle branch block). Sinus node dysfunction is considered present when the sinus node recovery time exceeds 1,600 to 2,000 ms and/or the corrected sinus node recovery time exceeds 525 ms. Similarly, His-Purkinje system dysfunction is considered present when the baseline HV interval is ≥100 ms or when His-Purkinje system block is demonstrated during rapid atrial pacing or after administration of intravenous procainamide. However, although EP testing has high specificity, it lacks sensitivity for diagnosing patients at risk for symptomatic bradycardia due to either sinus node dysfunction or His-Purkinje system disease. For example, with use of an implanted loop recorder, it has been possible to demonstrate that in a third of patients with bundle branch block (specifically, right bundle branch and fascicular block or left bundle branch block) recurrent syncope results from paroxysmal AV block, even though the EP study is "normal."

The disappointing yield of tilt testing and EP testing in patients with syncope in the absence of structural heart disease has necessitated the use of alternative diagnostic strategies. The most promising is the implantable loop recorder. This has been shown to be superior to a more conventional strategy of EP and tilt testing in making a definitive diagnosis (which is usually a form of bradycardia) in patients without structural heart disease presenting with syncope. The appeal of the implantable loop recorder has been greatly enhanced by the recent release of a second-generation device that offers an entirely wireless solution to ECG monitoring as well as extended 3-year battery longevity. The recorder, which is implanted subcutaneously in the left parasternal region, transmits ECG information to a PDA sized device that is carried by the patient. Transmission of data can be triggered by either the patient (in response to symptoms) or automatically if the heart rate falls below or exceeds a physician programmed detection rate. The captured data is transmitted to a central monitoring station via a base station that is connected to the patient's phone line. The physician is notified immediately if data meeting notification criteria is obtained (Fig. 5-3).

EP testing has greatest yield in patients with possible cardiac syncope. Patients with underlying structural heart disease, those in whom syncope occurs *during* exercise, those who experience chest pain or palpitations prior to syncope, and those with a family history of sudden death should be considered for EP testing. Sustained monomorphic ventricular tachycardia is inducible in approximately 40% of patients with an ischemic cardiomyopathy who present with unexplained syncope. Since these patients are at high risk for sudden cardiac death, an implantable cardioverter-defibrillator (ICD) is usually inserted. Within 15 months of ICD implantation, approximately 40% of these patients

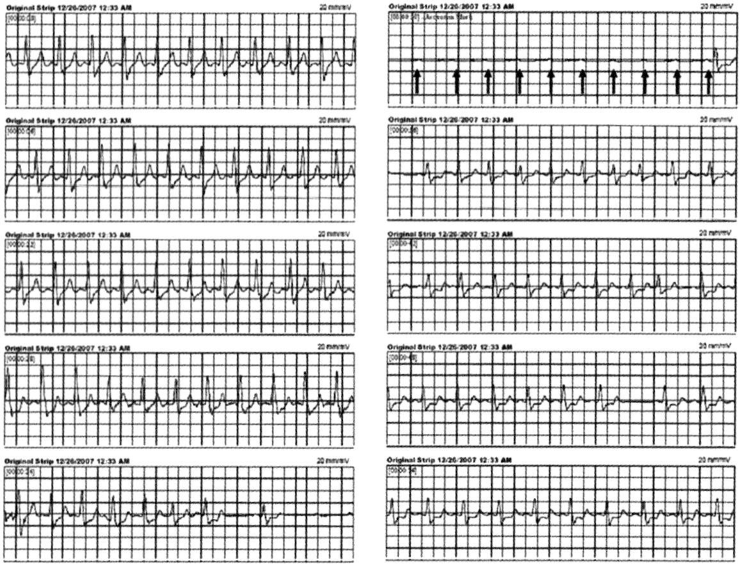

FIGURE 5-3. This 62-year-old male with no past medical history presented following an episode of syncope without prodrome. The episode was associated with marked facial trauma. ECG showed sinus rhythm with left bundle branch block; an echocardiogram showed normal left ventricular function. At EP study, the HV interval was less than 55 ms. A wireless implantable loop recorder was inserted. Several weeks later, the patient had another syncopal episode. Data from the loop recorder showed the abrupt onset of ventricular asystole. (The *arrows* show the P waves from underlying sinus rhythm.) The loop recorder was removed and a dual chamber pacemaker was implanted.

receive an appropriate therapy from the ICD for management of recurrent ventricular tachycardia or fibrillation. (The risk of recurrent events is greatest in patients with a prolonged QRS duration [≥120 ms]). Surprisingly, inducible patients, despite treatment with an ICD, have a higher overall mortality than noninducible patients.

An EP-guided approach is most effective for patients with an ischemic cardiomyopathy. In patients with a nonischemic cardiomyopathy, the negative predictive value of EP testing is poor. Patients with a nonischemic cardiomyopathy whose left ventricular ejection fraction is less than 30% appear to have particularly high mortality. Therefore, ICD implantation has been advocated in all of these patients who present with syncope, irrespective of the findings at EP testing. In practice, EP testing has been abandoned in patients presenting with unexplained syncope with underlying structural heart disease. Several randomized clinical trials (see Chapter 10) have shown that these patients benefit from an ICD on the basis of their underlying left dysfunction alone, irrespective of the history of syncope. A similar approach is probably warranted in patients with high-risk conditions such as hypertrophic cardiomyopathy, Brugada syndrome, and congenital short and long QT syndrome who present with syncope (Fig. 5-4).

Syncope is clearly an ominous marker in patients with structural heart disease. Recent data from the Sudden Cardiac Death in Heart Failure Trial (SCD-HeFT), a randomized trial of placebo, amiodarone, or single-chamber ICD implantation in patients with a left ventricular ejection fraction ≤35% irrespective of etiology, further highlight this concern. In this trial, after randomization, 356 (14%) patients had ≥1 episode syncope

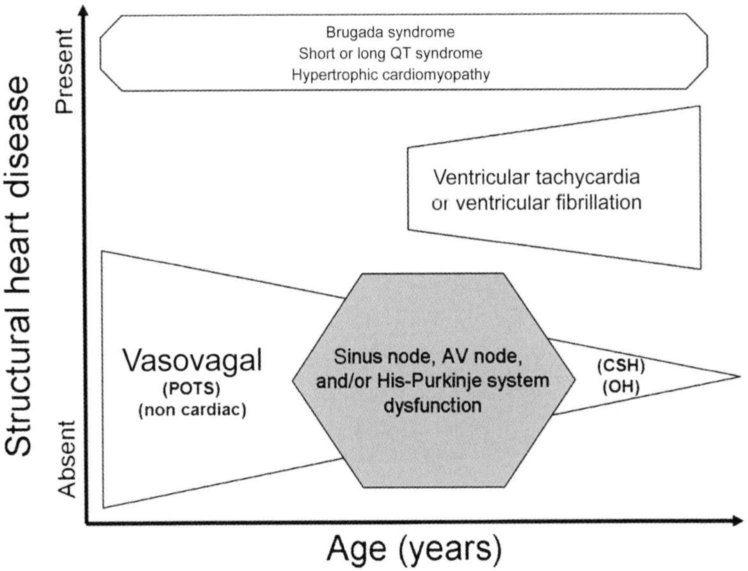

FIGURE 5-4. An algorithm for the evaluation of patients with suspected cardiac syncope. The likely diagnosis and subsequent treatment are heavily influenced by the patient's age and presence or absence of underlying structural heart disease. CSH, carotid sinus hypersensitivity; OH, orthostatic hypotension; POTS, postural orthostatic tachycardia syndrome.

at a median of 15 (5, 28) months. A QRS $d \geq 120$ ms (HR 1.30 [95% CI: 1.06 to 1.61, $p = 0.014$]) and lack of beta-blocker use (HR 1.25 [95% CI: 1.01 to 1.56, $p = 0.048$]) were more commonly observed in patients with an episode of syncope. Syncope after randomization was associated with increased risk of an appropriate ICD shock (HR 2.91 [95% CI: 1.89 to 4.47, $p = 0.001$]), increased risk of cardiovascular death (HR 1.55 [95% CI: 1.19 to 2.02, $p = 0.001$]), and all-cause mortality (HR 1.41 [95% CI: 1.13 to 1.76, $p = 0.002$]), *irrespective of randomization arm.*

NONCARDIAC SYNCOPE

Syncope due to a noncardiac etiology is associated with a benign prognosis. The most common noncardiac causes are seizures and psychiatric disorders, such as panic and anxiety attacks. Seizures may be difficult to distinguish from cardiac syncope since up to 12% of patients with syncope have an associated convulsive reaction ("convulsive syncope"). In fact, up to 30% of patients diagnosed with epilepsy may in fact suffer from convulsive syncope. Features suggestive of convulsive syncope include relationship to the upright posture, absence of tonic-clonic movements or automatisms, rapid recovery, *absence of postictal disorientation*, and a normal interictal electroencephalograpy (EEG). The entity of convulsive syncope should be considered in all patients with suspected epilepsy, especially when the history is atypical for epilepsy or when there is an inadequate response to anticonvulsant medication. However, a clinical practice of routinely performing neurologic evaluations (head CT or MRI, carotid Doppler examinations, and EEG) in patients presenting with unexplained syncope is not warranted given the high cost and extremely low yield of these diagnostic modalities.

CONCLUSIONS

Syncope remains a common clinical problem. Given the vast differential diagnosis, a uniform structured approach to the patient with unexplained syncope is useful. Toward this end, at our institution, we utilize the SELF clinical pathway to guide the evaluation and management of all patients admitted with unexplained syncope (Fig. 5-5), which is modeled according to current practice guidelines.

Patients in whom there is either not true loss of consciousness or prolonged loss of consciousness do not have cardiac syncope and should be managed accordingly. Patients with true syncope fulfill the four SELF criteria: (i) **S**hort period, **S**elf-limited, **S**pontaneous recovery, (ii) **E**arly (rapid) onset, (iii) **L**oss of consciousness (transient), and (iv) **F**ull recovery. In these patients, a diagnosis can be readily made on the basis of the initial

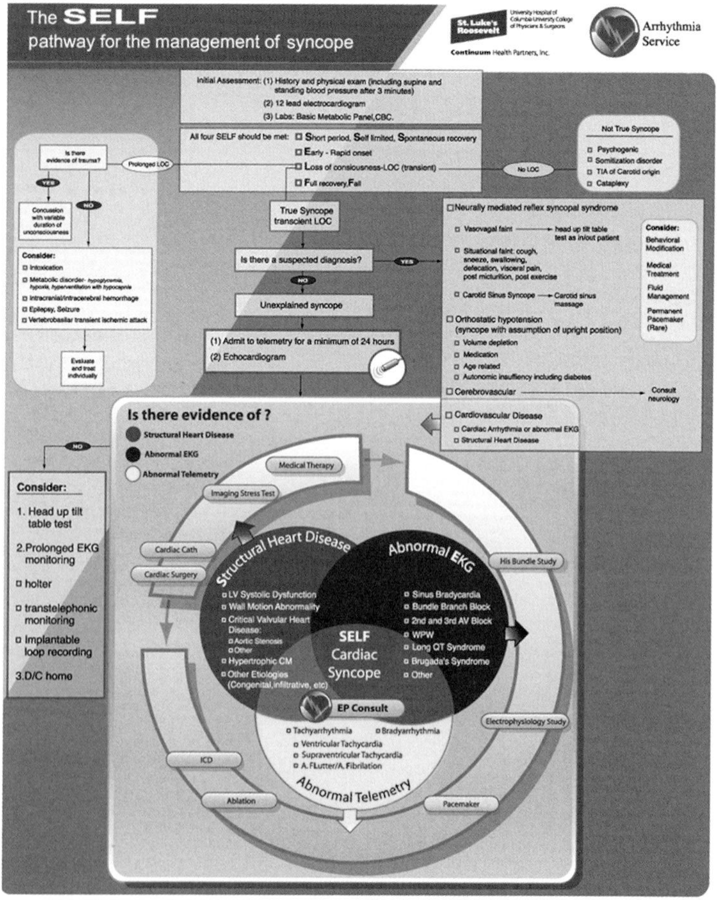

FIGURE 5-5. The SELF pathway for the management of syncope.

history and physical examination in conjunction with review of the patient's ECG and echocardiogram. In patients without structural heart disease, syncope is usually the result of bradycardia. In younger patients, this is most commonly due to a neurally mediated phenomenon, which is associated with excellent long-term prognosis. As a result, these patients can usually be managed with reassurance and behavioral/lifestyle modifications.

In patients in whom the diagnosis is uncertain, further diagnostic evaluation is necessary. Patients with abnormal telemetry and/or ambulatory ECG findings, an abnormal baseline ECG, and/or evidence of structural heart disease benefit from an evaluation by an electrophysiologist. In some cases, it may be necessary to exclude the presence of the underlying coronary artery disease. Patients with underlying structural heart disease who present with syncope are at high risk of death; these patients, in general, should be considered for ICD implantation.

The major challenge is to identify those middle-aged and older patients with underlying sinus node, AV node, or His-Purkinje system dysfunction who many benefit from permanent pacing. Although these patients have traditionally undergone ambulatory ECG monitoring (24-hour Holter, transtelephonic event/loop monitoring), tilt table testing, and "directed" EP testing (i.e., a sinus node and His-bundle evaluation), this approach appears to have poor sensitivity. Recent data suggest that loop recorder implantation may be a preferable initial strategy, especially in those patients in whom a definitive diagnosis is essential such as those in whom syncope is recurrent or associated with trauma.

KEY POINTS

1. The history and physical examination are the cornerstones in the evaluation and management of patients with unexplained syncope; in most cases, an ECG and echocardiogram should also be obtained.
2. An important question is whether the patient is at high-risk for future events and thus merits treatment. Toward that end, patients with bradycardia (due to sinus node dysfunction and/or heart block) should be treated with a pacemaker, and patients with underlying structural heart disease should be considered for ICD implantation.
3. Patients with recurrent syncope, traumatic syncope, or those in whom the ECG is abnormal should be considered for loop recorder implantation when the initial workup is not diagnostic.

SUGGESTED READINGS

Benditt DG, Ferguson DW, Grubb BP, et al. Tilt table testing for assessing syncope. *J Am Coll Cardiol.* 1996;28:263–275.

Brignole M, Alboni P, Benditt DG, et al. Guidelines on management (diagnosis and treatment) of syncope—Update 2004. The task force on syncope, European Society of Cardiology. *Europace.* 2004;6:467–537.

Brignole M, Menozzi C, Moya C, et al. Mechanism of syncope in patients with bundle branch block and negative electrophysiological tests. *Circulation.* 2001;104:2045–2050.

Connolly SJ, Sheldon R, Thorpe KE, et al. Pacemaker therapy for prevention of syncope in patients with recurrent severe vasovagal syncope. Second vasovagal pacemaker study (VPS II): A randomized trial. *JAMA.* 2003;289:2224–2229.

Krahn AD, Klein GJ, Yee R, et al. Randomized assessment of syncope trial: Conventional diagnostic testing versus a prolonged monitoring strategy. *Circulation.* 2001;104:46–51.

Mittal S, Iwai S, Stein KM, et al. Long-term outcome of patients with unexplained syncope treated with an electrophysiologic-guided approach in the implantable cardioverter-defibrillator era. *J Am Coll Cardiol.* 1999;34:1082–1089.

Moya A, Brignole M, Menozzi C, et al. Mechanism of syncope in patients with isolated syncope and in patients with tilt positive syncope. *Circulation.* 2001;104:1261–1267.

Olshansky B, Poole JE, Johnson G, et al. Syncope predicts the outcome of cardiomyopathy patients: Analysis of the SCD-HeFT study. *J Am Coll Cardiol.* 2008;51:1277–1282.
Soteriades ES, Evans JC, Larson MG, et al. Incidence and prognosis of syncope. *N Engl J Med.* 2002;347: 878–885.
Strickberger SA, Benson DW, Biaggioni I, et al. AHA/ACCF scientific statement on the evaluation of syncope: From the American Heart Association council on clinical cardiology, cardiovascular nursing, cardiovascular disease in the young, and stroke, and the quality of care and outcomes research interdisciplinary working group; and the American College of Cardiology Foundation in collaboration with the Heart Rhythm Society. *J Am Coll Cardiol.* 2006;47:473–484.

CHAPTER 6

Sudden Cardiac Death and the Cardiac Arrest Survivor

Jaimie Manlucu, Raymond Yee, Lorne J. Gula, George J. Klein, Allan C. Skanes, and Andrew D. Krahn

Sudden cardiac death (SCD) is defined as unexpected death that occurs within 1 h of the onset of symptoms or during sleep, most often attributed to cardiac arrhythmia. Although overall death from cardiovascular disease is falling, SCD remains a significant cause of mortality, accounting for over 400,000 deaths in the US annually. Therefore, for those at risk of cardiac arrest, the investigative workup necessitates a comprehensive and systematic approach that enables prompt identification of underlying structural heart disease, reversible causes, provides a phenotype and genotype for inherited causes, and leads to tailored treatment strategies. This chapter outlines an approach to the identification and management of patients who have experienced a cardiac arrest or are at risk for SCD.

CLINICAL CAUSES

Although the possible causes of SCD can be quite broad, 70% to 80% of cases are attributed to underlying coronary artery disease associated with either acute ischemia or chronic left ventricular (LV) dysfunction. Up to half of these cases present with SCD as the initial manifestation of their coronary disease. Autopsy findings reveal a high incidence of multivessel disease with acute changes in coronary plaque morphology in more than 50% of cases. In those with myocardial scar but no evidence of acute infarction, half will have active coronary lesions.

Hypertrophic and nonischemic dilated cardiomyopathies account for 15% to 20% of sudden death from cardiac causes. Dilated cardiomyopathy has innumerable secondary causes, including infection, endocrine disorders, tachycardia-induced cardiomyopathies, rheumatologic disorders, and nutritional deficiencies. Arrhythmogenic right ventricular cardiomyopathy (ARVC) is a special type of cardiomyopathy characterized by ventricular arrhythmias and right ventricular dilatation due to fibrofatty infiltration and progressive myocardial thinning. Patients may present with SCD as their initial symptom. Hypertrophic cardiomyopathy is a genetic defect of the cardiac sarcomere resulting in marked hypertrophy of the left ventricle. This population carries a well-defined risk of SCD, with an annual rate ranging from 2% to 4% depending on the patient's risk profile.

Less common causes of SCD include valvular or congenital heart diseases, coronary anomalies, and genetically determined channelopathies (e.g., long QT syndrome [LQTS], catecholaminergic polymorphic ventricular tachycardia [CPVT], and Brugada syndrome). In addition to a susceptible substrate, superimposed triggers such as ischemia, electrolyte imbalances, antiarrhythmic or QT-prolonging drugs, autonomic nervous system activation, and psychosocial factors are also thought to play a major role in precipitating an event and should be considered.

INITIAL INVESTIGATION STRATEGY

Given the spectrum of possible causes, a thorough history is of paramount importance, particularly if the etiology of cardiac arrest is not forthcoming. A previous history of heart disease, chest pain, or syncope, along with a family history of syncope or sudden death, may provide key historical insights that may be corroborated by subsequent investigations. As mentioned, the trigger for cardiac arrest is also informative. Exertion may trigger events in coronary artery disease as well as in less common inherited conditions such as LQTS and CPVT. A febrile illness may precipitate events in Brugada syndrome, and drugs that affect repolarization may unmask underlying Brugada syndrome or LQTS. A careful account of prescribed or over the counter drugs should also be obtained, including supplements and recreational drugs. A typical example would be the addition of a QT-prolonging agent resulting in torsade de pointes and cardiac arrest.

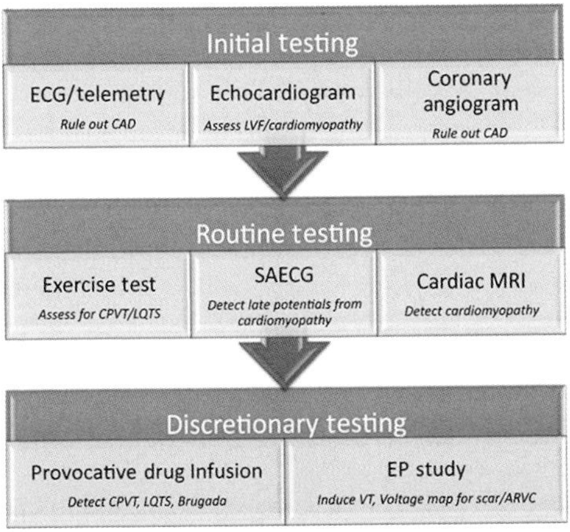

FIGURE 6-1. Diagnostic algorithm for the testing approach to the cardiac arrest survivor.

Routine blood work should also be performed to rule out contributing electrolyte disorders and to screen for toxins and drug overdose in the appropriate clinical circumstances. A summary of a systematic approach to investigation of the survivor of cardiac arrest is illustrated in Figure 6-1.

RESTING ELECTROCARDIOGRAM

Investigation begins with continuous ECG monitoring for recurrent arrhythmia and assessment of the ECG and biomarkers for evidence of acute or chronic myocardial ischemia. Consideration should be given to performance of high lateral and posterior leads when acute infarction is suspected. The QT interval should also be measured in cardiac arrest survivors, corrected for rate using Bazett formula. QT interval prolongation after cardiac arrest is common but is usually secondary to ischemic or systemic factors (Fig. 6-2). Some degree of QT prolongation is often evident in the patient with nonST elevation myocardial infarction or anoxic brain injury from the cardiac arrest without underlying LQTS. Transient QT prolongation and other repolarization changes may also be seen during induced hypothermia that resolves with warming. When genetic repolarization syndromes are suspected, obtaining previous ECGs of the patient or his/her first-degree relatives may assist in identifying repolarization abnormalities. In congenital LQTS, the degree of QT interval prolongation is associated with a higher risk of SCD and is often profoundly increased in the context of LQTS-related cardiac arrest.

QT interval prolongation has also been postulated to predict mortality in patients with acute myocardial infarction. Cohort studies have shown an association between QT interval prolongation and cardiac mortality; however, these were population-based studies with no defined subgroups. In the setting of LV dysfunction, QT interval prolongation is not a reliable predictor of SCD.

CARDIAC FUNCTION ASSESSMENT

The majority of cardiac arrest survivors have significant systolic LV dysfunction, which is usually assessed by echocardiography, nuclear imaging, or contrast ventriculography. Left ventricular ejection fraction (LVEF) has been shown to be the strongest predictor of cardiovascular mortality in patients with either ischemic or nonischemic cardiomyopathy.

In patients who have survived a cardiac arrest, a reduced LVEF provides evidence for a potential substrate for arrhythmia. If LV dysfunction is documented, the etiology should be established to identify reversible causes and optimise cause-specific therapy. Of note,

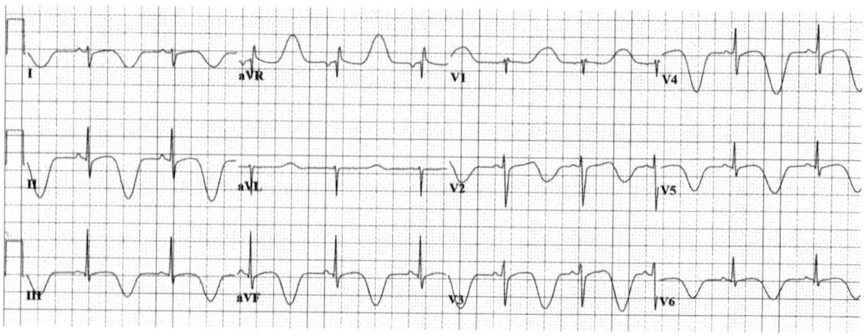

FIGURE 6-2. Dramatic QT prolongation after cardiac arrest in a 73-year-old male with evidence of anterior ischemia with T wave inversion in conjunction with biochemical evidence of non-ST elevation myocardial infarction. The T wave morphology returned to near normal after 10 days, and the QT interval shortened.

transient mild to moderate LV dysfunction is common after resuscitation, particularly if the "down time" is prolonged. This is presumably related to tissue hypoxia and acidosis with transient myocardial stunning. This may be difficult to distinguish from an acute myocarditis, which typically presents with a preceding febrile illness and other findings including arrhythmia and conduction system involvement. Serial LV function assessment is indicated when this is suspected.

CORONARY ANGIOGRAPHY

Coronary angiography is indicated in virtually all cardiac arrest survivors. On occasion, young patients with normal heart function and suspected primary arrhythmia may warrant consideration of noninvasive imaging with perfusion studies or CT angiography to exclude coronary artery disease or coronary artery anomalies. Regardless of the approach, careful exclusion of coronary disease is important. Coronary vasospasm is an eclectic cause of cardiac arrest that should be considered in unusual circumstances (Fig. 6-3). These patients are typically smokers with evidence of mild coronary luminal narrowing along with a chest pain history, at times in conjunction with the index event. The role of provocative testing with ergonovine in this population is controversial and not without risk but may warrant consideration in highly select cases.

FURTHER TESTING TO DETECT UNUSUAL CAUSES OF CARDIAC ARREST

The preceding section describes standard testing that applies to all cardiac arrest patients and explains the vast majority of cases. Further testing is not typically performed unless the cause remains unclear. Beyond the usual diagnoses of coronary artery disease and overt cardiomyopathy, the clinician is faced with a broad differential diagnosis for cardiac arrest, including an unrecognised cardiomyopathy such as ARVC or latent electrical disease such as LQTS, CPVT, or Brugada syndrome. Testing for these causes can be divided into routine noninvasive testing and discretionary provocative or invasive testing (Fig. 6-1).

EXERCISE TESTING

Treadmill or bicycle exercise testing should be performed in unexplained cardiac arrest to unmask evidence of exercise-induced arrhythmia such as polymorphic VT in CPVT and QT prolongation in LQTS (Fig. 6-4). At the authors' institution, treadmill testing is performed with continuous ECG monitoring; ST segment and QT intervals are measured every minute on a 12-lead ECG. Intravenous beta-blocking agents are available in the event that exercise precipitates ventricular arrhythmia. Detection of marked QT prolongation in conjunction with T wave morphology changes during exercise should prompt consideration of genetic testing and family screening for LQTS.

SIGNAL-AVERAGED ECG

The signal-averaged ECG (SAECG) is used to detect late potentials at the terminal portion of the QRS and signifies the presence of areas of slow conduction that serve as potential substrate for reentrant arrhythmias. These low-amplitude, high-frequency signals are caused by fractionated signals arising from infarcted or fibrosed myocardium. Although arrhythmia has already manifested in a SCD survivor, an abnormal SAECG may identify an abnormal arrhythmogenic substrate. A number of parameters are used when analyzing the SAECG; however, a filtered QRS duration greater than 114 ms is the most sensitive at predicting risk of SCD. Other parameters that are considered abnormal are low-amplitude signal duration greater than 38 ms and a root mean square voltage of the terminal 40 ms of the QRS complex less than 20 μV at 40 Hz filter settings. A positive SAECG should prompt consideration of an occult myocardial process such as ARVC or myocarditis or an infiltrative process such as sarcoidosis or amyloidosis.

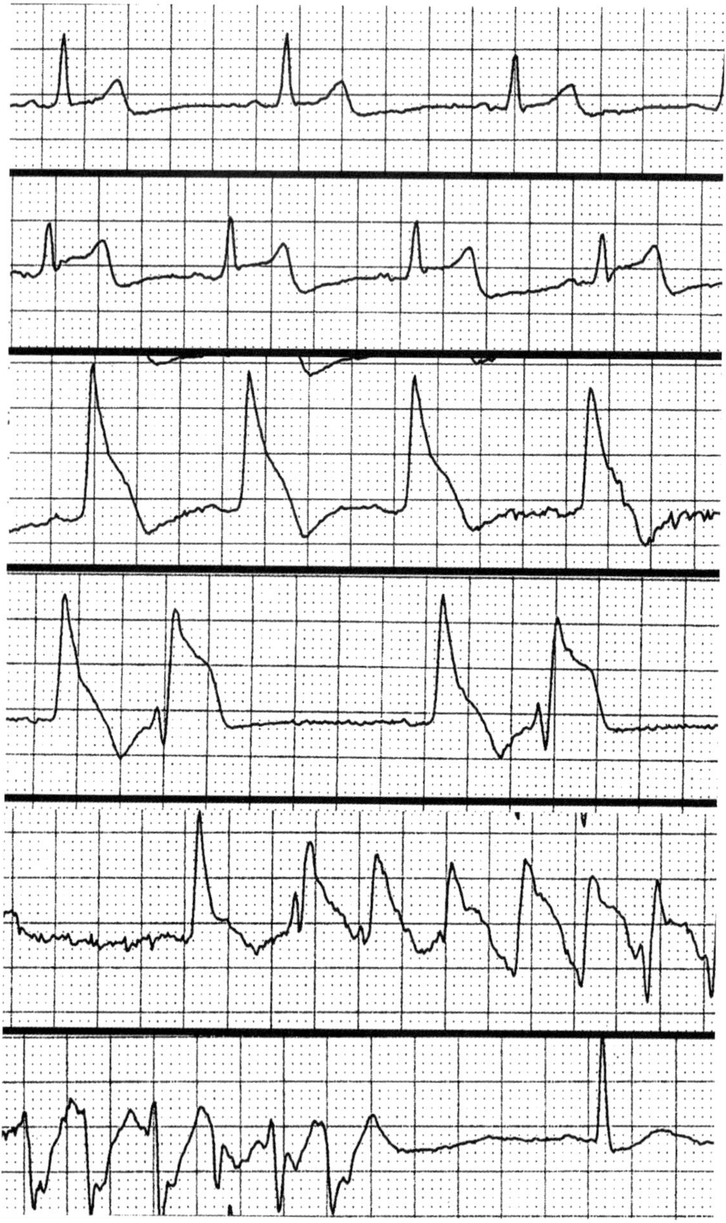

FIGURE 6-3. Serial rhythm strips over 2 min in a 46-year-old male with recent cardiac arrest. Mild luminal irregularity was noted on coronary angiography, with a normal LV function. Routine telemetry 72 h after presentation demonstrated asymptomatic dramatic ST segment changes in conjunction with ventricular ectopy and nonsustained polymorphic VT resulting in a diagnosis of vasospasm induced cardiac arrest.

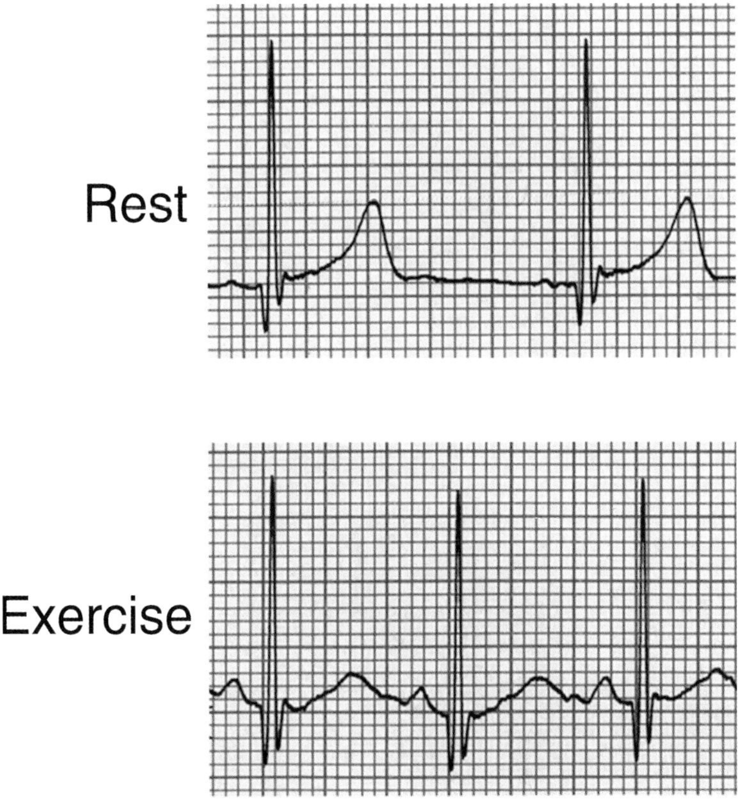

FIGURE 6-4. Rest and exercise lead II in a young patient with resuscitated cardiac arrest and borderline resting QT interval. Early in exercise she fails to shorten the QT interval, which is consistent with the diagnosis of LQTS. (See text for discussion.)

CARDIAC MRI

Cardiac magnetic resonance (CMR) imaging has emerged as a highly valuable tool for the diagnosis of cardiovascular disease associated with cardiac arrest. This is largely through recognition of its ability to identify disease substrate at the tissue level as well as identify more subtle structural and functional abnormalities. Conditions such as hypertrophic cardiomyopathy, acute myocarditis (Fig. 6-5), ARVC, or infiltrative processes such as amyloidosis and sarcoidosis are most appropriately evaluated using this imaging modality. The accurate identification and characterization of anomalous coronary arteries is also afforded through current MRI techniques, avoiding radiation exposure. Careful "prescription" of CMR scanning protocols in collaboration with a CMR expert is crucial to screen for these conditions and should include consideration of functional imaging, edema (T2 weighted), and fat (T1 weighted) imaging, as well as delayed enhancement using gadolinium.

ARVC is a diagnosis that is often entertained in the context of an unexplained cardiac arrest, particularly when there is a family history of sudden death or anterior T wave changes are present. CMR aims to identify both abnormal tissue characteristics and functional abnormalities in this condition. Although the specificity and interobserver

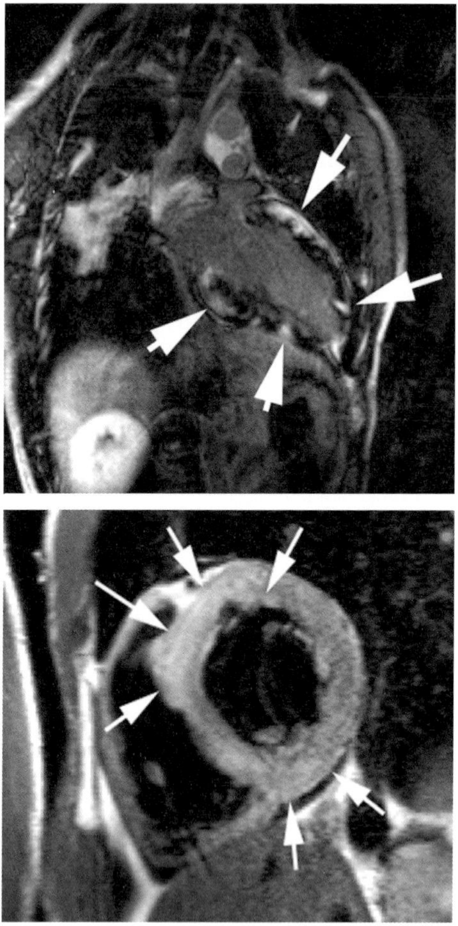

FIGURE 6-5. Cardiac MR images in a 23-year-old woman with resuscitated cardiac arrest showing evidence of acute myocarditis. Delayed enhancement imaging following gadolinium shows epicardial-based enhancement in the inferolateral wall consistent with acute myocyte injury (**upper panel**—white rim, *arrows*). An SSFP-based, T2-weighted image demonstrates corresponding edema in the same region (**lower panel**, *arrows*). These findings are typical for acute myocarditis.

variability appear to be a limitation, CMR remains the gold standard for right ventricular functional assessment; it is the imaging modality of choice in patients with suspected ARVC. It is important to stress that a normal MRI scan does not exclude ARVC, and that careful expert interpretation is crucial in the context of the clinical presentation.

DISCRETIONARY TESTING

Beyond the previously mentioned systematic testing, further testing should be considered on a case-by-case basis before a diagnosis of unexplained cardiac arrest or idiopathic ventricular fibrillation (VF) is made. This testing can either be provocative (through drug infusions or electrophysiologic [EP] testing), invasive (through voltage mapping in conjunction with EP testing), or myocardial biopsy. Pharmacologic challenge targets latent repolarization or related conditions that are unmasked in the context of channel or function stress. Best known is the response of Brugada syndrome patients to sodium channel blockers, unmasking or amplifying the severity and type of ST segment changes. The yield of this form of testing in a patient with no suggestion of pretest ST changes is unknown but is presumably low. Placing precordial ECG leads in a higher intercostal space enhances the sensitivity of the test.

Epinephrine challenge has been used to unmask or enhance QT prolongation in patients with diagnostic uncertainties that are ultimately diagnosed with LQTS. The yield of this form of testing in patients with unexplained cardiac arrest is currently being studied in a Canadian registry, where the preliminary yield was 16% in 51 patients. The other utility of epinephrine challenge is in unmasking CPVT (Fig. 6-6). Limited data suggest that epinephrine may be more sensitive than exercise testing for diagnosis of CPVT, with no comparative data to isoproterenol, which has also been used. Further forms of provocative infusions are likely to develop, as our understanding of the mechanism of occult life-threatening arrhythmias evolves. One such example is the preliminary report of use of erythromycin to unmask LQT2 in patients with borderline QT intervals.

As most survivors of SCD now routinely receive implantable cardioverter–defibrillators (ICDs) for secondary prevention, the role of cardiac EP studies in the identification of patients at high risk of recurrent SCD has largely been negated. EP testing may still be considered in select patients to tailor ICD programming (typically through the device at implant). Although inducibility of ventricular tachycardia (VT) confers a greater risk of SCD, noninducibility provides little prognostic value, especially in the context of hypertrophic or nonischemic cardiomyopathy.

The exception to this is when an occult cardiomyopathy such as ARVC is suspected based on prior testing. In these cases, EP studies are performed to assess for an inducible substrate such as VT arising from the right ventricle or a region of the left ventricle where imaging has suspected an abnormality. Voltage mapping is also often performed in conjunction with EP testing, to assess for evidence of scar to support the diagnosis of

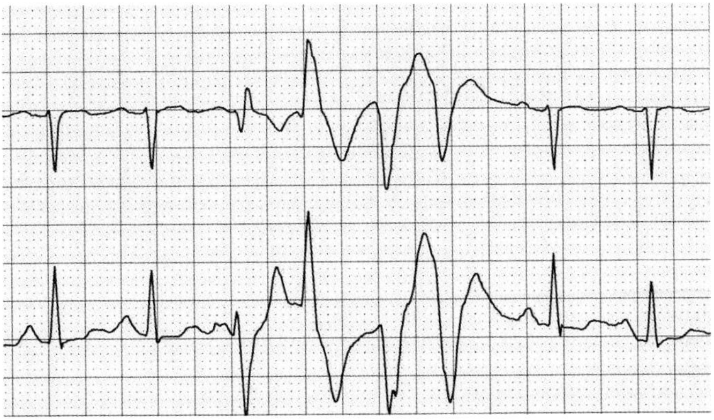

FIGURE 6-6. Leads V1and III during adrenaline challenge in a 42-year-old female with cardiac arrest and a structurally normal heart. Polymorphic VT in salvos was noted during infusion, which was stopped when tachycardia sustained for 8 s. Intravenous metoprolol was administered postinfusion and the diagnosis of CPVT was established.

an underlying cardiomyopathy. Though this process is both expensive and invasive, it warrants consideration in select circumstances such as in the younger patient, where a diagnosis is crucial to family screening.

OTHER CONSIDERATIONS

Preliminary data in a modest number of patients with apparent unexplained cardiac arrest suggests that a diagnosis can be obtained based on the testing algorithm in Figure 6-1 in 50% of patients. Rare circumstances lead to consideration of certain testing based on clinical suspicion. Endomyocardial biopsy may be considered to obtain a tissue diagnosis to correlate with other evidence of a myocardial process such as myocarditis or ARVC. Ergonovine challenge may be considered for coronary spasm. Other ancillary testing could include a catecholamine screen when pheochromocytoma is suspected.

THE GENETICS OF SUDDEN DEATH

Genetic testing of repolarization-related genes in the cardiac arrest survivor should be reserved for situations where a phenotype emerges from clinical testing that can both direct genetic testing and provide a correlate to assist in interpretation. Given the frequency of polymorphisms in most of the known culprit repolarization genes and the difficulty with obtaining expression models to ascertain the disease causing nature of many findings, routine screening is not indicated outside of a research environment.

TREATMENT

The management of SCD begins with acute resuscitation and continues with chronic preventative therapy. Acute management of cardiac arrest focuses primarily on rhythm stabilization and detecting and treating reversible causes or triggers. Once the patient is stable, efforts can be focused on minimizing the risk of future events (secondary prevention). In those without a history of aborted SCD, measures are taken to reduce the risk of an initial life-threatening arrhythmic event (primary prevention). In either circumstance, the main therapeutic options include implantable ICDs or antiarrhythmic medications. Though outside of the scope of this discussion, standard medical therapy for underlying heart disease including revascularization and proven medical therapy has clearly been shown to reduce risk of sudden death.

ACUTE MANAGEMENT OF SUDDEN CARDIAC DEATH

The electrical mechanisms of SCD include VF, pulseless VT, pulseless electrical activity, or asystole. Pulseless VT and VF are most common, accounting for 25% to 35% of all out-of-hospital SCD events. The acute management of SCD is guided by the underlying rhythm, with a rapid response time being the main determinant of survival. Advanced cardiac life support protocols are well established and are the cornerstone of resuscitative efforts. Survival from cardiac arrest falls 7% to 10% per minute without prompt initiation of resuscitative efforts. Following initial stabilization with asynchronous electrical shocks, normalization of potassium and magnesium levels, and the prophylactic use of beta-blockers may help reduce the incidence of recurrent arrhythmia. Resistant or recurrent ventricular arrhythmias in the setting of an acute infarct may respond to amiodarone or lidocaine infusion.

For cardiac arrests due to polymorphic VT in the context of a prolonged QT interval (i.e., torsade de pointes), withdrawal of offending medications and correction of electrolyte imbalances are of paramount importance. Cases with underlying congenital LQTS respond well to beta-blocker therapy, and overdrive pacing may be used in cases of pause-dependent torsade de pointes. Isoproterenol infusion is effective in bridging to either temporary or permanent pacing. Polymorphic VT with a normal QT interval during intervening episodes of sinus rhythm is most often seen in the setting of acute ischemia which should be identified and treated promptly. It is also rarely seen in idiopathic polymorphic VT or catecholaminergic polymorphic VT. Both respond well to intravenous beta-blockers or Amiodarone. Once the patient is stabilized and reversible causes have been identified and addressed, the extent of preventative measures will depend on neurologic recovery and the spectrum of comorbidities.

PRIMARY PREVENTION

The risk of the first episode of SCD is highly dependent on the underlying disease process predisposing the individual to arrhythmogenic death. From a population perspective, cardiac arrest happens most often in individuals with atherosclerotic risk factors or mild established disease without LV dysfunction. These individuals are at a very low overall risk but represent such a large pool of the adult population that they contribute the most to the societal burden of sudden death. In contrast, patients with established LV dysfunction are at markedly higher relative risk, but represent a smaller proportion of the overall burden of the disease. Lastly, the highest risk individuals are those that have been fortunate to survive a cardiac arrest (2 degree prevention), who represent a very tiny fraction of the sudden death population. LV dysfunction, regardless of the cause, is a universal marker of elevated risk, particularly when the ejection fraction falls below 30%. In addition to a susceptible substrate and appropriate triggers, the predisposition to arrhythmic death is also thought to have genetic influences.

MEDICAL THERAPY

For many years, beta-blockers were the only class of medication that demonstrated any reduction in SCD, particularly in those with low ejection fractions postinfarction. Recent evidence has shown that, in addition to optimal medical therapy, aldosterone antagonists such as eplerenone or spironolactone can reduce the risk of sudden death in the setting of reduced LV function. Antiarrhythmic medications, on the other hand, have been universally disappointing, demonstrating an increase in mortality, primarily from proarrhythmic effects. Despite a lower incidence of arrhythmic complications relative to other antiarrhythmics, treatment with Amiodarone also lacks any substantive mortality benefit relative to controls. This was most recently confirmed in the Sudden Cardiac Death Heart Failure Trial (SCD-HeFT). In those with nonischemic cardiomyopathy, there is new evidence that standard optimal medical therapy for heart failure significantly improves survival. Both ACE inhibitors and beta-blockers have been shown to reduce the rate of sudden death in this population. Moreover, unlike the setting of ischemic cardiomyopathy, there is some evidence that amiodarone may also provide some survival benefit in these patients.

DEVICE THERAPY

Unlike the relatively disappointing results from pharmacologic studies, several multicenter primary prevention studies have demonstrated that ICDs result in a significant reduction in mortality in patients with LV dysfunction of either ischemic or nonischemic causes. Mortality reductions are estimated at 23% to 55% (depending on the risk group), with the majority of this benefit being due to a reduction in SCD. Based on these findings, the ICD has become the preventative therapy of choice. Consistent with current national guidelines, most patients with LVEFs less than 35% on optimal medical therapy with a reasonable prognosis and good functional capacity are offered an ICD. In those with very poor systolic function (i.e., LVEF < 20%), the magnitude of device therapy is less clear because of the competing risk of nonarrhythmic death from progressive heart failure. Therefore, careful consideration regarding end of life issues should be discussed when contemplating ICD therapy in this population.

Optimal timing of device implantation in patients with recent myocardial infarctions also remains uncertain. Recent evidence suggests that ICD implantation within the first 40 days after infarction does not confer a survival benefit and therefore should not be offered during that period. Another point of contention is the lack of gold standard for the measurement of LVEF. All methods lack precision and may vary significantly between modalities, centers, and operators. Current guidelines recommend that clinicians choose the most accurate and appropriate modality offered at their center.

SECONDARY PREVENTION

The risk of recurrence of SCD in cardiac arrest survivors is high, particularly in the first 6 to 18 months. The 1-year mortality in this population is estimated at 32%, with the risk escalating with the severity of LV dysfunction. The first step in the process is to address reversible causes. This may include revascularization for ischemic precipitants and the appropriate treatments for the various reversible causes of LV dysfunction such as endocrine disorders, tachycardia-induced cardiomyopathies, infiltrative diseases, rheumatologic disorders, and nutritional deficiencies. For patients with persistent LV dysfunction and/or on-going risk of SCD, further measures are required to minimize recurrence. Although most will likely receive an ICD, a variety of other therapeutic options including medication, catheter ablation, or even surgery, may be considered depending on the cause.

DEVICE THERAPY

The mortality benefit of the ICD in patients who have survived a life-threatening arrhythmic event is well established. Their superiority to antiarrhythmics agents in reducing the incidence of recurrent SCD was confirmed in three major randomized trials (CASH, CIDS, and AVID). A subsequent meta-analysis of these trials showed that the relative benefit of these devices is most prominent in those with a LVEF of less than 35%, conferring an estimated 28% reduction in SCD. In contrast, little difference was noted between the two treatment strategies in those with an LVEF greater than 35%.

There are also several heritable and infiltrative conditions that are not amenable to medical therapy, leaving ICDs as their only preventative measure. Heritable arrhythmias such as Brugada syndrome and infiltrative cardiomyopathies at high risk for SCD such as ARVC, hypertrophic cardiomyopathy, Sarcoidosis, and amyloidosis all fall into this category. Despite the presence of effective prophylactic medical therapies for heritable arrhythmias such as LQTS and CPVT, those who present with SCD are considered at higher risk for recurrence and guidelines recommend an ICD for secondary prevention.

MEDICAL THERAPY

Medical therapy is rarely used in isolation for secondary prophylaxis, unless ICD implantation is refused or inappropriate. Several antiarrhythmics agents have been studied in randomized trials in patients with a history of aborted SCD in the context of reduced LV function due to either ischemic or nonischemic etiologies. Most had equivocal results, at best, with significant potential for adverse events related primarily to proarrhythmia. The only possible exception is Amiodarone, which demonstrated a survival benefit that was later noted to be modest compared to that of the ICD. Therefore, although Amiodarone may be associated with a mild protective effect, the magnitude of benefit is unclear.

Amiodarone is an effective adjunctive therapy to ICDs in the management of arrhythmia-prone patients. This may help reduce shocks due to frequent ventricular arrhythmia or atrial tachyarrhythmias with rapid ventricular response. Other classes of drugs have also been shown to help reduce the risk of recurrent SCD. In survivors of SCD due to coronary disease, statins have been associated with a reduction in recurrent ventricular arrhythmias. As seen in the primary prevention trials, beta-blockers also have a well-established role in patients at risk for recurrent arrhythmic death. Moreover, arrhythmias driven by sympathetically mediated triggers such as LQTS and CPVT also respond well to beta-blockers.

ABLATION

Although catheter ablation is usually reserved for more benign, focal tachyarrhythmias, it may be considered as adjunctive therapy in patients with frequent ICD shocks due to recurrent ventricular arrhythmias not manageable by reprogramming or adjunctive medical therapy. This is discussed in the section on ventricular arrhythmias. Initial studies suggest that a reduction in incidence of VT improves quality of life, which should be viewed as a morbidity intervention, predominantly targeting reduced shocks in ICD patients.

SURGERY

Surgical ablation or resection of an arrhythmogenic focus for patients with recurrent ventricular tachyarrhythmias may be considered when patients are undergoing concomitant cardiac surgery or rarely when drug therapy or ablation is unsuccessful. The outcome of this relatively uncommon approach is not well described in the ICD and catheter ablation era. Left cervicothoracic sympathetic ganglionectomy is suited to adrenergically triggered life-threatening ventricular arrhythmias associated with LQTS or CPVT. This approach may be useful as an adjunctive therapy in patients with aborted SCD despite combined ICD and beta-blocker therapy.

CONCLUSION

Cardiac arrest is a prevalent problem with a potentially devastating outcome. Consequently, those at risk warrant careful attention to determine the underlying cause in order to guide appropriate preventative therapy. Preliminary testing will detect coronary artery disease and/or LV dysfunction in the majority of cases. Various modes of noninvasive imaging and provocative testing may assist in diagnosing the more unusual causes. Although the treatment of choice remains ICD implantation, a variety of adjunctive therapies including optimal medical therapy and perfusion are important.

ACKNOWLEDGMENT

Dr Krahn is a Career Investigator of the Heart and Stroke Foundation of Ontario, and is supported by a grant from the Heart and Stroke Foundation of Ontario (NA3397).

KEY POINTS

CLINICAL CAUSES OF SCD

1. Susceptible substrate
   (a) Ischemic cardiomyopathy
   (b) Nonischemic dilated cardiomyopathy
   (c) Hypertrophic cardiomyopathy
   (d) Congenital heart disease
   (e) Valvular heart disease
   (f) Heritable channelopathies

(Continued)

2. Triggers
   (a) Ischemia
   (b) Electrolyte imbalances
   (c) QT-prolonging drugs
   (d) Congestive heart failure/hypoxia
   (e) Psychosocial factors

PRIMARY AND SECONDARY PREVENTION STRATEGIES

1. Optimal perfusion
2. Optimal medical therapy
3. ICD

CLASS I INDICATIONS FOR ICD IMPLANTATION (ACC/AHA/NASPE GUIDELINES)

1. NYHA I to III and
   (a) Nonischemic cardiomyopathy with an LVEF ≤ 35% or
   (b) Ischemic cardiomyopathy with an LVEF ≤ 35% and ≥40 days postinfarct
2. Previous cardiac arrest not due to a transient or reversible cause
3. Structural heart disease with spontaneous or induced sustained ventricular arrhythmia

SUGGESTED READINGS

Connolly SJ, Hallstrom AP, Cappato R, et al. Meta-analysis of the implantable cardioverter defibrillator secondary prevention trials. AVID, CASH and CIDS studies. Antiarrhythmics vs Implantable Defibrillator study. Cardiac Arrest Study Hamburg. Canadian Implantable Defibrillator Study. *Eur Heart J*. Dec 2000;21(24):2071–2078.

Krahn AD, Gollob M, Yee R, et al. Diagnosis of unexplained cardiac arrest: Role of adrenaline and procainamide infusion. *Circulation*. Oct 2005;112(15):2228–2234.

Myerburg RJ, Kessler KM, Castellanos A. Sudden cardiac death: epidemiology, transient risk, and intervention assessment. *Ann Intern Med*. Dec 1993;119(12):1187–1197.

Nanthakumar K, Epstein AE, Kay GN, et al. Prophylactic implantable cardioverter-defibrillator therapy in patients with left ventricular systolic dysfunction: A pooled analysis of 10 primary prevention trials. *J Am Coll Cardiol*. Dec 2004;44(11):2166–2172.

Subbiah R, Gula LJ, Klein GJ, et al. Workup of the cardiac arrest survior. *Prog Cardiovasc Dis*. Nov–Dec 2008;51(3):195–203. Review.

Zipes DP, Camm AJ, Borggrefe M, et al. ACC/AHA/ESC 2006 Guidelines for management of patients with ventricular arrhythmias and the prevention of sudden cardiac death: A report of the American College of Cardiology/American Heart Association Task Force and the European Society of Cardiology Committee for Practice Guidelines (Writing Committee to Develop Guidelines for Management of Patients With Ventricular Arrhythmias and the Prevention of Sudden Cardiac Death). *J Am Coll Cardiol*. Sep 2006;48(5):e247–e346.

SECTION II
The Electrophysiology Laboratory

CHAPTER 7

Electrophysiology Equipment

Mark W. Preminger

Cardiac electrophysiology is based upon the recording of electrical potentials from within the heart. More specifically these potentials are recorded from electrode pairs on catheters positioned along the endocardial surface of the cardiac chambers, from within surrounding vascular structures (coronary sinus, pulmonary veins, and aortic cusps) and less commonly from its epicardial surface accessed through the pericardium. The timing of these signals from one catheter in relation to others, the stability of the recorded signal at a specific target site, and the sequence of cardiac activation based on the signals have prompted the development of diagnostic and mapping catheters, as well as three-dimensional mapping systems and advanced physiologic recording systems capable of storing and displaying these signals.

MULTICHANNEL PHYSIOLOGIC RECORDERS

The process of recording signals from the various electrode catheters is accomplished by means of a data acquisition system or physiologic recorder. This system is comprised of a junction box where the electrode pins from the catheters are connected. The signals then pass to an amplifier that filters and amplifies the signals and then to a multichannel physiologic recording system. These computerized systems are capable of selecting which pairs of electrode poles in the junction box are paired to record a bipolar signal and of displaying these signals in real-time on an LCD screen as well as storing them for subsequent review. Most systems will have a real-time and a review screen that allows for the physician conducting the study to analyze the information as it is being obtained (Fig. 7-1). Typically the endocardial signals undergo amplification, high pass (30 to 40 Hz) and low pass (400 to 500 Hz) filtering and analog to digital conversion for subsequent display on an LCD screen and storage. A notch filter is also often available to help reduce 60 cycle noise; however, its use can potentially result in some loss of information. Bipolar electrograms are recorded from two closely spaced electrode pairs approximately 2 to 5 mm apart and are highly filtered. They are used primarily to time

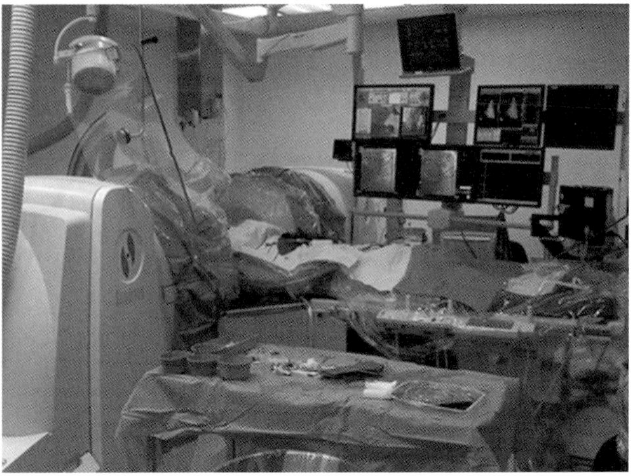

A

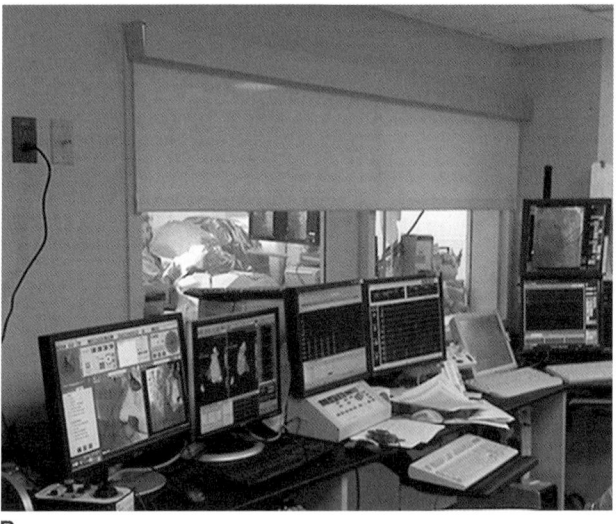

B

FIGURE 7-1. A: A modern electrophysiology laboratory demonstrating a moveable fluoroscopy table, an image intensifier, two large magnets used for remote magnetic navigation and LCD displays for viewing fluoroscopic images, real time-electrograms and electroanatomic maps from tableside. **B:** A typical control booth with physiologic recording equipment, LCD displays for viewing real time and stored electrograms, fluoroscopic images, a stimulator, an electroanatomic mapping system, and the controls for remote magnetic catheter navigation. A control panel for remote control of the RF generator is also shown in the forefront.

the wave front of electrical depolarization of cardiac cells as it passes by this electrode pair. Bipolar electrograms are useful for providing information regarding the timing and locations of a signal. Unipolar electrograms are less highly filtered and are recorded from a single electrode to a widely spaced distant or "indifferent" electrode. The unipolar signal provides additional information regarding the direction that the wave front is traveling either toward (in which case a +R wave is inscribed) or away from (QS complex) the electrode that is recording it. This is of particular use in mapping the site of origin of focal tachycardias or the insertion of accessory pathways where a QS signal is indicative of the catheter being at the site of origin of the signal.

STIMULATORS

The stimulator delivers a constant current output through one or more output channels in order to pace the heart and deliver at least four coupled extrastimuli. The stimulator can be connected directly to the junction box where pacing poles are used to connect electrode pairs for pacing, or as is more commonly done today, the stimulator output is connected to the recording system where the computer controls which electrode pairs are used for pacing. This allows for different stimulation protocols to be set up using a multitude of specific electrode sites for stimulation. Often integrally connected to the physiologic recording system, the stimulator allows for pacing stimuli to be delivered to the specific electrode pairs on the electrophysiology catheters. An input from the recorder allows the stimulator to synchronize its output with a signal sensed from another catheter. By convention, pacing stimuli are delivered at twice late diastolic threshold or 2 mA at a pulse width of 2.0 ms. Pacing at higher outputs is often used to improve capture when the electrodes are not in direct contact with the tissue, for example, within the coronary sinus, however higher outputs can be pro-arrhythmic and can result in "far-field" capture remote from the catheter tip. This can result in inaccuracy when "pace mapping" at high outputs during ablation procedures. In general, pace mapping should be performed at the lowest current that results in continuous capture. Conversely, the inability to pace the heart at high pacing outputs (10 mA and 2.0 ms) has been used to define areas on "unexcitable scar" during substrate mapping of arrhythmias.

CATHETERS

Electrophysiology catheters are typically made of woven Dacron, a woven copolymer, polyurethane, or plastic. The electrodes are usually silver or platinum based. Electrode pairs are usually closely spaced approximately 2 mm apart and with varying amounts of space between the pairs. Typical diagnostic catheters will have four electrodes (a proximal pair and a distal pair spaced approximately 5 mm apart) and a fixed curve at the distal end. The catheter is rotated at its proximal end by the physician as it is inserted from a vascular access site and is advanced under fluoroscopic imaging and precisely positioned within the heart so as to record the desired signal (Fig. 7-2). Quadripolar fixed curve diagnostic catheters are usually positioned at the high right atrium, just across the tricuspid valve in order to record a His bundle potential and at either the right ventricular (RV) apex or RV outflow tract (RVOT). Specially designed multipolar catheters are sometimes added in order to record signals from multiple sites from within a structure such as the coronary sinus or a pulmonary vein or adjacent to an anatomic structure such as the tricuspid annulus (Halo catheter) or the crista terminalis (Crista catheter). Steerable catheters incorporate a "pulley" mechanism that allows the operator to vary the curve at the end of the catheter. This is most useful in positioning catheters in specific locations, such as the coronary sinus from a femoral approach or for mapping and ablation. Mapping catheters can bend in one direction (unidirectional) or two directions (bidirectional) and deflect along a specific radius of curvature. Finally, the size of the distal electrode on ablation catheters through which radiofrequency (RF) energy is delivered can be varied. Most catheters have 4 mm tips; however, larger tips of 5, 8, and 10 mm have also been produced. Larger sized electrodes will produce larger lesion sizes during ablation and have been shown to reduce recurrence rates for arrhythmias such as atrial flutter where creation of a long contiguous line of scar is desired, as compared with conventional 4 mm tip catheters. This increase in lesion formation with an increase in electrode size comes at the expense of decreased electrogram signal resolution. Thus smaller electrode sizes are preferable for detailed mapping procedures.

Irrigated saline tip catheters provide continuous cooling of the distal electrode during RF energy delivery. "Closed" loop systems circulate saline within the catheter to the tip whereas "open" irrigation catheter rinse the outside of the catheter tip with a controlled flow rate of saline allowing it to remain cool while large amounts of RF energy are delivered to the adjacent tissue. Irrigated catheters also produce larger and deeper lesions and potentially more durable results.

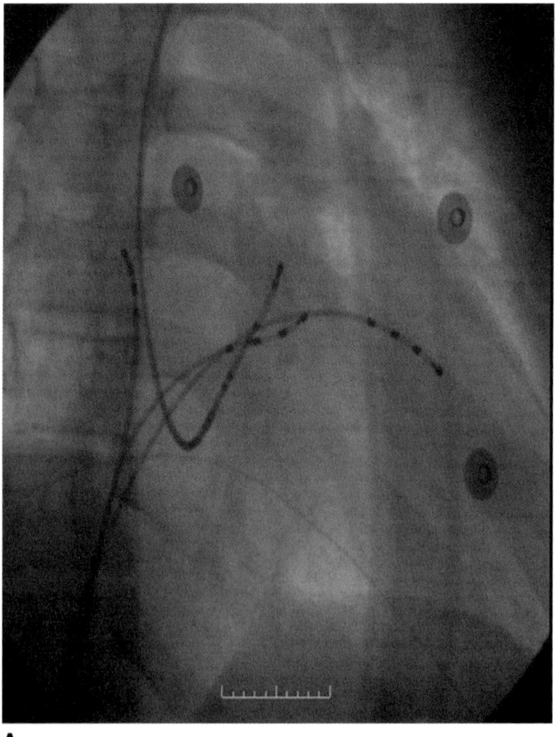

A

FIGURE 7-2. A, B: RAO and LAO images of diagnostic catheters positioned for a typical electrophysiologic study. Quadripolar electrode catheters are placed at the high right atrium, across the tricuspid valve so as to record a His bundle potential and at the right ventricular apex. A decapolar catheter is positioned within the coronary sinus.

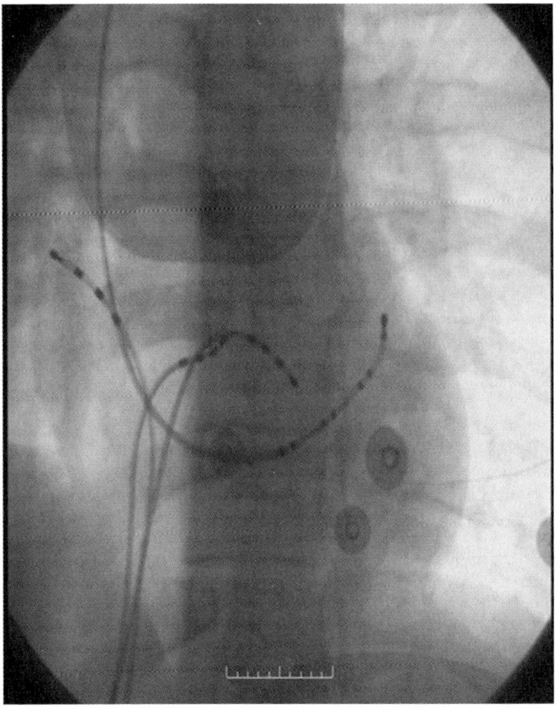

B

FIGURE 7-2. Cont'd.

FLUOROSCOPY

Cardiac electrophysiology studies are usually performed either in modified cardiac catheterization suites or dedicated electrophysiology laboratories. Fluoroscopy is essential for positioning electrophysiology catheters within the heart. While basic electrophysiology studies and simple device implantation can be performed using portable fluoroscopy equipment, advanced mapping and ablation as well as accurate positioning of pacing leads in the coronary sinus call for the use of high quality fixed image intensifiers. *Biplane fluoroscopy* further adds to the efficiency of complex procedures allowing the heart to be sequentially imaged in orthogonal views. In our lab, we use biplane fluoroscopy routinely for transseptal catheterization, for mapping of accessory pathways, and for pulmonary vein angiography during ablation of atrial fibrillation.

Mapping and ablation procedures involve considerable doses of radiation to the patient and scatter radiation to the electrophysiologist. The use of "pulse" fluoroscopy combined with proper shielding and good radiation techniques can minimize this risk to both the patient and the lab personnel.

ENERGY SOURCES FOR ABLATION

A. Radiofrequency Generators. While a variety of energy sources have been used experimentally to create lesions in cardiac tissue, RF energy has remained the standard form of energy used for catheter ablation since it supplanted the use of DC ablation in the late 1980s. RF energy, as it is used clinically, involves the delivery of alternating current at a frequency of 300 to 1,000 kHz from the small tip of the ablation catheter to a large patch applied to the patient's skin. The RF current heats the tissue in close proximity (1 to 2 mm) to the electrode by resistive heating whereas the heat that develops by this process is then conducted to deeper tissue where "thermal" injury occurs. The lesions produced by RF energy are homogenous and develop in a predictable fashion. Lesion size increases in proportion to current density, the surface area of the electrode, the degree of contact pressure between the tissue and the catheter as well as the temperature at the catheter tip/tissue interface. Maximum lesion growth is usually achieved within approximately 40 s. At temperatures above 100°C, boiling occurs resulting in a sudden rise in electrical impedance, reflecting the formation of "char" or coagulum from denaturation of proteins in blood and tissue. This further insulates the catheter tip preventing energy delivery to the adjacent tissue. Steam pops also occur with boiling and may result in tissue injury. Safety features on current RF generators will terminate energy delivery if a sudden rise in impedance occurs. A maximum temperature of 50°C to 60°C can also be programmed which will reduce the power delivered so as not to exceed the maximum temperature at the catheter tip as measured by a thermistor that is located on the catheter.

B. Irrigated tip catheters cool the surface of the electrode tip, allowing for more RF energy to be delivered without increasing the tissue at the electrode/tissue interface to the boiling point. More energy is delivered to the tissue by resistive heating, and deeper lesions are therefore created by conductive thermal injury at a distance from the catheter tip, resulting in the creation of larger and deeper lesions. Closed loop systems pump saline through a lumen that passes to the tip of the catheter and back. Open irrigation systems pump saline out the tip of the catheter cooling the exterior surface of the distal electrode at a controlled flow rate. The latter system is more effective in creating larger lesion sizes however significant volumes of fluid can be delivered during prolonged ablation procedures.

CRYOABLATION

Cryoablation involves the destruction of tissue by freezing. Catheter based cryoablation involves circulating a nitrous oxide based refrigerant through a "closed loop" system. Temperatures at the catheter tip/tissue interface as low as –85°C are reached resulting in permanent tissue destruction. Freezing to an intermediate temperature of –30°C will result in reversible injury to the tissue "temporarily" eliminating cardiac conduction. This allows for "cryomapping" in order to avoid potentially serious complications such as the inadvertent creation of heart block during ablation of the AV nodal slow pathway or para-hisian accessory pathway. As compared with RF ablation, cryoablation results in less damage to surrounding structures and therefore may provide added safety. While acute success rates in treating most arrhythmias approach those seen with RF ablation, the long-term success rates appear to be significantly lower. Cryoablation is therefore usually reserved for higher risk patients with AV node reentry undergoing slow pathway ablation and patients with anteroseptal and midseptal accessory pathways where the risk of creating inadvertent heart block is high. For these reasons, cryoablation is often used in the pediatric electrophysiology laboratory. Because of the time needed to thaw the catheter between each ablation, before mapping can be resumed, the length of the procedure time and in some types of ablation, the total fluoroscopy times may be adversely affected.

New technologies that involve a balloon containing the refrigerant placed at the ostia of the pulmonary veins in order to produce circumferential isolation of the veins are being investigated in the treatment of atrial fibrillation.

THREE-DIMENSIONAL MAPPING SYSTEMS

Three-dimensional mapping systems create a three-dimensional representation of the chamber being mapped and allow for real-time localization of a mapping catheter within that chamber. Electrogram data can be displayed on the three-dimensional reconstruction and can be cataloged for later review. Several mapping systems exist and utilize different technologies as described below.

CARTO ELECTROANATOMIC MAPPING (BIOSENSE WEBSTER)

With three small electromagnetic field generators placed equidistant from one another below the patient, and a reference patch positioned on the patient's back, a small sensor embedded within the tip of the mapping catheter can be localized in three dimensions. Thus a computerized three-dimensional map of a chamber can be created by placing the catheter at multiple sites in that chamber. At each location the catheter is positioned, the endocardial (or epicardial in the case of epicardial mapping) signal is collected and attached to that position. Maps can then be displayed based on the timing of the signal (activation maps) at each point as compared to a reference point (usually the QRS complex on a surface lead or a stable electrogram in the coronary sinus) or as voltage maps based on the voltage amplitude of the signal at each site. The timing or amplitude of each signal is recorded from each point on the map and can then be displayed in color as either an activation map (usually obtained during tachycardia) or a voltage map. Activation maps can be used to precisely localize the earliest site of electrical activation during a tachycardia (Fig. 7-3). This is most useful in mapping automatic tachycardias such as atrial tachycardias or RVOT tachycardias. Different patterns of activation are seen with reentrant tachycardias such as macroreentrant atrial tachycardias or atrial flutters. Voltage maps are often made during sinus rhythm in order to define areas of diminished voltage

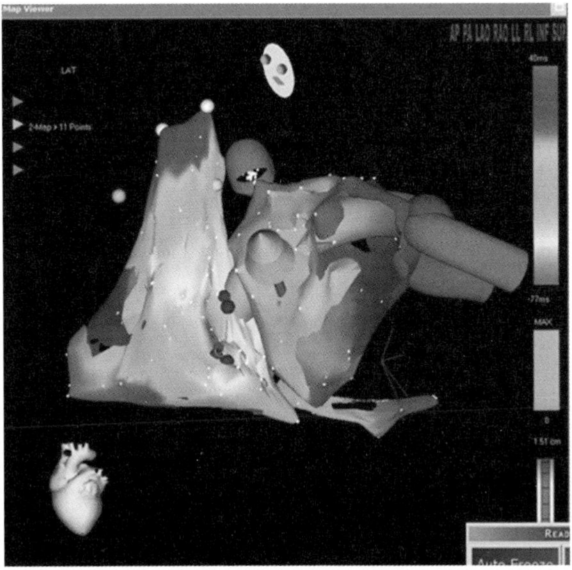

FIGURE 7-3. Electroanatomic activation maps of the right and left atria in a patient with a focal left atrial tachycardia tachycardia (see color insert).

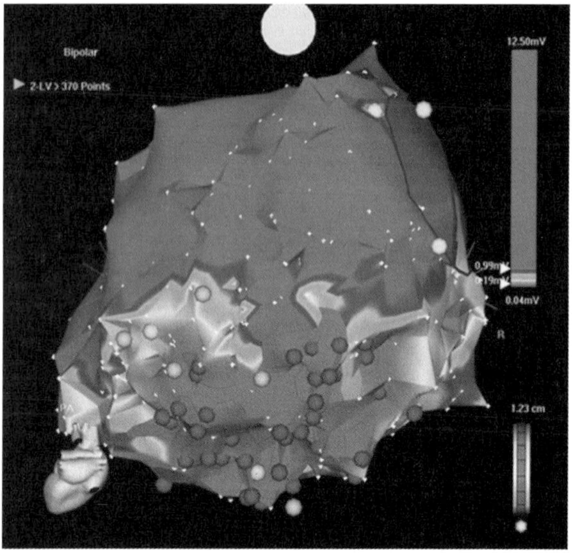

FIGURE 7-4. Voltage map obtained in normal sinus rhythm of the left ventricle in a patient with extensive scar and ventricular tachycardia. Areas displayed in purple are healthy tissue with local electrogram voltages >1.5 mV. Whereas areas displayed in red demonstrate voltages less than 0.5 mV. Areas displayed in gray demonstrate no appreciable electrograms and are electrically unexcitable (see color insert).

representing scar tissue that may serve as the substrate for the development of reentrant arrhythmias (Fig. 7-4). Others have defined areas within the scar where pacing cannot be achieved even at high pacing output as "dense scar" to further differentiate this tissue from areas of viable but low voltage channels of excitable tissue within the scar capable of providing the isthmus of slow conduction necessary for the development of reentry.

Three-dimensional mapping systems can also be used to catalog and display specific types of points such as those where RF energy has been delivered, area of anatomic or electrical interest (double potentials or fractionated electograms), or areas to be avoided (His bundle recording).

IMPEDANCE-BASED MAPPING SYSTEMS: THE NAVEX MAPPING SYSTEM (ST JUDE MEDICAL)

Six cutaneous patches generate electromagnetic fields around the patient's chest in order to generate voltage gradients that are used to localize the electrodes of the mapping catheter as well as other catheters within the heart. The mapping catheter is then used to create a three-dimensional anatomic map of the cardiac chamber being mapped. The electrograms from the mapping catheter can be timed in reference to a reference electrode and activation maps can be created similar to those seen with the CARTO system. One advantage to this system is the ability to display and localize multiple electrode pairs on the same map and thereby show the relationship of one catheter to another during mapping.

NONCONTACT MAPPING

The Ensite Mapping System (St Jude Medical) is based on an elegant concept whereby a multielectrode basket or array (MEA) containing 64 electrodes on eight splines is deployed within a cardiac chamber. Unlike standard basket catheters that are rarely

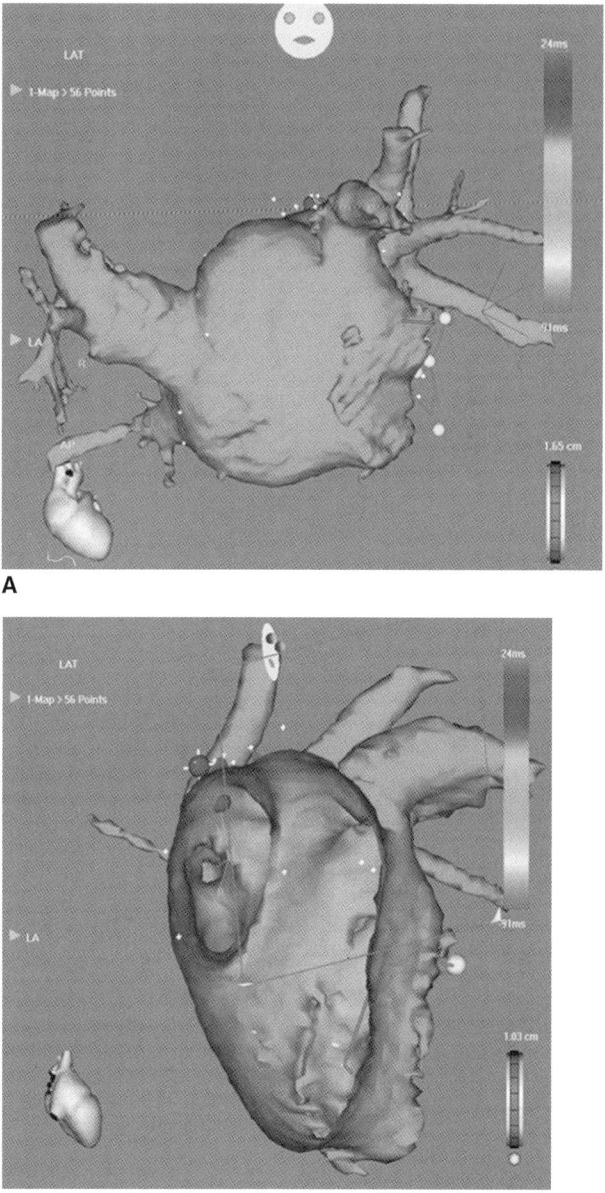

A

B

FIGURE 7-5. A: Three-dimensional image of the left atrium registered to the electroanatomic map of the left atrium and used to demonstrate the left atrial anatomy and guide catheter positioning during ablation of atrial fibrillation. **B:** Open "clipped" view demonstrating the pulmonary vein ostia around which RF lesions will be placed (see color insert).

used, the MEA sits within a chamber without making contact with the endocardium. A balloon inside of the MEA inflates to expand the array once it is in position. Each of the 64 electrodes on the MEA records a unipolar electrogram to a common ring electrode located at a distance on the shaft of the catheter outside of the heart. The intracavitary unipolar electrograms then undergo filtering and mathematical manipulation using an inverse solution to the Law of La Place in order to extrapolate what signals would look like if they were recorded on the endocardial surface. The boundaries of that endocardial surface are defined by moving any standard mapping catheter around the cardiac chamber of interest. A 5.68 kHz signal delivered through any standard mapping catheter is recorded by two ring electrodes positioned just above and below the MEA basket in order to localize the catheter and a three-dimensional volume is created by sweeping the mapping catheter around the cardiac chamber of interest. The arrhythmia is then induced and the signal from a single cardiac cycle can generate over 3,000 virtual electrograms that are updated over 1,000 times per second. The ability of this system to "map" an arrhythmia circuit in as little as one cardiac cycle makes it ideal for activation mapping of hemodynamically unstable rhythms as well as ectopic beats. Because the MEA basket is potentially thrombogenic, the patient is heparinized to an ACT of 250 to 300 s for right-sided procedures and 300 to 350 s for left-sided procedures. Dynamic Substrate Mapping allows for the display of voltage maps and similar to the CARTO system, and new software improvements allow for the simultaneous display and registration of previously acquired three-dimensional MR and CT images. The ability to localize multiple electrode pairs from many catheters simultaneously and display them in real time on the three-dimensional shell is of particular value in correlating the position of the ablation catheter with the positions of the other catheters within the heart.

Three-dimensional image integration software allows for a three-dimensional image of the heart reconstructed from a CT angiogram or an MRI, obtained prior to the study, to be integrated into the real-time anatomic map of the heart used for mapping. The CT or MRI data are reconstructed into a three-dimensional model. Software tools allow this image to be segmented into individual chambers of the heart and the chamber of interest is then registered to anatomic points on the electroanatomic (CARTO) or noncontact (St Jude) maps. This allows for great anatomic detail to be incorporated into the map improving the physician's ability to locate specific anatomic structures (Fig. 7-5) and deploy RF lesions with more accuracy (such as around anterior portion of the left superior pulmonary vein between the vein and the left atrial appendage).

ECHOCARDIOGRAPHY IN THE EP LAB

Ultrasound technologies play an important role in the electrophysiology lab both prior to, during and sometimes following electrophysiology procedures. Ready access to echocardiographic equipment is essential for a smooth running electrophysiology lab.

TRANSTHORACIC ECHOCARDIOGRAPHY (TTE)

While cardiac emergencies are uncommon during diagnostic electrophysiology procedures, perforation of the heart with catheters or during transseptal catheterization remains a much feared complication. Timely recognition and treatment of cardiac tamponade is the best way of ensuring a good outcome for the patient. Access to transthoracic echocardiography (TTE) is essential for diagnosis and management of this complication. For high-risk procedures, such as laser lead extraction, an ultrasound machine should be available on standby in the lab throughout the procedure. In addition, TTE remains the echocardiographic method of choice in diagnosing left ventricular thrombus and is therefore part of the preoperative evaluation of patients undergoing left ventricular tachycardia ablation in the setting of structural heart disease.

TRANSESOPHAGEAL ECHOCARDIOGRAPHY (TEE)

Transesophageal echocardiography (TEE) plays an important role in preparing patients with atrial flutter or atrial fibrillation for both electrical cardioversion and for left atrial ablation procedures. It is our practice to perform TEE prior to cardioversion in patients with atrial fibrillation undergoing cardioversion without documentation of at least 4 to 6 weeks of adequate anticoagulation prior to the procedure (INR ≥ 2). It is also often used to exclude the presence of left atrial appendage thrombus in patients with persistent atrial fibrillation undergoing left atrial ablation. Irrespective of whether the patient was fully anticoagulated prior to restoring sinus rhythm or whether thrombus is excluded by TEE, it is essential that the patient be fully anticoagulated following the procedure as resumption of electromechanical function may be delayed by several days, leaving the patient at risk for developing new atrial appendage thrombus.

INTRACARDIAC ULTRASOUND (ICUS)

Advances in miniaturization of ultrasound technology has permitted the creation of catheters with both mechanical and more recently phased array transducers that can be advanced from the femoral vein and positioned within the cardiac chambers. Mechanical transducers image from a forward angled tip and have relatively small fields of view with little depth penetration. They are useful in guiding transseptal punctures and for assessing local tissue contact. Current phased array systems allow imaging at 5.5 to 10.5 MHz and provide a 90 degree sector scan perpendicular to the shaft of the catheter. By rotating the catheter, a full 360 degree view of the heart and its surrounding structures can be obtained. In general, increasing imaging frequency will increase axial resolution but will decrease the depth of penetration. Thus in order to view far field structures (such as the left-sided pulmonary veins or the left atrial appendage) from the ultrasound catheter positioned in the right atrium, the frequency should be decreased to 5.5 to 7.5 MHz. Two-dimensional, three-dimensional, and Doppler imaging are now feasible. Intracardiac ultrasound (ICUS) imaging has greatly added to the safety of transseptal catheterization which is routinely used to gain access to the left atrium and left ventricle for mapping

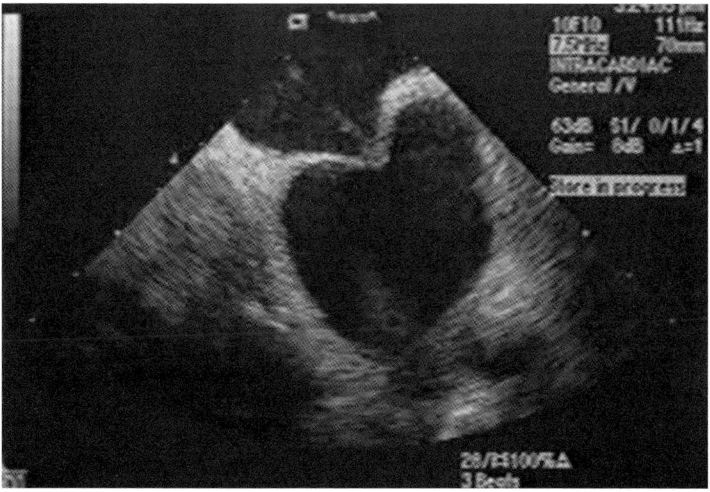

FIGURE 7-6. Intracardiac ultrasound demonstrating "tenting" of the interatrial septum during transseptal puncture.

and ablation procedures (Fig. 7-6). In addition ICUS allows for real-time assessment of the patient's anatomy during electrophysiology procedures. In our lab it remains the primary method used to confirm the proper position and orientation of multipolar Lasso catheters at the ostium of the pulmonary veins. We routinely measure both the diameter of the pulmonary veins at their ostia as well as the Doppler flow velocities within the veins prior to and following pulmonary vein isolation to exclude pulmonary vein stenosis. Although its predictive value has not been proven, a rise in velocity to greater than 100 m/s raises the concern of possible injury to the pulmonary vein and thereby a potential for the development of pulmonary vein stenosis.

Other uses of ICUS during ablation procedures include the assessment of catheter contact with the endocardium which has proven useful in ablating in areas of complex anatomy such as the superior portion of the crista terminalis during ablation of sinus nodal reentrant tachycardia and during ablation within the coronary cusps during ablation of left ventricular outflow tract tachycardias. Real-time ICUS monitoring during RF energy delivery with nonirrigated catheters can demonstrate the presence of microbubbles allowing energy to be titrated in order to avoid steam pops.

New three-dimensional mapping software (CARTOSOUND, Biosense Webster) allows the creation of three dimension reconstructions from ICUS imaging which can be incorporated into the CARTO electroanatomic mapping system. Unlike the CT or MRI images that must be obtained prior to the study, these real-time images can be updated during the study. We have found this technology particularly useful in imaging the course of the esophagus in real time as it passes behind the left atrium, a structure to be avoided during RF ablation of the posterior wall of the left atrium (Fig. 7-7).

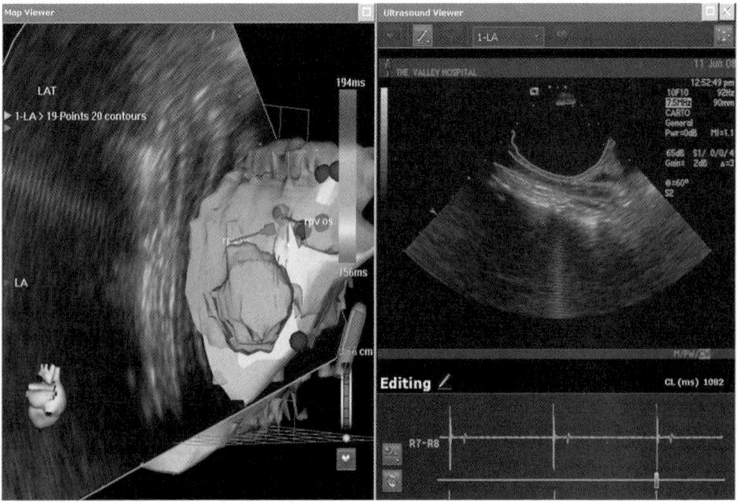

FIGURE 7-7. Three-dimensional imaging of the left atrium during an ablation procedure for atrial fibrillation. The left panel shows the three-dimensional shell created with ultrasound imaging in gray, the color represents points obtained with the mapping catheter and displayed on the shell and registered to a three-dimensional CT image in blue. The two-dimensional ultrasound fan demonstrates the real time position of the esophagus behind the posterior wall of the right atrium near the right sided pulmonary veins. The right panel shows the two-dimensional echocardographic image with the left atrium and esophagus outlined in green (see color insert).

REMOTE NAVIGATION SYSTEMS

Mapping and ablation require the precise manipulation of an electrode, positioned at the tip of a catheter and positioned within the heart. Conventional mapping is performed with a relatively stiff, deflectable catheter. A pullstring mechanism deflects the catheter tip along a specific radius of curvature and the tip is then steered in a given direction by rotating the shaft of the catheter while advancing it, thus transmitting torque along its length to the distal tip. This adds a certain inherent inaccuracy to the mapping procedure. During complex mapping procedures, a second physician will usually collect and analyze the recorded electrograms and direct the operator at the bedside where to move the catheter. Remote navigation systems allow the physician at the recording console and work station to collect and analyze the electrogram data, simultaneously directing the mapping catheter to the next desired location. At the present time, there are two available systems that employ very different technologies.

MAGNETIC NAVIGATION

The Remote Magnetic Navigation System (RMS-Stereotaxis Inc.) uses two large static magnets that are positioned on either side of the patient. The magnets are rotated and they generate a magnetic field of approximately 0.08 T (or 1/10th that of an MRI unit). The RMS catheter is a soft, very flexible catheter with a pair of electrodes at its distal end and three small magnets aligned along its distal shaft. These magnets align the catheter in the direction of the magnetic field that is being applied by the magnets. The physician, at the workstation, changes the desired vector on the Navigant workstation through a software link on the CARTO three-dimensional mapping screen, and the magnets rotate to apply the new magnetic field which aligns the catheter with the new applied vector. The difference between the applied vector and the actual vector of the catheter is seen as "contact" with an interposing structure or wall of the heart and is used as a measure of tissue-catheter contact. A mechanical cable drive attached to the proximal end of the catheter at the patient's groin is used to advance or retract the catheter and is operated by the computer keyboard or by a manually driven "joystick." Once the catheter has been positioned at a specific location, the vector coordinates from the mapping system can be stored so that the catheter can be navigated back to that location at a later time. The soft catheter virtually eliminates the risk of catheter-induced trauma and perforation and the magnetic field maintains the contact between the catheter tip and the endocardium ensuring significant electrogram stability. The RMS system is of particular use in mapping both focal and reentrant atrial tachycardias, RVOT tachycardias, and accessory pathways. Early studies have suggested its utility in the ablation of atrial fibrillation which will become more apparent with the release of an irrigated saline catheter.

ROBOTIC NAVIGATION

At least one robotic navigation system (Hansen Medical) is currently available and others are in various stages of development. They incorporate a mechanical drive system at the bedside with a computer-based interface controlled by a "joystick". The Hansen system uses a two-sheath system with a fairly large 14 Fr outer supporting sheath and a smaller 8 Fr robotic inner sheath that is manipulated by a "joystick" which is capable of manipulating the sheath in three dimensions including advancing and retracting movements. The mapping catheter is positioned within the inner guide sheath, although it is the inner sheath that is mechanically rotated and advanced by the joystick. While the sheaths and catheters are both large and quite stiff, a sensitive pressure sensor prevents excessive force to be applied at the catheter tip and has proven quite reliable in preventing catheter tip trauma and perforation. A recent presentation found no increase in pericardial effusions/tamponade with the Hansen system as compared with conventional mapping techniques during ablation of atrial fibrillation. The advantages of the robotic system over the magnetic navigation system are its portability and affordability while potential disadvantages are the relatively large size of its sheaths.

CARDIOVERTER DEFIBRILLATORS

Unstable rhythms are frequently induced intentionally during programmed stimulation in the course of electrophysiolgic studies, and during defibrillation threshold testing. Therefore, a well functioning cardioverter as well as a back-up unit are essential to the safe performance of electrophysiologic procedures. R-2 pads are routinely applied to the patients prior to the study. Synchronized cardioversion of atrial fibrillation is an integral part of many ablation procedures for atrial fibrillation. This can be accomplished either through external cardioversion through the R-2 pads or via internal cardioversion using either a special catheter that is positioned within the coronary sinus and that incorporates a coil along its length or through the proximal and distal sets of electrodes on a 20 pole duodeca catheter positioned with the distal electrodes positioned in the coronary sinus and the proximal electrodes positioned along the right atrial free wall. Internal cardioversion energies 10 to 30 J are usually sufficient to terminate atrial fibrillation.

KEY POINTS

EP LABORATORY EQUIPMENT

1. Physiologic data recorder
2. Stimulator
3. Fluoroscopy
4. Three-dimensional mapping system
5. RF energy generator
6. Ultrasound equipment
   (a) Transthoracic echo availabililty
   (b) Intracardiac ultrasound
7. External defibrillator
8. Advanced cardiac life support medications and airway equipment

SUGGESTED READINGS

Bhakata D, Miller JM. Prinicples of electroanatomic mapping. *Ind Pacing Electrophysiol J*. 2008;8910:32–50.

Calkins H, Jais P, Steinberg J. *A Practical Approach to Catheter Ablation of Atrial Fibrillation*. Philadelphia, PA: Lippincott Williams & Wilkins; 2008.

Chinitz L, Sethi JS. How to perform non-contact mapping. *Heart Rhythm*. 2006;3(1):120–123.

Kort S. Intracardiac echocardiography: Evolution, recent advances and current applications. *J Am Soc Echocardiogr*. 2006;19(9):1192–1201.

Lemola K, Dubuc M, Khairy P, Transcatheter cryoablation part II: Clinical utility. *Pacing Clin Electrophysiol*. Feb 2008;31(2):235–244.

Ren JF. *Practical Intracardiac Echocardiography in Electrophysiology*. Malden, MA: Blackwell Futura; 2006.

CHAPTER 8

Electrophysiologic Testing: Indications and Limitations

Aman Chugh and Fred Morady

Electrophysiologic (EP) testing has evolved substantially from its origins in the 1970s when it was primarily a diagnostic tool for elucidating the mechanisms of supraventricular and ventricular arrhythmias and for drug testing. The early experience was critical to our understanding of these mechanisms and laid the foundations for a therapeutic procedure, that is, catheter ablation. Today, an EP study is usually performed in the context of a catheter ablation procedure aimed at curing various arrhythmias, such as paroxysmal supraventricular tachycardia (PSVT), atrial fibrillation (AF), atrial flutter, and ventricular tachycardia (VT). This chapter will review the current indications for EP testing in patients with these arrhythmias, in patients with bradycardia and unexplained syncope, and in patients who may be at risk of sudden death. It is also meant to serve as an introduction to clinical cardiac electrophysiology for the trainee in general cardiology.

DIAGNOSTIC EP STUDY

Electrophysiology testing is usually performed using a femoral vein and/or artery. Some laboratories prefer to cannulate into the coronary sinus from either the internal jugular or subclavian vein. An atrial catheter is typically placed in the right atrial appendage for determining atrial activation and for atrial pacing. A multielectrode catheter is placed at the His position near the anterior aspect of the tricuspid valve. A catheter is also placed in the right ventricular apex for recording and pacing. The following data are acquired from the surface electrocardiogram (ECG): heart rate, PR, QRS, and QT intervals. Pacing threshold, defined as the minimum output required to consistently capture the myocardium, is then determined for each pacing site.

The following basic intervals are measured by analysis of the intracardiac electrograms (Fig. 8-1): the atrial-His (AH) interval (the conduction time from the septal aspect of the right atrium through the atrioventricular [AV] node and to the bundle of His) and His-ventricular (HV) interval (the conduction time from the His bundle to the earliest ventricular activation on the ECG). Atrial and ventricular pacing are performed to determine the AV (Fig. 8-2) and ventriculoatrial block cycle lengths. Thereafter, the various refractory periods are determined, defined as the longest coupling interval during extrastimulus testing that fails to capture the myocardium (the atrial and ventricular effective refractory periods) or fails to conduct to the bundle of His (the AV nodal effective refractory period). Further maneuvers and investigations depend upon the precise indication for the EP study.

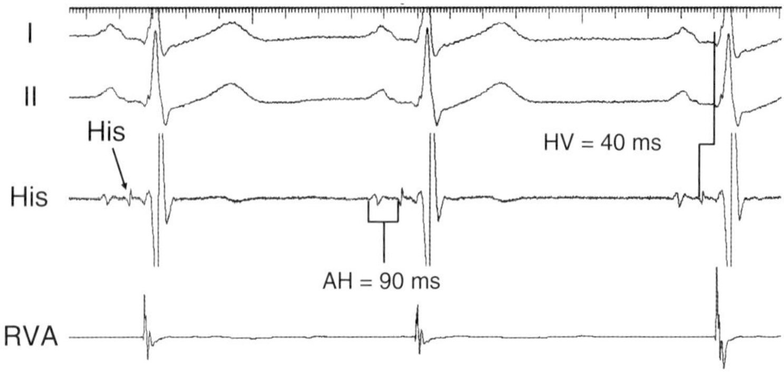

FIGURE 8-1. Measurement of basic intervals in a patient undergoing an EP study for SVT. Also shown are electrocardiographic leads (I and II) and bipolar electrograms recorded by catheters placed at the His position and the right ventricular apex (RVA). AH, atrial-His interval; HV, His-ventricular interval.

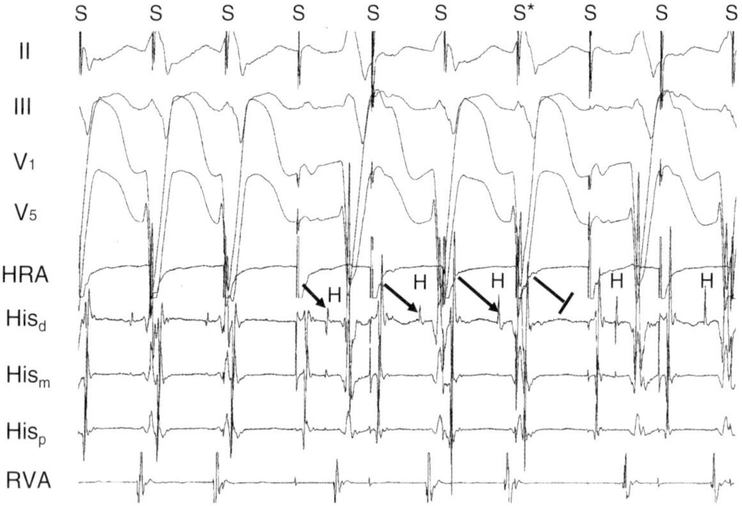

FIGURE 8-2. Determination of AV block cycle length during atrial pacing. Note the gradual prolongation of the AH interval during rapid atrial pacing at 400 ms, consistent with AV nodal Wenckebach phenomenon. The stimulus marked with an asterisk results in AV block above the His bundle, and hence no His potential is seen. This is consistent with normal AV nodal physiology and no pacemaker is required. HRA, high right atrium; RVA, right ventricular apex.

PAROXYSMAL SUPRAVENTRICULAR TACHYCARDIA

A common indication for an EP study is a history of recurrent PSVT. Patients with PSVT typically report symptoms of rapid palpitations, dyspnea, chest discomfort, lightheadedness, and rarely syncope. Patients may also report that they are able to terminate the arrhythmia with vagal maneuvers. The ECG usually shows a regular, narrow complex tachycardia without obvious P waves (Fig. 8.3). Patients seeking medical attention in the

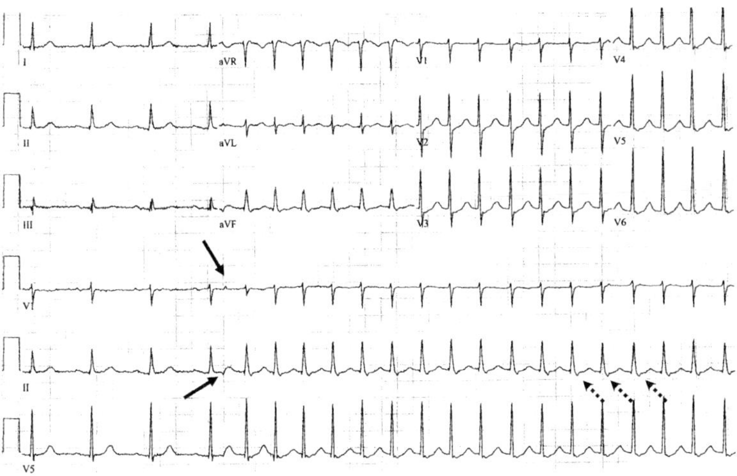

FIGURE 8-3. Spontaneous initiation of SVT. Note after 3 beats of sinus rhythm, an atrial premature complex (*solid arrows*) conducts with a long PR interval, and initiates a sustained tachycardia. The *dashed arrows* point to a pseudo S-wave, consistent with the diagnosis of typical atrioventricular nodal reentrant tachycardia.

emergency room are usually hemodynamically stable. Intravenous adenosine terminates the tachycardia in most cases.

Patients with an initial episode of supraventricular tachycardia (SVT) without serious symptoms such as angina or syncope may be reassured and are instructed to avoid possible triggers and to employ abortive maneuvers in case of recurrent symptoms. Electrophysiology study and catheter ablation is a class I indication for patients with recurrent SVT. During the EP study, determination of baseline EP data as described above may help in elucidating the mechanism of the tachycardia. AV nodal reentrant tachycardia (AVNRT), orthodromic reciprocating tachycardia (ORT) utilizing an accessory pathway, and atrial tachycardia (AT) account for more than 95% of cases of PSVT.

The ECG during tachycardia may offer clues that help to narrow the differential diagnosis. During AVNRT, atrial and ventricular activation occur nearly simultaneously, resulting in a retrograde P wave at the end of the QRS complex. Electrocardiographically, this results in a pseudo R' in lead V1 or a pseudo S wave in the inferior leads (Fig. 8.3).

In patients with AVNRT, one is able to demonstrate the presence of dual ("slow" and "fast") AV nodal pathways in the EP laboratory. The fast pathway typically is associated with a longer refractory period and therefore blocks at a longer coupling interval during extrastimulus testing. After anterograde block in the fast pathway, conduction may proceed down the slow pathway resulting in a long AH (or PR) interval. Given adequate time for recovery, the fast pathway then may be engaged retrogradely, resulting in an AV nodal echo beat. If this sequence of events repeats itself, the result is AVNRT (Figs. 8-4 and 8-5). The endpoint of the procedure is to render AVNRT noninducible by eliminating or significantly altering conduction over the slow pathway. Catheter ablation of the slow pathway is performed by delivering radiofrequency energy outside the ostium of the coronary sinus, that is, inferior and posterior to the bundle of His.

Patients with a history of SVT and evidence of pre-excitation on the ECG should undergo EP evaluation and catheter ablation to eliminate symptoms and the small risk of sudden death. The presence of a delta wave on the ECG (Fig. 8-6) suggests that the mechanism of the tachycardia is ORT. During ORT, anterograde conduction proceeds down

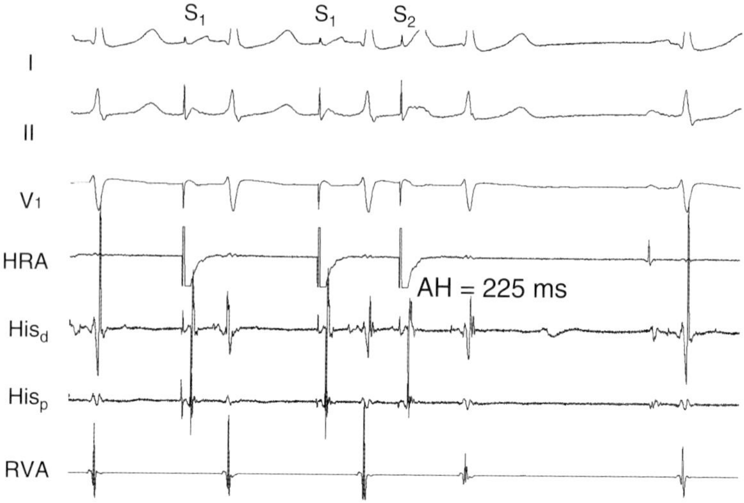

FIGURE 8-4. Extrastimulus testing in a patient with recurrent SVT. After a drive train of 700 ms, an atrial extrastimulus is delivered at 250 ms, resulting in an AH interval of 225 ms. No tachycardia is induced. See Fig. 8-4. HRA, high right atrium; RVA, right ventricular apex.

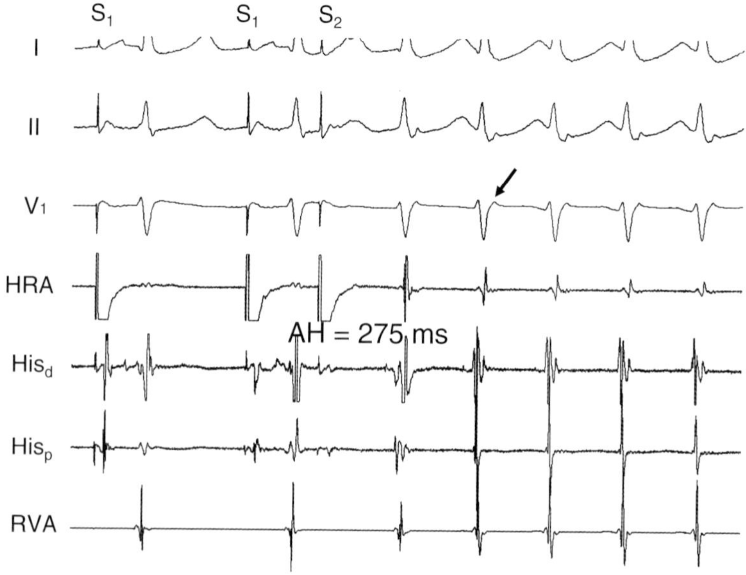

FIGURE 8-5. Extrastimulus testing in the same patient as in Figure 8-3. The extrastimulus is delivered at 340 ms after the drive train, yielding a long AH interval (consistent with anterograde conduction over the slow pathway) and tachycardia during which the retrograde activation occurs over the fast pathway. Note that the ventricular and atrial activation (per the HRA electrogram) are nearly simultaneous consistent with typical AV nodal reentrant tachycardia. Also, note the pseudo R′ wave in lead V_1 (*arrow*). HRA, high right atrium; RVA, right ventricular apex.

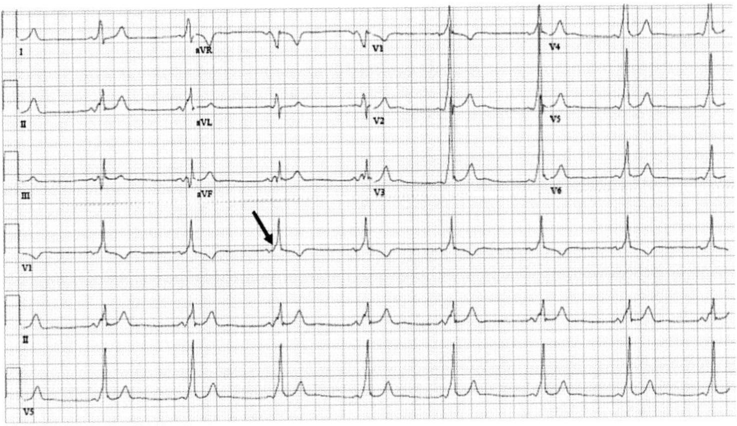

FIGURE 8-6. An ECG from a patient with a history of SVT. Note the presence of a delta wave (*arrow*), consistent with a left free-wall accessory pathway. The patient underwent a successful ablation of the pathway, which inserted at the lateral aspect of the mitral valve.

the AV node and retrograde conduction occurs over the accessory pathway. The result is a narrow QRS-complex tachycardia with retrograde P waves that may be seen within the ST segment. In some patients, the reentry circuit may consist of anterograde conduction over the accessory pathway and retrograde conduction over the AV node, resulting in a wide QRS-complex tachycardia referred to as antidromic reciprocating tachycardia. Some patients with ORT may not demonstrate pre-excitation on the 12-lead ECG owing to absence of or very slow anterograde conduction over the accessory pathway. The end point of the procedure is elimination of pathway conduction during radiofrequency energy delivery at the atrial or ventricular insertion of the accessory connection (Fig. 8.7).

ATs may arise from the right or left atrium or from the musculature of the coronary sinus. Common sites of origin of focal ATs include the crista terminalis, pulmonary veins, tricuspid or mitral annuli, and the interatrial septum. The site of origin is determined by mapping the earliest activation with respect to the P wave on the ECG.

The success rate for ablation of PSVT is greater than 95% and the recurrence rate is extremely low. The risk of a serious complication such as perforation or thromboembolism is less than 1%. The risk of AV block requiring a pacemaker is approximately 0.5% in patients with AVNRT.

RISK STRATIFICATION IN PATIENTS WITH STRUCTURAL DISEASE

In the recent past, an EP evaluation was routinely used to risk stratify patients with coronary artery disease and left ventricular (LV) dysfunction. It was also performed to determine an effective antiarrhythmic regimen for patients with sustained VT in the setting of structural heart disease. After the publication of MADIT II (Mulitcenter Automatic Defibrillator Implantation Trial) and SCD-HeFT (Sudden Cardiac Death in Heart Failure Trial), EP evaluation in patients with advanced heart disease has become less common. The MADIT II study randomized patients with a prior myocardial infarction and a LV ejection fraction ≤30% to conventional medical therapy or an implantable cardioverter-defibrillator (ICD). The all-cause mortality rate was significantly lower in the ICD group, and as a result, ICD implantation in such patients has become standard

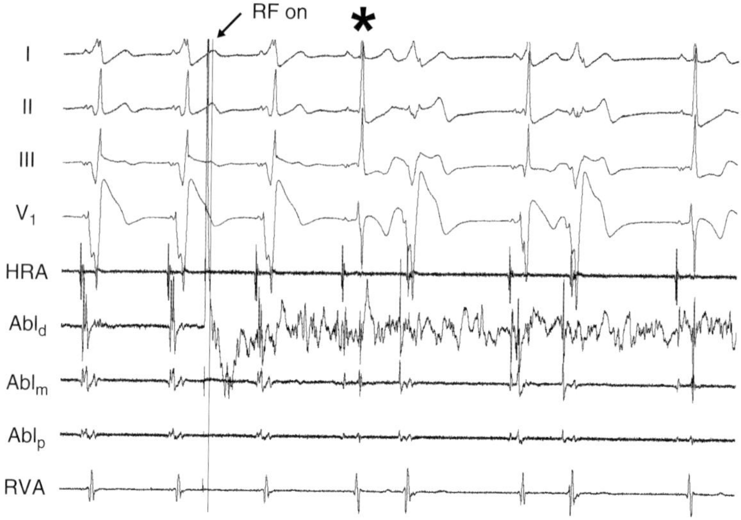

FIGURE 8-7. Effect of radiofrequency (RF) energy delivery in a patient with a right free wall accessory pathway. Energy delivery (*arrow*) results in elimination of pre-excitation (*asterisk*), which is followed by wide QRS complexes, resembling the pre-excited QRS, consistent with pathway automaticity related to heating. HRA, high right atrium; RVA, right ventricular apex.

clinical practice. Due to the clear benefit of device therapy in patients with coronary disease and severe LV dysfunction, EP risk stratification is not needed.

Results from the SCD-HeFT study have been helpful in the management of patients with nonischemic cardiomyopathy (ejection fraction ≤35%) and a history of New York Heart Association's class II or III congestive heart failure. In this randomized trial, ICD therapy was associated with a higher survival rate than optimal medical therapy or optimal medical therapy plus amiodarone. As in the MADIT II study, an EP testing was not required as an entry criterion.

Since MADIT II and SCD-HeFT have streamlined the management of patients with ischemic and nonischemic cardiomyopathy, one may question whether there is any role for invasive EP testing in ascertaining the risk of sudden death in this population. In patients who do not qualify for an ICD by way of these landmark studies, EP testing may still be helpful in risk assessment. For example, a patient with a history of myocardial infarction, nonsustained VT, and an ejection fraction of 35% but no history of heart failure would not meet the criteria for an ICD according to the aforementioned studies. The results of the MADIT I and MUSTT (Mulitcenter Unsustained Tachycardia Trial) may be invoked in the management of such patients. In these randomized studies, patients with a history of ischemic cardiomyopathy and nonsustained VT underwent a diagnostic EP study to evaluate for the possibility of inducible, monomorphic VT. Patients who had inducible sustained, monomorphic VT were randomized to therapy with antiarrhythmic medications or an ICD. In both of these studies, there was a clear benefit of device therapy. Therefore, EP testing may be useful in patients with structural heart disease who otherwise would not qualify for a prophylactic ICD.

Survivors of a cardiac arrest and patients with sustained VT in the setting of structural heart disease should undergo implantation of an ICD for secondary prevention given the demonstrated superiority of device therapy.

LIMITATIONS OF ELECTROPHYSIOLOGIC RISK-STRATIFICATION

Although EP testing has a role in risk stratification in patients with coronary disease and moderate LV dysfunction, its negative predictive value is less than ideal. For example, in the MUSTT trial, the 5-year rate of cardiac arrest or arrhythmic death was still 24% in patients who were noninducible for VT. Although the event rates were lower than those in patients with inducible VT who were assigned to no therapy, lack of VT inducibility is not necessarily indicative of a low risk of mortality. Also, patients in MUSTT who were inducible for VT were randomized to EP-guided therapy (consisting of antiarrhythmic therapy or possible ICD after drug failure) or no therapy. The results showed that there was no difference in mortality between patients in the EP-guided group who were treated with antiarrhythmic medications and those randomized to no treatment. In fact, a survival benefit was seen only among patients in the EP-guided group who received an ICD. Thus, medical treatment of patients with inducible VT guided by EP testing has little role as stand-alone therapy in patients with structural heart disease.

TECHNICAL ASPECTS OF PROGRAMMED VENTRICULAR STIMULATION

Although there are various protocols for ventricular stimulation, they all include the introduction of one or more ventricular extrastimuli. In our laboratory, we typically begin with an introduction of four extrastimuli delivered after a drive train (Fig. 8-8). This protocol has been shown to more quickly induce sustained monomorphic VT than

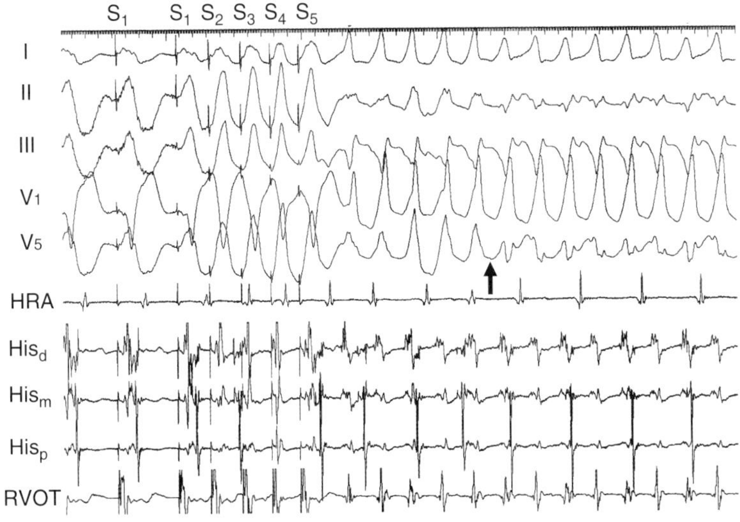

FIGURE 8-8. Induction of VT during programmed ventricular stimulation in a patient with a prior myocardial infarction and unexplained syncope. After a drive train at 450 ms, four extrastimuli are delivered (240, 230, 220, and 210 ms) from the right ventricular outflow tract (RVOT). A few beats of polymorphic VT are followed by sustained, monomorphic VT (*arrow*) at cycle length of 220 ms. The VT is characterized by a right bundle branch block pattern and superior axis in the frontal plane. Note that ventriculo-atrial dissociation is present, consistent with VT. The patient was treated with an implantable defibrillator for secondary prevention. HRA, high right atrium.

protocols that call for less extrastimuli. Sometimes programmed ventricular stimulation induces ventricular fibrillation (VF). VF may be inducible even in normal hearts particularly when multiple extrastimuli are delivered close to the ventricular refractory period. Thus, inducibility of VF in a patient undergoing an evaluation for monomorphic VT may be a nonspecific finding in the setting of an aggressive stimulation protocol. On the other hand, induction of VF during a less aggressive protocol, e.g., two extrastimuli, may be of clinical import depending upon the clinical context.

EP EVALUATION IN PATIENTS WITH BRUGADA SYNDROME

Patients with Brugada syndrome demonstrate characteristic ECG findings including an incomplete right bundle branch block and ST-segment elevation in the right precordial leads (Fig. 8.9). Although these patients typically are young and have no obvious structural cardiac abnormalities, they are at risk for sudden death due to VF. While it is widely accepted that patients with Brugada syndrome who experience unexplained syncope or cardiac arrest should undergo implantation of an ICD, the management of asymptomatic individuals is controversial. Some experts in the field advocate close follow-up since the absolute risk of death may be low in this group, while other experts recommend an EP study for risk stratification. The latter also recommend an ICD for patients who are inducible for VT or VF. An ongoing randomized study will hopefully lead to an evidence-based approach in this challenging group of patients.

SYNCOPE IN PATIENTS WITH A NORMAL HEART

The management of patients with structural heart disease who present with syncope has been greatly facilitated by publication of the landmark ICD trials mentioned previously. However, patients with a normal heart and ECG who present with syncope are at extremely low risk for sudden death. Thus, if noninvasive testing has failed to reveal an obvious cause in such a patient, an EP study is unlikely to be helpful.

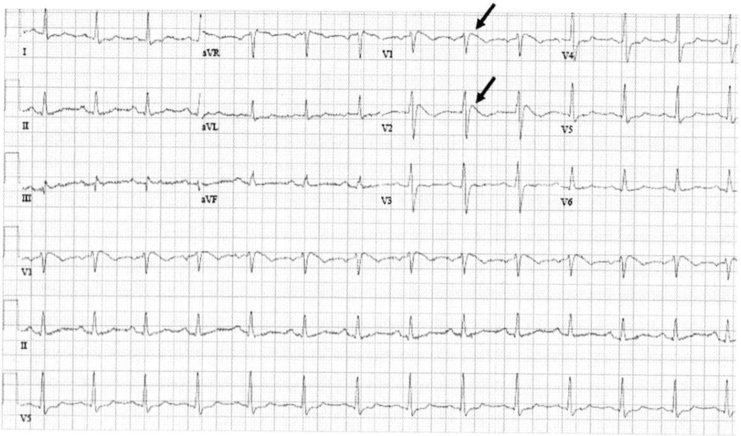

FIGURE 8-9. An ECG from a patient with Brugada syndrome. Note the incomplete right bundle branch block pattern and J-point elevation (*arrows*) in the right precordial leads. The patient underwent implantation of a defibrillator because of a history of unexplained syncope and a family history (mother) of sudden death.

The diagnostic yield of an EP study in a patient with syncope, in whom sinus node dysfunction is suspected, is also suboptimal. Although measures such as the sinus node recovery time have been used to assess sinus node function, the existence of various reference ranges and the confounding effects of sedation and autonomic tone make it difficult to use on a routine basis. Instead, a detailed and focused history along with the findings from exercise testing or ambulatory monitoring may be more helpful in making the diagnosis of sinus node dysfunction.

It is reasonable to perform a diagnostic EP study in a patient with unexplained syncope and a left bundle branch block on the ECG. One may observe findings such as infra-hisian AV block or split His potentials (Fig. 8-10), which call for implantation of a permanent pacemaker. An implantable loop recorder may be considered in such patients if the EP study is nondiagnostic, because long-term monitoring may eventually reveal AV block responsible for syncope. Patients with a bifascicular block (right bundle branch block with a left anterior or posterior fascicular block) should be considered for permanent pacing if the following are found during an EP study: HV > 100 ms or infra-hisian or intra-hisian block. In these patients, involvement of the distal His-purkinje conduction system may be progressive and may eventually culminate in advanced AV block and

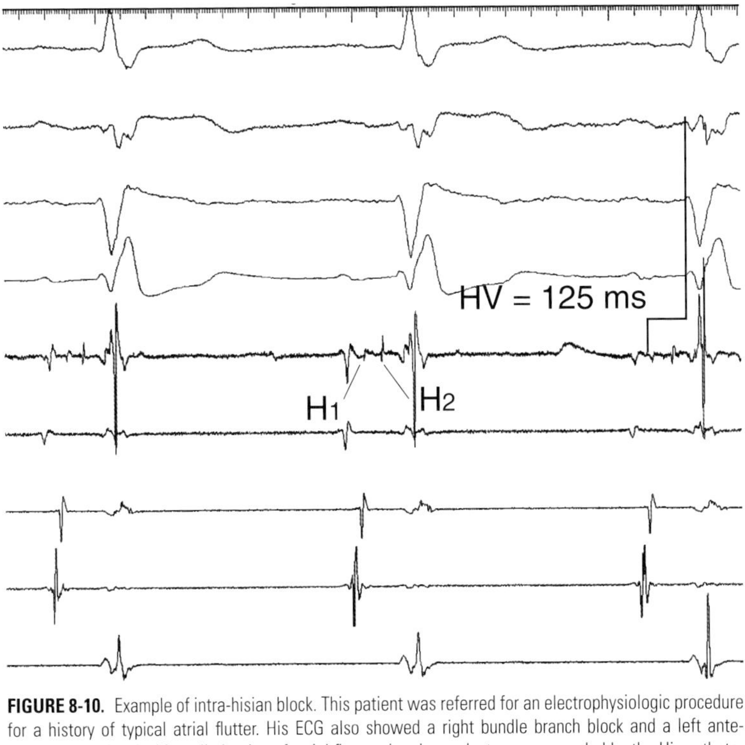

FIGURE 8-10. Example of intra-hisian block. This patient was referred for an electrophysiologic procedure for a history of typical atrial flutter. His ECG also showed a right bundle branch block and a left anterior fascicular block. After elimination of atrial flutter, the above electrogram recorded by the His catheter was observed. Note the split His potentials and the extremely prolonged HV interval (125 ms). Because of the potential for complete AV block and syncope, the patient underwent implantation of a dual chamber pacemaker.

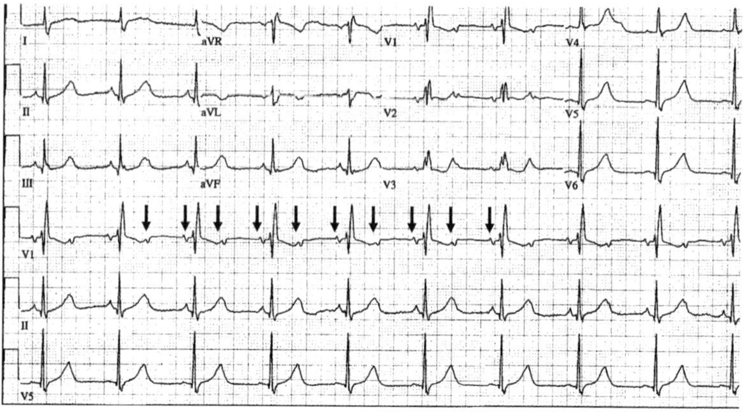

FIGURE 8-11. An ECG from a 70-year-old man with unexplained falls. Sinus tachycardia (*arrows*) is present with 2:1 AV block. The presence of a right bundle branch block suggests that the level of block is at or below the His, and hence pathologic (Mobitz II). This patient was referred for implantation of a permanent pacemaker.

syncope. Patients with clear evidence of type II AV block (Mobitz II) should undergo implantation of a permanent pacemaker without EP testing (Fig. 8-11).

There is little role for an invasive EP evaluation for patients presenting with vasodepressor syncope. Prodromal symptoms, such as warmth, diaphoresis, nausea and vomiting, light-headedness or dizziness, followed by postevent fatigue are consistent with the diagnosis. In some patients, especially the elderly, these "classic" symptoms may not be present and upright tilt table testing can be helpful in making the diagnosis. Orthostatic hypotension, particularly in the elderly population, is an under-appreciated cause of syncope. Patients in whom carotid sinus hypersensitivity is suspected need not undergo an EP study, because a carotid massage, the diagnostic maneuver, can be performed in the office setting or during tilt testing.

ELECTROPHYSIOLOGIC STUDY AND CATHETER ABLATION OF SPECIFIC ARRHYTHMIAS

ATRIAL FLUTTER

Typical atrial flutter is due to a large reentrant circuit in which activation proceeds around the atrial aspect of the tricuspid valve in a counterclockwise manner. Although typical atrial flutter may occasionally be seen in patients without heart disease, it usually occurs in patients with various cardiovascular disorders, e.g., hypertension, during antiarrhythmic treatment of AF, congestive heart failure, following cardiac surgery, and also right-heart enlargement related to a variety of respiratory disorders. Clinical manifestations range from an absence of symptoms to dyspnea, exercise intolerance, palpitations, fatigue, cardiomyopathy, and heart failure. The flutter waves on the ECG resemble a sawtooth pattern, with a large negative initial component, followed by terminal positivity of varying degree in the inferior leads (Fig. 8.12). Although transthoracic cardioversion is acutely effective in restoring sinus rhythm, many patients with typical flutter without a reversible cause will experience a recurrence. While the medical management of AF and flutter is very similar and although both arrhythmias are amenable to catheter ablation,

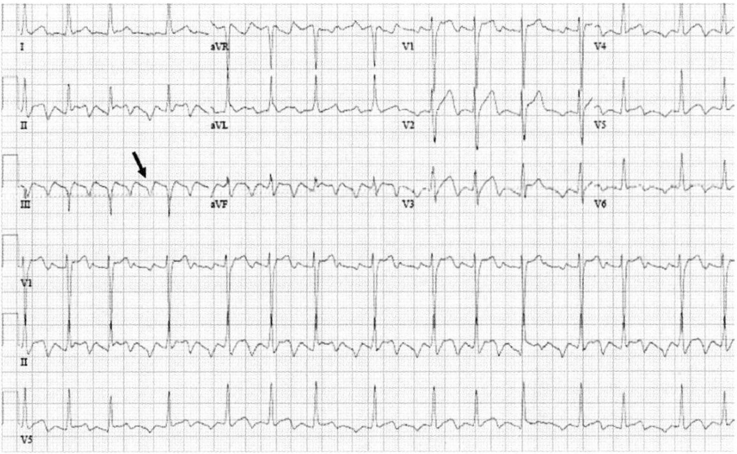

FIGURE 8-12. An example of typical flutter from a patient without any obvious heart disease. Note the sawtooth pattern of the flutter waves (*arrow*) in the inferior leads.

it is helpful to make a distinction between the two since the latter is readily curable with an outpatient procedure with minimal risk to the patient.

Catheter ablation is the preferred mode of treatment of patients with typical atrial flutter. Although documentation of the classic findings on ECG is highly specific as to the anatomic origin of the tachycardia, prior to radiofrequency ablation, it is useful to prove *isthmus dependence*. The *cavotricuspid* isthmus is defined as the rim of atrial tissue extending from the inferior aspect of the tricuspid valve to the inferior vena cava. Isthmus dependence is determined by pacing from this area at a rate slightly faster than that of the atrial flutter, which is typically 200 to 300 ms (Fig. 8-13). If the myocardium is captured with each pacing stimulus, the tachycardia is said to be "entrained." If the tachycardia persists after cessation of pacing, the *postpacing interval* is measured. The postpacing interval is the time from the last paced beat to the first return beat of the flutter and is a measure of proximity of the pacing site to the reentry circuit. The postpacing interval incorporates the time required for the paced impulse to enter the reentrant circuit, plus the time needed for one revolution around the circuit (i.e., the flutter cycle length), and the time for the impulse to return to the pacing site (Fig. 8-13). If the maneuver is performed from the cavotricuspid isthmus during typical flutter, the postpacing interval will closely approximate the flutter cycle length since the time needed to engage and return from the circuit is negligible. However, if pacing is performed from an area remote from the isthmus, the postpacing interval will be significantly longer than the flutter cycle length due to the time required to engage and return from the circuit.

Once isthmus dependence has been demonstrated, radiofrequency energy is delivered from the inferior tricuspid valve (6 o'clock in the left anterior oblique view) to the inferior vena cava, which results in the termination of the flutter (Fig. 8.14). Additional lesions are deployed to ensure that conduction block across the ablation line is complete. The procedure requires approximately 1 h and patients are discharged on the same day. The success rate for typical flutter is 95% and the recurrence rate is low. The risk of serious complications such as perforation or AV block is less than 1%. Although catheter ablation for typical atrial flutter is very safe and effective, some patients may develop AF during follow-up (see below).

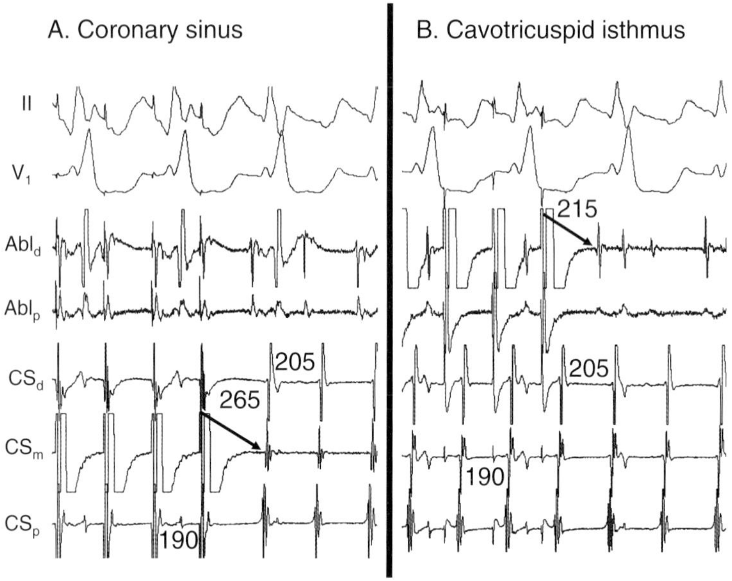

FIGURE 8-13. Entrainment mapping for atrial flutter. **A:** Pacing 15 ms shorter than the flutter cycle length (205 ms) from the mid coronary sinus (CS) accelerates the tachycardia, and upon cessation of pacing, the "postpacing interval" is 265 ms. Since the postpacing interval exceeds the flutter cycle length by more than 20 ms, the CS is not part of the circuit. **B:** Pacing at the same cycle length as in (**A**) but now from the cavotricuspid isthmus yields a return cycle of 215 ms, which closely approximates the flutter cycle length, proving isthmus dependence. Radiofrequency energy delivery here terminated atrial flutter. See text for details.

CATHETER ABLATION OF ATRIAL FIBRILLATION

AF is the most common arrhythmia encountered in clinical practice. Like atrial flutter, it usually occurs in the setting of cardiovascular disease but may be seen in patients without heart disease (idiopathic or lone AF). Patients with AF may be entirely unaware of rhythm status or may complain of fatigue, palpitations, chest discomfort, dyspnea, or dizziness. The course of patients with AF may also be complicated by stroke or LV dysfunction and heart failure.

AF is usually classified into three subtypes. Paroxysmal AF is defined as episodes that self-terminate within 7 days. Persistent AF is defined as episodes of AF lasting for more than 7 days or requiring cardioversion. Patients with AF continuing for at least one year are said to have long-lasting persistent AF.

For patients with symptomatic AF, medical therapy consisting of an antiarrhythmic and rate-controlling agent is appropriate. However, pharmacologic therapy is often ineffective and may be limited by serious side effects such as proarrhythmia and end-organ toxicity. Given these limitations along with the increasing incidence of AF, the number of patients undergoing a catheter ablation procedure for AF has greatly increased in recent years. In fact, during a typical month in the electrophysiology laboratory at the University of Michigan, 50% of the EP procedures are dedicated to catheter ablation of AF.

Patients with symptomatic AF who have failed one course of medical therapy are appropriate candidates for catheter ablation. Patients with decompensated heart failure,

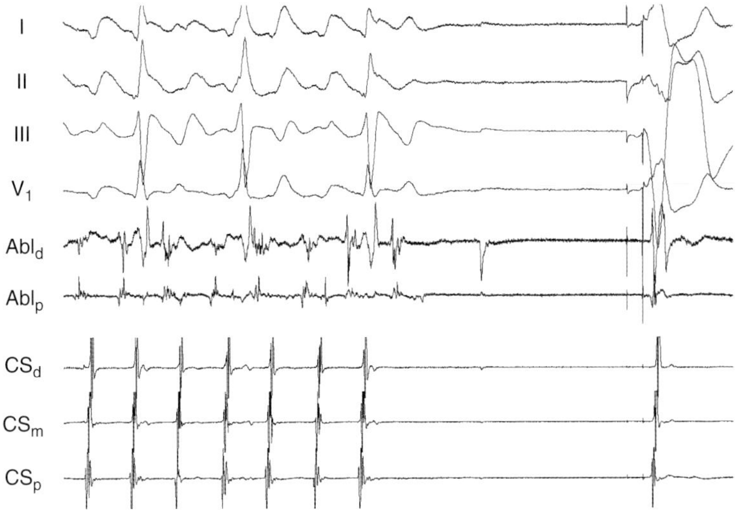

FIGURE 8-14. Termination of typical atrial flutter during radiofrequency ablation at the cavotricuspid isthmus. Shown are electrocardiographic leads I, II, III, and V_1, and also bipolar electrograms recorded by the ablation catheter (Abl), and a catheter placed in the coronary sinus (CS).

left atrial diameter greater than 6.5 cm, multiple comorbidities, or a bleeding diathesis are poor candidates for the procedure. A history of prior thromboembolic complication related to AF or heart failure is not a contraindication.

The left atrium plays a major role in the pathogenesis of AF in almost all patients with the arrhythmia. Left atrial access is obtained by transseptal catheterization. The fossa ovalis is first identified either by intracardiac echocardiography or fluoroscopy and then pierced with the transseptal needle. This portion of the procedure is also guided by contrast injection and pressure monitoring. Thereafter, a ring catheter is inserted sequentially into each of the four pulmonary veins. Radiofrequency energy is delivered with an ablation catheter outside the ostium of the pulmonary veins with the end point of complete electrical disconnection or isolation of the pulmonary veins. In patients with paroxysmal AF without significant left atrial enlargement, isolation of the pulmonary veins is sufficient to eliminate AF in about 85% of patients without the use of antiarrhythmic medications. The procedure requires about 3 to 3.5 h in most cases. Approximately, 30% of patients will require a repeat procedure, most commonly due to reconnection of the pulmonary veins. Serious complications such as perforation/pericardial tamponade, transient ischemic attack/stroke, or pulmonary vein stenosis occur in approximately 1% of patients.

Whereas the pulmonary veins play a dominant role in the pathophysiology of paroxysmal AF, the left atrium proper, and occasionally the right atrium, is the target in patients with persistent or chronic AF. In these patients, one begins with isolation of the pulmonary veins, followed by ablation of sites exhibiting complex electrograms and also linear ablation (Fig. 8.15). This stepwise approach requires about 4 to 5 h. Repeat procedures for more organized arrhythmias, such as left atrial flutter, are required in about 50% of patients. Although persistent AF is a much more complex and challenging arrhythmia to ablate than paroxysmal AF, it can be eliminated in about 85% of patients without the need for antiarrhythmic medications.

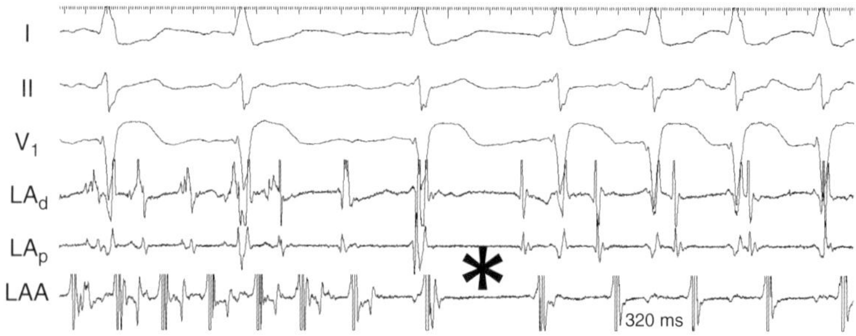

FIGURE 8-15. Termination of long-lasting, persistent atrial fibrillation (AF) in a 72-year-old man with ischemic cardiomyopathy who had not responded to amiodarone therapy. After isolation of the pulmonary veins, and ablation of fractionated electrograms in the left atrium (LA), linear ablation at the roof finally terminated AF (*asterisk*). As is usually the case, AF termination was followed by atrial flutter, which was successfully ablated at the cavotricuspid isthmus, finally yielding sinus rhythm. LAA, left atrial appendage.

ABLATION OF THE AV JUNCTION

One of the goals of treatment in patients with AF is rate control with AV nodal blocking agents in order to improve symptoms and prevent tachycardia-related LV dysfunction and heart failure. If this goal cannot be met, the patient may be considered for an AV junction ablation and pacemaker implantation. This strategy has been shown to improve symptoms and LV function. The "ablate and pace" approach is better suited for elderly patients and those with significant comorbidities, e.g., chronic obstructive lung disease, who can not tolerate medical therapy. Younger patients with symptomatic AF should undergo left atrial ablation in order to eliminate the arrhythmia itself since AV junction ablation is a palliative procedure. Another disadvantage is that ablation of the AV junction renders the patient pacemaker-dependent, which is not an attractive option in younger patients who will need multiple procedures for generator changes and lead failure over their lifetime. Indeed, with the advent of AF ablation, AV junction ablation is much less likely to be performed than it was a decade ago.

VENTRICULAR ARRHYTHMIAS

Another indication for an EP evaluation and ablation is a history of symptomatic premature ventricular complexes (PVCs) or VT. PVCs are common and are usually thought to be benign in the setting of a normal heart. However, patients with frequent ventricular ectopy are at risk of developing cardiomyopathy and heart failure. Patients whose quality of life or LV function is impaired by frequent PVCs are candidates for catheter ablation. The right ventricular outflow tract is a common source of PVCs. The PVCs originating from this site have a left bundle branch block pattern, with an inferior axis on the 12-lead ECG. Other sites of origin include the conduction system of the LV, mitral annulus, ventricular myocardium associated with one of the cusps of the aortic valve, and the epicardium, which may be targeted via the coronary sinus or a pericardial puncture. Catheter ablation results in elimination of PVCs in about 80% to 85% of cases, with a low risk of complication (perforation, thromboembolic complications, and severe bleeding). Importantly, cardiomyopathy owing to frequent PVCs may be completely reversible after successful ablation. Idiopathic VT, that is, sustained ventricular arrhythmias in the absence of structural heart disease, also originates from the aforementioned areas and can be safely eliminated in about 90% of patients (Fig. 8.16).

As mentioned above, patients with frequent VT in the setting of ischemic or nonischemic cardiomyopathy are best treated with an ICD and an antiarrhythmic agent for

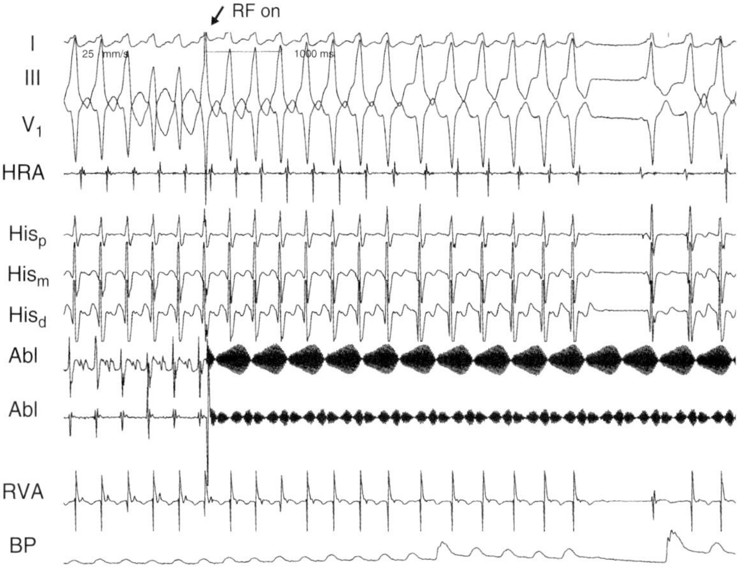

FIGURE 8-16. Termination of ventricular tachycardia originating from the right ventricular outflow tract during radiofrequency energy delivery in a patient with a normal heart. BP, blood pressure.

arrhythmia suppression. However, VT frequently recurs despite medical therapy, which may result in frequent ICD shocks and electrical storm. Catheter ablation has been shown to result in reduction in the number of ICD shocks in most patients and may even have a favorable impact on mortality in this challenging group of patients. Importantly, the reduction in the frequency of ICD therapy is also associated with an improvement in the patient's quality of life and psychological well-being.

Patients with scar-related VT frequently have multiple inducible VTs, many of which are hemodynamically unstable. Detailed activation mapping during tachycardia cannot be performed in such situations. Mapping of the LV in patients with infarct-related VT may be performed during sinus rhythm. Areas exhibiting no detectable voltage (scar), low voltage (infarct border), and fragmented electrograms (consistent with slow conduction) are tagged on a three-dimensional map. Pacing is performed during sinus rhythm to determine whether the paced QRS closely resembles that of one of the induced VTs. If so, radiofrequency energy is delivered at the site, which may be extended to an anatomical obstacle (mitral valve) or scar. Since scar-related VTs are usually due to macroreentry, well-tolerated VTs may be explored by entrainment techniques described above. Not uncommonly, epicardial mapping and ablation may be required if an endocardial procedure has failed. Percutaneous epicardial access is obtained using a subxyphoid approach. Coronary angiography may be required to ensure that the target site is at a safe distance from the coronary arteries.

SUMMARY

The pace at which electrophysiology procedures have evolved from offering only mechanistic and diagnostic information to allowing cure of even complex arrhythmias has been astonishing and inspiring. Despite many advances, important questions remain unanswered, opening up numerous opportunities for investigation and contribution. For example, in spite of our ability to eliminate AF in most patients, its mechanisms remain poorly understood. Also, better tools are required for catheter ablation of complex arrhythmias. Better measures of risk stratification of sudden death are sorely needed to ensure that patients at high risk are adequately treated and those at low risk may be safely followed without ICD implantation. As these issues are likely to be clarified in the next several years, the practice of clinical cardiac electrophysiology will continue to fuel intellectual curiosity and provide personal satisfaction by making a meaningful impact in the lives of patients.

KEY POINTS

1. Common indications for electrophysiology study and catheter ablation
   (a) Recurrent PSVT
   (b) PSVT in patients with evidence of pre-excitation on the ECG (Wolff-Parkinson-White syndrome)
   (c) Atrial flutter
   (d) Symptomatic paroxysmal or persistent AF despite antiarrhythmic therapy
   (e) AV junction ablation for AF with rapid ventricular rates despite medical therapy in patients who are not good candidates for a curative procedure for AF
   (f) Frequent PVCs with symptoms or with evidence of LV dysfunction
   (g) Idiopathic VT
   (h) Recurrent VT associated with frequent ICD discharges in patients with structural heart disease
2. Common indications for a diagnostic electrophysiology study
   (a) Evaluation for inducible VT in a patient with a prior myocardial infarction, moderate LV dysfunction, and nonsustained VT
   (b) Unexplained syncope in patients with a left bundle branch block on ECG
3. Areas of controversy/lack of consensus
   (a) Programmed ventricular stimulation in asymptomatic patients with Brugada's pattern on ECG
4. Situations in which electrophysiology testing is unlikely to be helpful
   (a) Patients with vasodepressor syncope
   (b) Unexplained syncope in a patient with a normal heart and ECG
   (c) Carotid sinus hypersensitivity

SUGGESTED READINGS

Bardy GH, Lee KL, Mark DB, et al. Amiodarone or an implantable cardioverter–defibrillator for congestive heart failure. *N Engl J Med.* 2005;352(3):225–237.

Blomstrom-Lundqvist C, Scheinman MM, Aliot EM, et al. ACC/AHA/ESC Guidelines for the management of patients with supraventricular arrhythmias—executive summary: A report of the American College of Cardiology/American Heart Association Task Force on Practice Guidelines and the European Society of Cardiology Committee for Practice Guidelines (Writing Committee to Develop Guidelines for the Management of Patients With Supraventricular Arrhythmias). *Circulation.* 2003;108(15):1871–1909.

Buxton AE, Lee KL, DiCarlo L, et al. Electrophysiologic testing to identify patients with coronary artery disease who are at risk for sudden death. Multicenter Unsustained Tachycardia Trial Investigators. *N Engl J Med.* 2000;342(26):1937–1945.

Buxton AE, Lee KL, Fisher JD, et al. A randomized study of the prevention of sudden death in patients with coronary artery disease. Multicenter Unsustained Tachycardia Trial Investigators. *N Engl J Med.* 1999;341(25):1882–1890.

Hummel JD, Strickberger SA, Daoud E, et al. Results and efficiency of programmed ventricular stimulation with four extrastimuli compared with one, two, and three extrastimuli. *Circulation.* 1994;90(6):2827–2832.

Moss AJ, Hall WJ, Cannom DS, et al. Improved survival with an implanted defibrillator in patients with coronary disease at high risk for ventricular arrhythmia. Multicenter Automatic Defibrillator Implantation Trial Investigators. *N Engl J Med.* 1996;335(26):1933–1940.

Moss AJ, Zareba W, Hall WJ, et al. Prophylactic implantation of a defibrillator in patients with myocardial infarction and reduced ejection fraction. *N Engl J Med.* 2002;346(12):877–883.

CHAPTER 9

Principles of Mapping and Ablation

Eric Buch, Noel G. Boyle, and Kalyanam Shivkumar

Successful treatment of a cardiac arrhythmia with catheter ablation requires a clear understanding of the arrhythmia mechanism. Further, the location of the circuit or focus must be determined using cardiac mapping techniques. This then allows for the successful ablation of the arrhythmia focus or interruption of the arrhythmia circuit, most commonly with radiofrequency (RF) energy. For the majority of supraventricular and ventricular arrhythmias, RF catheter ablation is a safe and effective alternative to drug therapy and, in many cases, offers an opportunity to cure the arrhythmia.

The purpose of this chapter is to discuss general principles of mapping and ablation for both supraventricular and ventricular arrhythmias. After a brief discussion of the historical development of catheter ablation and the biophysics of ablation, various mapping techniques and their application in the ablation of specific arrhythmias will be reviewed.

CATHETER ABLATION: HISTORICAL DEVELOPMENT

The first nonpharmacologic therapy for cardiac arrhythmias was surgery. In the late 1960s the development of intraoperative epicardial mapping allowed effective treatment of Wolff-Parkinson-White syndrome by surgical disruption of accessory pathway fibers. As in catheter ablation procedures, the goal was to interrupt electrical conduction to prevent recurrent arrhythmia. A successful ablation precisely targets critical tissue, creating permanent lesions there while minimizing damage to surrounding structures.

Building on the success of arrhythmia surgery and the development of transvenous recording of intracardiac signals using electrode catheters, Scheinman et al. performed the first catheter-based ablation in 1982. They used high-energy direct-current shocks to create complete atrioventricular (AV) block for rate control in patients with atrial arrhythmias, a strategy which also required implantation of a permanent pacemaker. Energy was delivered between the tip of a catheter located near the His bundle and a grounding pad on the skin, creating a plasma arc and steam bubble that destroyed AV junctional tissue and caused permanent AV block. Though effective, the force of the energy discharge frequently resulted in damage to surrounding structures, and sometimes caused cardiac perforation or even death. In-hospital mortality rates approached 6%, which prevented widespread application of the technique.

The use of RF energy for catheter ablation was first reported for AV nodal ablation by Huang et al. in 1987. By 1991, RF energy had supplanted direct-current shock due to its improved safety profile. Adapted from surgical electrocautery, RF ablation uses high-frequency alternating current of 500 to 1,000 kHz, delivering energy between the catheter tip and a large dispersive grounding pad on the skin. This results in an electrical burn of the targeted arrhythmogenic tissue due to resistive heating and thermal conduction. Since lesion size depends on delivered power and tissue temperature, both of which can be controlled by the operator, this method offers more precise control over the tissue ablated. A wide variety of ablation catheters and guiding sheaths allow access to virtually any part of the heart. Due to the safety and efficacy of RF catheter ablation, it has become one of the most commonly used treatments in managing cardiac arrhythmias.

BIOPHYSICS OF CATHETER ABLATION

When a sustained tissue temperature of 50°C is achieved, the result is tissue desiccation and protein denaturation, leading to irreversible loss of conduction, the goal of catheter ablation (Fig. 9-1). With temperature-controlled energy delivery, the RF generator automatically reduces power when a preset temperature is exceeded, as measured from the tip of the ablation catheter. This minimizes the risk of coagulum formation and steam pops from excessive heating. Damage is generally limited to within a few millimeters of the catheter tip, since heat generated by resistive heating decreases as the fourth power of distance from the catheter tip.

During an ablation procedure, the operator can manipulate various parameters to control lesion size and depth, including catheter contact, power, duration of RF delivery, and maximum temperature. Newer technologies have been developed to create larger lesions and improve ablation efficacy, including catheters with larger tips (8 mm instead of 4 mm), internally cooled catheters, and open-irrigated catheters that flush saline through holes at the tip of the catheter (Fig. 9-2). Internally cooled catheters permit the delivery of more power without excessive heating of the tissue-catheter interface, resulting in reliable energy delivery that creates deeper lesions with less coagulum formation. Open-irrigated catheters offer even greater tissue interface cooling and further reduce the incidence of thrombus formation and steam pops. However, with all of these technologies that increase lesion size and depth, the risk of collateral damage to surrounding structures also increases.

OTHER ENERGY SOURCES FOR ABLATION

Although RF energy is used in the vast majority of ablation procedures, other energy sources are also commercially available. In cryothermy, also called cryoablation, tissue is destroyed not by electrical heating, but rather by extreme cooling. The first transvenous

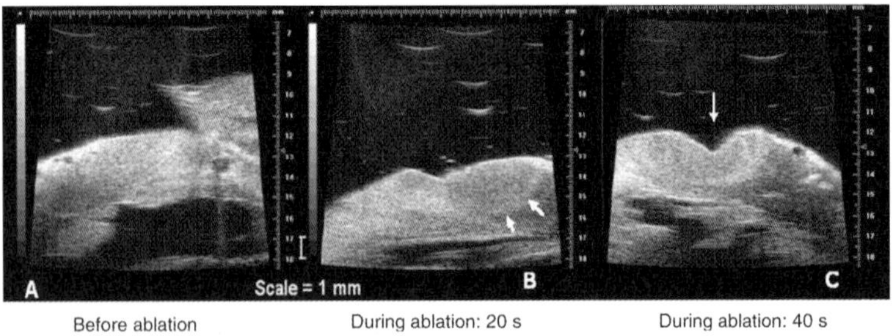

FIGURE 9-1. Lesion formation during RF delivery on the epicardial surface of a Langendorff-perfused rabbit heart. This heart was imaged using a 30-MHz ultrasound system (VisualSonic); **panel A** shows the tissue before ablation. The *arrows* indicate the border of the lesion in **panel B**, and evidence of tissue damage in **panel C**. (Courtesy of Aman Mahajan, MD, PhD, UCLA.)

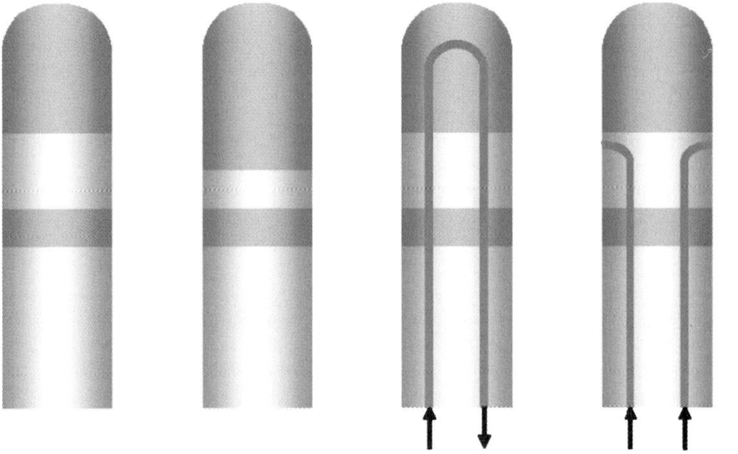

FIGURE 9-2. Currently available RF ablation catheter designs. Lesion depth increases with larger catheter tips and cooling the ablation electrode (irrigation) so more power can be delivered. The standard tip is 4 mm in length.

catheter ablation using cryothermy was reported by Khairy et al. in 1999. The cryoablation catheter is cooled by injection of liquid nitrous oxide into the catheter, which cools as it changes to the gas phase, resulting in temperatures of 75°C below zero centigrade. This damages tissue by creating extracellular ice crystals, drawing water out of cells. When the tissue thaws, hypotonic fluid flows back in, causing swelling and cell membrane rupture. A second mechanism of lesion formation from cryotherapy is vascular-mediated tissue injury.

The main advantage usually cited for cryoablation is enhanced safety. It offers the opportunity to create a "test lesion" at an intermediate low temperature of −30°C with reversible effects, avoiding permanent damage to vital structures. Once determined to be safe, this can be followed by cooling the catheter tip to −75°C for 4 min, producing a permanent lesion. Other reported advantages are increased catheter stability due to adherence of the catheter tip to frozen tissue, and creation of smaller, better demarcated lesions than those resulting from RF ablation. The disadvantage of cryoablation include lower acute efficacy and higher arrhythmia recurrence rate, likely due to incomplete tissue destruction.

Other methods of catheter-based energy delivery are currently in development. These include bipolar RF ablation, in which energy is delivered between two catheter electrodes, rather than between an electrode and skin pad as in traditional unipolar RF. Novel non-RF energy sources are also being tested in animal and human studies. These include laser, microwave, and high-intensity focused ultrasound, some of which will be delivered through newly developed catheters designed to increase the safety and efficacy of ablation.

CATHETER MAPPING AND ABLATION: ANATOMICAL APPROACHES

Catheter ablation is usually performed by the transvenous approach via the femoral vein. This allows direct access to the right atrium through the inferior vena cava for ablation of atrial flutter, right atrial tachycardia, or AV nodal modification. The ablation catheter can also be advanced across the tricuspid valve for right ventricular ablation and to the right ventricular outflow tract. Ablation within the left atrium, for treatment of atrial fibrillation, left atrial tachycardia, or left-sided accessory pathways, is usually performed by the transseptal approach. In this procedure, a long guiding sheath is placed transvenously into the right atrium, and a specialized needle is used to puncture the fossa ovalis for access to the left atrium, under fluoroscopic or echocardiographic guidance.

Access to the left ventricle, for ablation of ventricular tachycardia, can be obtained by the retrograde approach, advancing the catheter through the femoral artery to the ascending aorta and across the aortic valve. Alternatively, the atrial transseptal approach can be used to enter the left atrium; from there, the ablation catheter can be advanced across the mitral valve into the left ventricle. It must be emphasized that any mapping or ablation procedure on the left side of the heart requires systemic anticoagulation, usually with intravenous unfractionated heparin, to prevent thrombus formation and thromboembolic complications, including stroke. The activated clotting time (ACT) should be monitored frequently to ensure adequate anticoagulation for the duration of left heart access; typically the heparin infusion is adjusted to maintain ACT of at least 300 s.

Although all of the heart's chambers can be accessed with intravascular catheters, these approaches only allow mapping and ablation on the endocardial surface of the heart. Some arrhythmias, such as ventricular tachycardias in patients with nonischemic cardiomyopathy, can arise from an epicardial focus or reentrant circuit, and are best treated by epicardial ablation, applying energy to the outer surface of the heart. Until recently, this required sternotomy or thoracotomy by a cardiac surgeon. However, the technique of percutaneous subxiphoid puncture, described by Sosa et al. (1996), allows cardiac electrophysiologists to access the pericardial space for epicardial catheter ablation. Newer minimally invasive surgical epicardial ablation techniques have also been developed, and may turn out to be particularly useful for treatment of atrial fibrillation.

GOALS OF CARDIAC MAPPING

Electroanatomic mapping generally refers to correlation of anatomic location with electrophysiologic data, chiefly local electrograms. When gathered by catheter electrodes touching the myocardium, the technique is known as contact mapping, and can be performed on either the endocardial or epicardial surface of the heart. Less commonly, multielectrode array catheters within a chamber of the heart can be used to extrapolate the heart's electrical activity without actually touching the myocardium, a process known as noncontact mapping. Another method now under development is body surface mapping, in which hundreds of electrodes on the skin can be used to precisely infer activation of structures within the heart. Unless otherwise stated, topics in this chapter refer to contact mapping. Mapping can be performed either during sinus rhythm or during tachycardia; examples of both will be discussed.

The goal of most mapping techniques is to reveal an arrhythmia's mechanism or identify an anatomic site at which ablation can be used to treat the arrhythmia. For focal mechanisms such as automaticity, triggered activity, and microreentry, each beat of tachycardia arises from a single focus and spreads outward. Cardiac mapping aims to localize the site of impulse formation, usually by finding the earliest local activation during tachycardia. The onset of the "P" wave (for atrial tachycardias) or the "QRS" complex (for ventricular tachycardias) is taken as the reference point for local electrogram timing. This technique is most useful for focal atrial and ventricular tachycardias.

In reentrant arrhythmias, on the other hand, there are no true "early" sites, since tachycardia results from an activation front continually traveling around the reentrant circuit. Examples of these arrhythmias include atrial flutter, AV reentrant tachycardia, and most types of ventricular tachycardia. The initial goals of cardiac mapping in these arrhythmias are to prove a reentrant mechanism and identify the course of the circuit. The next step is to find critical areas of the circuit, such as the site of exit to normal myocardium or a critical isthmus between anatomic conduction barriers, where ablation might interrupt the circuit and terminate the tachycardia. Since reentry requires two limbs and an area of slow conduction, many reentrant arrhythmias occur in the setting of abnormal connections such as accessory pathways, after myocardial infarction or surgery, and in congenital malformations.

Finally, cardiac mapping can also be performed to localize arrhythmias when the exact mechanism of the tachycardia cannot be determined. Also called substrate modification or anatomic ablation, this approach targets sites that are likely to participate in the arrhythmia, yet, without definitive electrophysiologic evidence of their involvement. It is useful for ablation of atrial fibrillation, in which the exact mechanism is not well understood in most patients, but ablation of certain sites within the left atrium does offer clinical benefit. Another application is in the treatment of hemodynamically unstable ventricular tachycardia; targeting the anatomic substrate can be effective even when other mapping techniques cannot be safely employed.

TOOLS FOR CARDIAC MAPPING

At the most basic level, a cardiac mapping system stores and displays local electrograms and the locations at which they were recorded. Effective mapping requires high-fidelity unipolar or bipolar electrograms; their timing, amplitude, and morphology must be clearly and reproducibly recorded from each site. The simplest mapping system consists of fluoroscopic imaging with annotation of local electrograms as they are recorded. For successful ablation of many focal and reentrant arrhythmias, including typical atrial flutter, accessory-pathway mediated tachycardia, and others, these tools are often sufficient.

However, more advanced electroanatomic mapping systems have been developed, and are particularly useful for defining the circuits of complex arrhythmias such as atypical atrial flutter and hemodynamically unstable ventricular tachycardias. These systems use magnetic or electric fields to accurately locate the position of a mapping catheter within the heart. The operator can create a three-dimensional model of a cardiac chamber, and associate each stored electrogram with a point on that model. Some systems allow the user to import cardiac imaging from CT, MRI, or ultrasound to aid in construction of chamber geometry. These intracardiac positioning systems, which are usually more precise than fluoroscopic localization, can offer assistance with navigation and catheter movement, as well as the opportunity to return to any given point of interest. Finally, they can allow a procedure to be performed with less fluoroscopy time, limiting radiation exposure for both the patient and the medical team. All of these technologies have limitations such as imperfect fidelity of the chamber geometry, but are important adjunctive tools in treating more complex arrhythmias, especially in hearts with variant anatomy.

SPECIFIC MAPPING TECHNIQUES: ACTIVATION MAPPING

For patients with inducible, sustained, and well-tolerated tachycardias that have a focal mechanism, activation mapping is the most precise method of determining the arrhythmia's origin. It can also be used to locate the exit site of a reentrant tachycardia or the source of monomorphic ectopic beats, provided they occur with sufficient frequency. The key observation made during activation mapping is the exact time local myocardium is depolarized, as compared to a constant reference. This reference, sometimes called a fiducial marker, can be the onset of the surface P wave or QRS complex, or the local electrogram from a stable intracardiac recording electrode such as the coronary sinus electrogram.

By searching for the earliest local electrogram during tachycardia, the operator can precisely locate the site from which the tachycardia originates. Combining relative activation time with the location of each point on an electroanatomic map creates a three-dimensional map of cardiac activation (Fig. 9-3). Color-coded isochrones (lines or colors

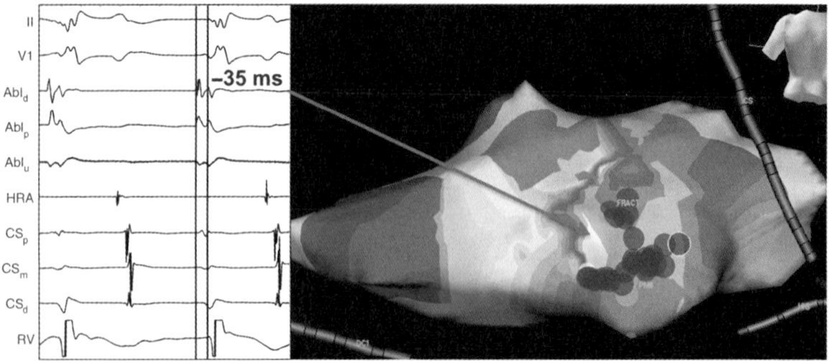

FIGURE 9-3. Activation map of ventricular tachycardia. Local activation time at hundreds of individual sites are recorded and displayed on an electroanatomic map, with colors to indicate timing as compared to a constant reference. The earliest local activation is at the white area, latest at the purple area. Local electrogram recorded from the site indicated by the *arrow* showed local activation 35 ms before onset of QRS complex in a beat of ventricular tachycardia. After ablation lesions at early sites (*brown circles*) with abnormal electrograms, the tachycardia was not inducible. Abl end, endocardial ablation catheter; HRA, high right atrial catheter; CS, coronary sinus catheter (p, proximal; m, middle; d, distal); RV, right ventricular catheter; HIS, His bundle catheter; FRACT, fractionated local EGM; PM5; pace map 5 (see color insert).

indicating points with simultaneous activation) can be used to display the tachycardia's propagation pattern. Successful ablation sites show *presystolic potentials*, which are local electrograms occurring before the onset of the P wave for atrial tachycardia or the QRS complex for ventricular tachycardia. Activation mapping has been proven superior to pace mapping for precise determination of a tachycardia's origin.

Although most often applied in the setting of focal tachycardias, the principles of activation mapping can also be used in treating some reentrant arrhythmias. An example cited previously is locating the exit site of a scar-related ventricular tachycardia, which can be an important site for ablation. Sometimes the entire circuit of a macroreentrant arrhythmia can be sampled, creating a map in which "early meets late" activation. Activation mapping can also be used in ablation of accessory pathways. For manifest pathways with overt preexcitation, the earliest local ventricular electrograms during sinus rhythm (or atrial pacing) identify the ventricular insertion site of the pathway. Similarly, for concealed accessory pathways, the earliest atrial activation during ventricular pacing or orthodromic AVRT can be used to locate the atrial insertion site. Targeting these sites usually results in successful ablation, leading to accessory pathway conduction block and noninducibility of accessory-pathway-mediated tachycardias.

SPECIFIC MAPPING TECHNIQUES: PACE MAPPING

Pace mapping, most frequently used in ablation of ventricular tachycardia, is performed in sinus rhythm by positioning the distal electrode of the ablation catheter near the suspected origin of the tachycardia and pacing from that site. The resulting captured QRS complex is compared in all 12 surface leads to the QRS complex during tachycardia (Fig. 9-4). If the match between paced and tachycardia complexes is not perfect, the catheter is adjusted slightly and the process repeated until the resulting QRS complex appears identical. This allows the operator to identify a site close to the origin of a focal arrhythmia or the exit site of a reentrant arrhythmia, provided a 12-lead electrocardiogram of the tachycardia is available. Studies have shown that in the absence of major differences in any of the 12 leads, the two sites are likely to be within 5 mm of each other.

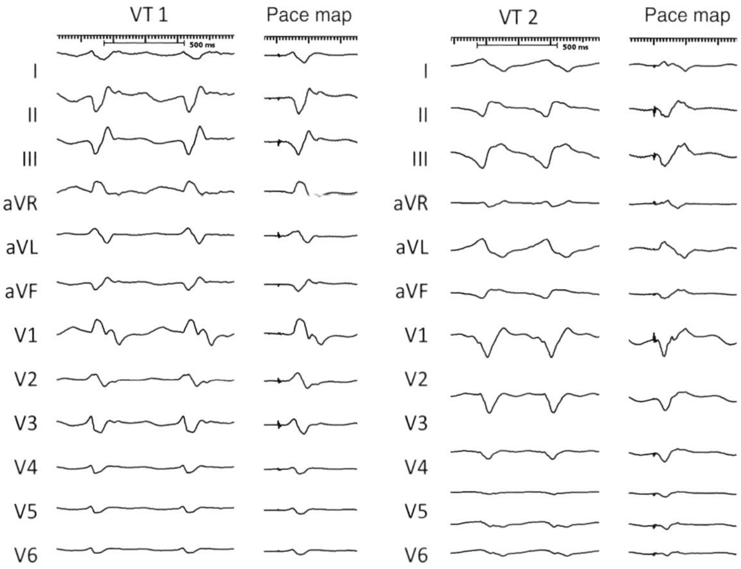

FIGURE 9-4. Pace mapping during ventricular tachycardia (VT) ablation. This patient with ischemic cardiomyopathy had two distinct tachycardias, and pace mapping was performed from different sites. The pace map for VT 1 more closely matches the 12-lead electrocardiogram of the clinical tachycardia than the pace map for VT 2. This indicates proximity of the ablation catheter to the origin of a focal tachycardia or the exit site of a reentrant tachycardia. (Courtesy of Shiro Nakahara, MD, PhD, UCLA.)

The best results are achieved by pacing at the same cycle length as the index tachycardia, since functional conduction delay or block could alter QRS configuration at different pacing rates. Also, the lowest possible pacing output should be used; higher output could capture a larger volume of myocardium and change QRS morphology. Finally, every effort should be made to ensure that the surface electrodes are placed in exactly the same position as they were when the tachycardia was recorded. Even minor differences can result in subtle changes in the electrocardiographic appearance of ventricular activation. In theory, the same principle could be applied to localize a focal atrial tachycardia, but the smaller amplitude of the P wave (which is sometimes obscured by a T wave) makes this application of pace mapping less practical.

The main advantage of pace mapping is that it can be employed even when tachycardia cannot be induced or is not tolerated. The disadvantages are that it does not establish the mechanism of the tachycardia, localizes only the exit site of a reentrant arrhythmia (which might not be the best ablation site), and is often not precise enough to allow effective ablation, even for focal tachycardias. Still, pace mapping is useful in identifying the general location of an arrhythmia and, when used in combination with other mapping techniques, often aids in successful ablation.

SPECIFIC MAPPING TECHNIQUES: ENTRAINMENT MAPPING

Entrainment mapping can be used to locate areas within the circuit of a reentrant arrhythmia and choose promising sites for effective ablation. By pacing at a cycle length 10 to 40 ms less than the tachycardia cycle length (TCL) (i.e., slightly faster), the arrhythmia can be continuously reset by each pacing stimulus. Entrainment mapping is used to study reentrant tachycardias such as ventricular tachycardia, atrial flutter, AV nodal reentrant tachycardia, and accessory-pathway mediated AV reentrant tachycardia. One crucial measurement made during entrainment mapping, relevant if the tachycardia continues after cessation of pacing, is the *postpacing interval* (*PPI*). This is defined as the time from the last pacing stimulus to the first return beat of tachycardia, measured at the same site as pacing. The PPI is then compared to the *TCL*. The smaller the difference between these two measurements, the closer is the pacing site to the tachycardia circuit. If the PPI is within 30 ms of TCL, the site is likely to be close to the tachycardia circuit, and ablation there may be successful in terminating the tachycardia.

Other features of entrainment mapping can help define whether a particular site is located in a critical isthmus, an outer loop, or a bystander site (Fig. 9-5). A critical isthmus location is ideal for ablation. It shows (i) ventricular tachycardia accelerated to the paced cycle length with no change in QRS morphology (known as entrainment with concealed fusion), (ii) the PPI is nearly identical to the TCL, (PPI = TCL) (within 30 ms), and (iii) the stimulus to QRS interval is equal to the electrogram to QRS interval during tachycardia, (Stim to QRS = local EGM to QRS) (within 20 ms).

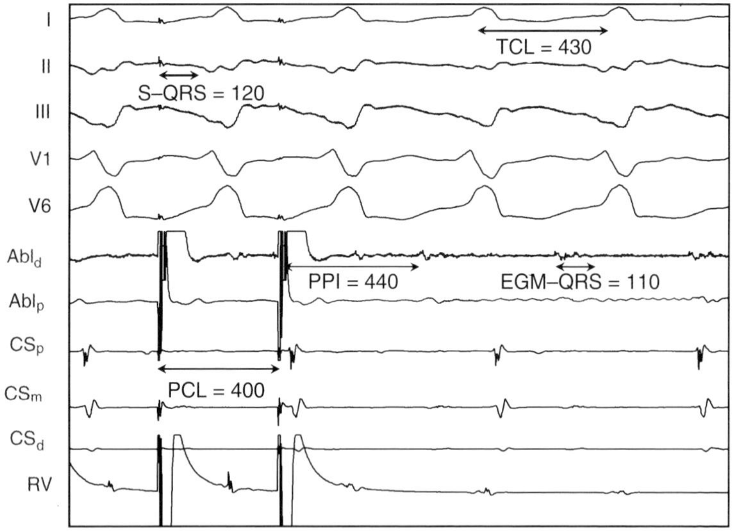

FIGURE 9-5. Entrainment mapping during ventricular tachycardia ablation. If the tachycardia is hemodynamically tolerated, entrainment mapping can be performed by overdrive pacing at a rate slightly faster, (cycle length slightly shorter), than the TCL. In this example, overdrive pacing is performed at 30 ms faster than the TCL. This results in entrainment with concealed fusion, since the tachycardia is accelerated to the paced cycle length but the QRS morphology is identical in all 12 leads (only 5 are shown). The PPI, measured from the last pacing stimulus to local activation at the same site in the first beat of tachycardia, is within 10 ms of the TCL, indicating that the ablation catheter was in the tachycardia circuit. The stimulus–QRS interval is also close to the local electrogram–QRS interval during tachycardia. Ablation at this site terminated the tachycardia. S–QRS, stimulus to QRS interval; EGM–QRS, local electrogram to QRS interval; PCL, paced cycle length. (Courtesy of Roderick Tung, MD, UCLA.)

For sustained reentrant arrhythmias, entrainment mapping is the most powerful way of characterizing the tachycardia mechanism and circuit and choosing the optimal ablation strategy.

SPECIFIC MAPPING TECHNIQUES: SUBSTRATE MAPPING

For some arrhythmias, careful characterization of the cardiac substrate is the first step in planning an ablation strategy. This is especially true of hemodynamically unstable arrhythmias, such as ventricular tachycardia causing hypotension, which makes mapping during tachycardia unsafe or impossible. An alternative approach is to gather electroanatomic information during baseline rhythm, whether sinus or paced. The most common form of substrate mapping is measuring electrogram amplitude (voltage) at each point in the area of interest. This information is then displayed on a three-dimensional electroanatomic model to create a "*voltage map*" of the heart, and can be performed for both the endocardial and epicardial surfaces (Fig. 9-6). Low-voltage areas often correspond to fibrosis, or scar, and can result from

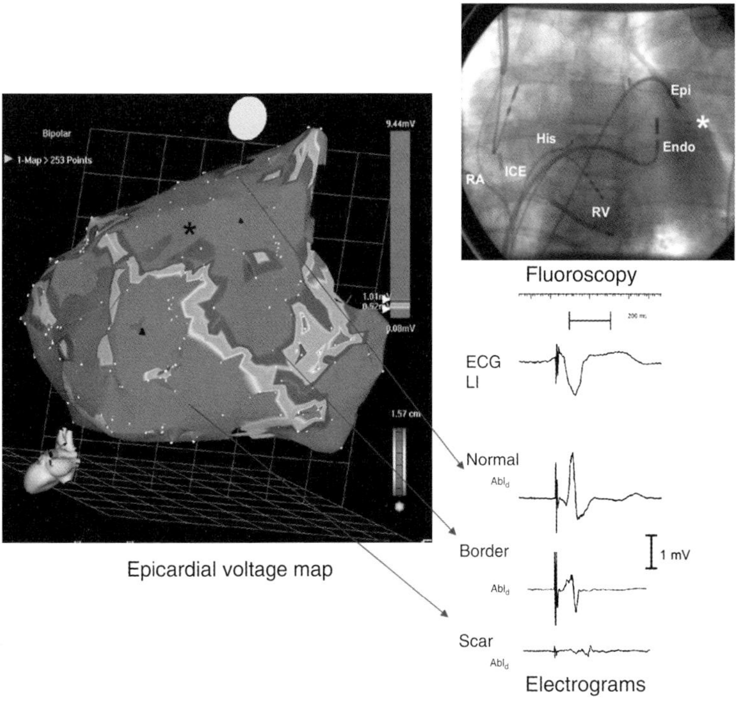

FIGURE 9-6. Electroanatomic map of the epicardial surface in a patient with nonischemic cardiomyopathy and a large epicardial scar. Also shown are fluoroscopy of catheter positions, and representative local electrograms from normal tissue, border zone, and dense scar regions. RA, right atrial catheter; ICE, intracardiac echocardiogram catheter; RV, right ventricular catheter; Endo, endocardial left ventricular mapping catheter; Epi, epicardial left ventricular mapping catheter; ECG LI, electrocardiogram lead I; Abl d, ablation distal bipole. (Courtesy of David Cesario, MD, PhD, University of Southern California.) (See color insert.)

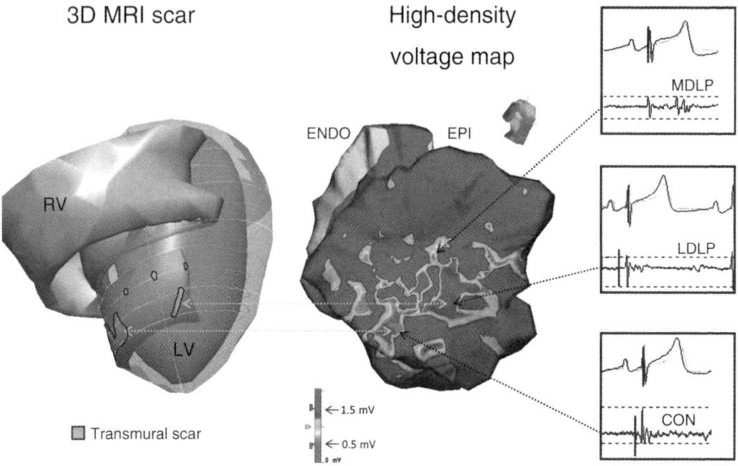

FIGURE 9-7. Substrate mapping correlating magnetic resonance imaging (MRI) with electroanatomic voltage map. Areas of scar on MRI correlate with low-voltage areas on electroanatomic map. Late potentials are recorded within scar and in scar border zones. RV, right ventricle; LV, left ventricle; ENDO, endocardial surface; EPI, epicardial surface; MDLP, mid-diastolic late potential; LDLP, late-diastolic late potential; CON, continuous electrical activity. (Courtesy of Shiro Nakahara, MD, PhD, UCLA.) (See color insert.)

previous infarction, surgery, or ablation, or from inflammation due to myocarditis or transplant rejection. This technique is sometimes referred to as scar mapping. Since scarred areas are often associated with conduction slowing or block, a voltage map can be helpful in suggesting pathways for potential reentrant circuits, even without inducing the arrhythmia.

Besides low-voltage areas, substrate mapping can also display other electrophysiologic characteristics of interest. One example is *fractionated electrograms* with multiple deflections, which are thought to result from anisotropic local conduction. These are often recorded in scar border areas, zones of interface between disparate tissues, and sites of cardiac innervation/denervation. Fractionated sites can be annotated on the electroanatomic map. Another example of substrate mapping is *late potentials*, or sites of low-amplitude local activation recorded during cardiac electrical diastole, corresponding to areas of slowed local conduction. Again, marking the location of these late potentials on the electroanatomic map can be useful for planning ablation (Fig. 9-7).

KEY POINTS

1. Catheter ablation has become the preferred method of treating many cardiac arrhythmias.
2. It has an excellent safety profile and is highly effective in treating many types of tachycardia. RF energy is most commonly used, but other energy sources are also in clinical use and experimental development.
3. Using the various mapping techniques described here (compared in Table 9-1) can help the operator precisely target sites where ablation is most likely to be successful in treating the arrhythmia.

TABLE 9-1 Comparison of Mapping Techniques

	Rhythm Required for Mapping	Advantages	Disadvantages	Useful for Ablation in
Activation mapping	Tachycardia	Precisely localizes focus or exit site	Requires sustained tachycardia or frequent beats of tachycardia	Focal, well-tolerated tachycardia (VT or AT)
Pace mapping	Baseline rhythm (sinus or paced)	Does not require sustained tachycardia	Imprecise (only localizes within 5 mm) Only finds exit site	VT that is not tolerated hemodynamically
Entrainment mapping	Tachycardia	Provides strong evidence that a site is within tachycardia circuit	May be difficult to capture and entrain tachycardia PPI may be hard to measure	Sustained, stable reentrant tachycardia (VT or SVT)
Voltage (scar) mapping	Baseline rhythm (sinus or paced)	Does not require sustained tachycardia	Does not prove a given site participates in tachycardia	Unstable tachycardias (especially VT) Complex tachycardias with multiple circuits

VT, ventricular tachycardia; AT, atrial tachycardia; SVT, supraventricular tachycardia.

SUGGESTED READINGS

Bogun F, Taj M, Ting M, et al. Spatial resolution of pace mapping of idiopathic ventricular tachycardia/ectopy originating in the right ventricular outflow tract. *Heart Rhythm*. 2008;5:339–344.

Cobb FR, Blumenschein SD, Sealy WC, et al. Successful surgical interruption of the bundle of Kent in a patient with Wolff-Parkinson-White syndrome. *Circulation*. 1968;38:1018–1029.

Edgerton JR, Edgerton ZJ, Weaver T, et al. Minimally invasive pulmonary vein isolation and partial autonomic denervation for surgical treatment of atrial fibrillation. *Ann Thorac Surg*. 2008;86:35–38; discussion 39.

Evans GT Jr, Scheinman MM, Bardy G, et al. Predictors of in-hospital mortality after DC catheter ablation of atrioventricular junction. Results of a prospective, international, multicenter study. *Circulation*. 1991;84:1924–1937.

Haines DE, Watson DD. Tissue heating during radiofrequency catheter ablation: A thermodynamic model and observations in isolated perfused and superfused canine right ventricular free wall. *Pacing Clin Electrophysiol*. 1989;12:962–976.

Huang SK, Bharati S, Graham AR, et al. Closed chest catheter desiccation of the atrioventricular junction using radiofrequency energy—a new method of catheter ablation. *J Am Coll Cardiol*. 1987;9:349–358.

Jackman WM, Wang XZ, Friday KJ, et al. Catheter ablation of accessory atrioventricular pathways (Wolff-Parkinson-White syndrome) by radiofrequency current. *N Engl J Med*. 1991;324:1605–1611.

Kadish AH, Childs K, Schmaltz S, et al. Differences in QRS configuration during unipolar pacing from adjacent sites: Implications for the spatial resolution of pace-mapping. *J Am Coll Cardiol*. 1991;17:143–151.

Khairy P, Novak PG, Guerra PG, et al. Cryothermal slow pathway modification for atrioventricular nodal reentrant tachycardia. *Europace*. 2007;9:909–914.

Ramanathan C, Ghanem RN, Jia P, et al. Noninvasive electrocardiographic imaging for cardiac electrophysiology and arrhythmia. *Nat Med*. 2004;10:422–428.

Scheinman MM, Morady F, Hess DS, et al. Catheter-induced ablation of the atrioventricular junction to control refractory supraventricular arrhythmias. *JAMA*. 1982;248:851–855.

Sosa E, Scanavacca M, d'Avila A, et al. A new technique to perform epicardial mapping in the electrophysiology laboratory. *J Cardiovasc Electrophysiol*. 1996;7:531–536.

Stevenson WG, Khan H, Sager P, et al. Identification of reentry circuit sites during catheter mapping and radiofrequency ablation of ventricular tachycardia late after myocardial infarction. *Circulation*. 1993;88:1647–1670.

Yokoyama K, Nakagawa H, Wittkampf FH, et al. Comparison of electrode cooling between internal and open irrigation in radiofrequency ablation lesion depth and incidence of thrombus and steam pop. *Circulation*. 2006;113:11–19.

Zipes DP, Jalife J. *Cardiac Electrophysiology: From Cell to Bedside*. 5th Ed. Philadelphia, PA: W. B. Saunders/Elsevier; 2009.

CHAPTER 10

Indications for Cardiac Rhythm Management Devices

Gautham Kalahasty and Kenneth Ellenbogen

Understanding the indications for device therapy for cardiac arrhythmias should be one of the primary goals of any Cardiology fellow during his or her electrophysiology (EP) rotation. The ACC/AHA/HRS 2008 Guidelines for Device-based Therapy provide an excellent framework on which to base the patient management. These guidelines are based on a combination of clinical trial data (with emphasis on randomized control trials when available) and expert consensus opinion (when data are limited). A class I indication means that the benefits far outweigh the risks and the procedure should be performed. A class IIa indication means that the benefits outweigh the risks and it is reasonable to perform the procedure. A class IIb indication means that the benefits may outweigh the risks or be equivalent and that the procedure can be considered. A class III indication means that the risks outweigh benefits and that the procedure should not be performed. The use of pacemakers and defibrillators for class I and IIa indications is well supported by clinical data or consensus opinion. Rigid application of the guidelines is not always appropriate or productive, and judicious use of devices for what are considered IIb indications can be reasonable. The goals of this chapter are not to simply restate the guidelines for device implantation, but rather, to provide practical insights for appropriate patient selection and management. Although summarized throughout this chapter, a thorough reading of the ACC/AHA/HRS Guidelines is mandatory for any cardiologist. The currently available devices used for the management arrhythmias include pacemakers, implantable cardioverter-defibrillators (ICDs), cardiac resynchronizations pacemakers (CRT-P) and defibrillators (CRT-D), and implantable loop recorders (ILRs).

PHYSIOLOGIC PACING

A discussion about current indications for implantable devices for cardiac rhythm management is incomplete without addressing the importance of physiologic pacing. The function of a pacemaker is to, as much as possible, approximate normal cardiac function. Therefore, careful mode selection (AAI, VVI, DDI, DDD, etc.) and proper programming (atrioventricular [AV] delay, hysteresis, mode switch rates, etc.) are needed to optimize the beneficial effects and minimize the potentially detrimental effects of pacing. Although "demand" ventricular pacemakers have been in clinical use since the 1960s and it seems intuitive that dual chamber pacing would be superior to ventricular demand pacing, the body of clinical data needed to support this conclusion took almost 20 years to accumulate. The benefits of dual chamber AV synchronous pacing in patients with sinus node dysfunction (SND) and paroxysmal atrial fibrillation (AF) are now widely accepted. More recently, the potentially adverse effects of ventricular pacing (synchronous or asynchronous) have been recognized and are summarized in

TABLE 10-1 Potential Adverse Effects of Ventricular Pacing (RV) in SND

Ventricular dyssynchrony
Altered cardiac hemodynamics due to loss of "atrial kick"
Atrial proarrhythmia
Ventricular Proarrhythmia
Increased valvular regurgitation
Adverse electrical remodeling of the atria promoting AF
Pacemaker syndrome

Table 10-1. Some of these effects are not unique to ventricular pacing with AV dyssynchrony but may occur with dual chamber pacing and will be discussed below. Even ventricular proarrhythmia (ventricular tachycardia [VT] and ventricular fibrillation [VF]) has been described with both single chamber ventricular and dual chamber pacing. Ventricular remodeling, hemodynamic parameters, quality of life measures, and clinical end points such as incidence of AF, stroke, congestive heart failure (CHF), and mortality have all been investigated. Proper device selection and programming are needed to prevent some of the potentially detrimental effects of pacing. The important clinical trials in pacing and mode selection are summarized in Table 10-2.

In a secondary analysis of the MOST data, two important findings were reported. Increasing percentage of ventricular pacing was found to be associated with an increasing incidence of AF during both VVIR and DDDR pacing. Also, a greater percentage of ventricular pacing was associated with a greater risk of hospitalization for heart failure. If ventricular pacing occurred more than 40% of the time, there was a twofold increase in the risk of developing CHF. This study suggests that the relative benefits of AV synchronous pacing compared to only ventricular pacing are due to the deleterious effects of right ventricular (RV) pacing rather than the presumed advantages of AV synchronous pacing. The CTOPP and MOST studies had relatively few patients with true atrial based pacing (AAI) without the confounding effect of ventricular pacing. In the MADIT (Multicenter Automatic Defibrillator Implantation Trial) II study, patients who received an ICD had higher survival rates but also demonstrated a trend toward an increased rate of CHF; 73 patients (14.9%) in the conventional-therapy group and 148 in the defibrillator group (19.9%) were hospitalized with heart failure (p = 0.09). In the DAVID (Dual Chamber and VVI Implantable Defibrillator) Trial, a composite endpoint of time to death and first hospitalization for CHF was compared in ICD patients programmed to receive dual-chamber pacing (DDDR-70) or ventricular backup pacing (VVI-40). At 1 year, 83.9% of the patients in the VVI-40 group were free from the composite endpoint compared to 73.3% of patients in the DDDR-70 group. Hospitalization for CHF occurred in 13.3% of VVI-40 patients compared to 22.6% of DDD-70 patients trending in favor of the VVI-40 group. The VVI-40 group received very little ventricular pacing compared to the DDD-70 group. Although the DAVID study looked only at an ICD population, it had a major impact on the programming of dual chamber pacemakers. By highlighting the deleterious effects of RV pacing, it underscored the importance of mode selection in patients with SND and paroxysmal AF. When a physician programs a pacemaker or an ICD, he or she should minimize RV pacing. All major pulse generators have incorporated programming parameters/algorithms which allow for maximization of the AV delay to promote intrinsic ventricular conduction. Algorithms also exist that allow for dual chamber pacemakers to automatically switch from single chamber atrial based pacing (AAI/R) to dual chamber AV sequential pacing (DDD/R). When this algorithm is selected, the device operates in AAI/R mode until AV block occurs and then switches to DDD/R mode (Fig. 10-1).

TABLE 10-2 Important Clinical Trial in Pacing and Mode Selection

Trial	Year	Average Follow-up (years)	Design	Key Findings
Danish (Andersen et al.). *Lancet*. 1997;350: 1210–1216.	1994	5.5	AAI vs. VVI in 225 patients with SSS	At long-term follow-up (mean 5.5 years), the incidence of paroxysmal AF and chronic AF was reduced in the AAI group. Overall survival, heart failure, and thromboembolic events were reduced with atrial-based pacing.
PASE. *N Engl J Med* 1998; 338:1097–1104.	1998	2.5	Single blinded assignment of VVIR or DDDR mode in 407 patients with SSS, AV block, and other indications	Patients with SSS showed a trend towards a lower incidence of AF and all-cause mortality (AF: 19% vs. 28%, $p = 0.06$; mortality: 12% vs. 20%, $p = 0.09$). QOL was not different between the two pacing modes. 26% of patients developed pacemaker syndrome when paced in the VVIR mode.
Mattioli et al. *Clin Cardiol.* 1998 Feb; 21(2):117–122.	1998	2.0	VVI/VVIR vs. AAI/DDD/DDDR/ VDD pacing in patients with AV block (100) and SSS (110)	Incidence of AF was 10% at 1 year, 23% at 2 years, and 31% at 5 years. An increase in the incidence of chronic AF was observed in patients with SSS in the VVI/VVIR arm.
CTOPP. *N Engl J Med.* 2000; 342:385–1391.	2000	6.0	2568 patients randomized to ventricular pacing (VVI/R) vs. physiologic pacing (DDD/R or AAI/R) for any appropriate indication	The annual rate of AF was less with physiologic pacing. No difference was observed in stroke or cardiovascular death between the two groups. There was a 27% reduction in the annual rate of progression to chronic AF.
MOST. *Circulation.* 2003;107:2932–2937.	2002	4.5	2,010 patients with SND (only) randomized to VVIR vs. DDDR programming, >50% had prior AF	AF was reduced in patients randomized to physiologic pacing. No difference in mortality and stroke was observed between pacing modes. Thirty-one percent of patients crossed over from VVIR to DDDR mode, 49% of which was due to pacemaker syndrome.

(Continued)

TABLE 10-2 Important Clinical Trial in Pacing and Mode Selection (Cont'd)

Trial	Year	Average Follow-up (years)	Design	Key Findings
PAC-ATACH. *Circulation.* 1998;98:I-494.	2001	2.0	198 patients with SND and history of atrial arrhythmias randomized to DDDR pacing or VVIR pacing	Abstract only. Manuscript to be published. Mortality was lower in the dual chamber group. (3.2% vs. 6.8%, $p = 0.007$) There was no difference in the AF recurrence rate.
UKPACE. *Heart* 1997;78: 221–223.	2002	4.6	2,021 patients, age >70 years, randomly assigned to 3 arms: DDD (50%), VVIR (25%), and VVI (25%)	There was no difference in all-cause mortality, rate of stroke or incidence of AF between the dual chamber group and ventricular pacing group.
SAVEPACe. *N Engl J Med.* 2007;357(10): 1000–1008.	2007	1.7	530 patients in DDD mode, 535 patients in AAI ←→ DDD mode for symptomatic SND; nearly an equal number of patients in both groups (38%) had paroxysmal AF	Persistent AF occurred in 12.7% of patients in conventional pacing group and 7.9% of patients in minimal ventricular pacing group.

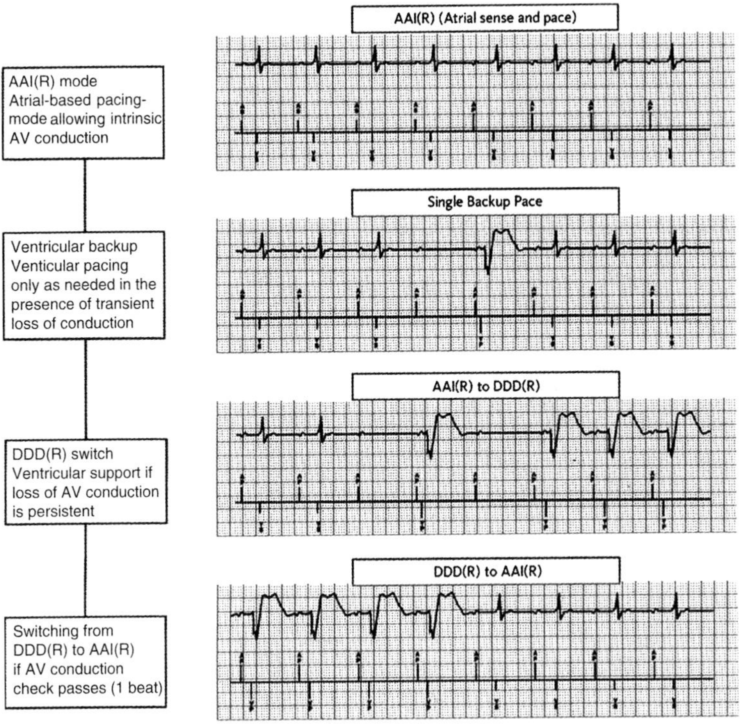

FIGURE 10-1. Managed ventricular pacing (MVPTM, Medtronic Inc., Minneapolis, MN) is an atrial-based pacing mode that significantly reduces unnecessary RV pacing by primarily operating in an AAI(R) pacing mode while providing the safety of a dual chamber backup mode if necessary. As shown in the figure, the algorithm allows for a single blocked beat before a backup ventricular paced beat is delivered. Mode switch will occur only if two out of four blocked beats occur. Two sequential blocked beats cannot occur due to backup ventricular pacing.

A prospective randomized trial (SAVE PACe) of an algorithm that minimizes ventricular pacing (Sweeney et al.) showed a 40% relative risk reduction in the development of persistent AF compared to conventional dual chamber pacing for patients with SND and normal left ventricular (LV) function when this algorithm was utilized. No difference was seen in mortality between the two groups of paced patients.

From the above discussion, it is clear that the definition of physiologic pacing has evolved. A single chamber ventricular based pacemaker should be avoided in patients with paroxysmal AF and SND. It is no longer enough to maintain AV synchrony with a dual chamber atrial based pacemaker. When possible, intrinsic AV conduction should be promoted to minimize the deleterious effects of RV pacing. Therefore, mode selection is important (AAI ←→ DDD, DDI, or DDD with long AV delays). Unresolved questions include the maximum hemodynamically acceptable AV delay and the optimal site for RV pacing.

Common indications for pacing are summarized in Table 10-3. Most of these are class I indications. Class II and Class III indications are discussed in the text.

TABLE 10-3 Indications for Pacing

SND

1. SND with documented symptomatic bradycardia
2. Symptomatic chronotropic incompetence
3. Symptomatic sinus bradycardia secondary to essential drug therapy

Acquired AV block

1. Third degree or advanced AV block associated with symptomatic bradycardia or ventricular arrhythmias secondary to AV block
2. Third degree or advanced AV block associated with symptomatic bradycardia due to essential medical therapy
3. Symptom free, awake patient with AF and pauses of at least 5 s
4. Symptom free, awake patient in sinus rhythm with asystole ≥3 s or an escape rate less than 40 bpm
5. AV block in association with AV junction ablation or postoperative AV block that is not expected to resolve
6. Third degree AV block or advanced AV block associated with neuromuscular diseases (i.e., myotonic muscular dystrophy, Kearns-Sayre syndrome, Erb dystrophy, peroneal muscular atrophy) with or without symptoms
7. Second or third degree AV block during exercise
8. Symptom free patient with second degree type II AV block and a wide QRS (bundle branch block)

Pacing for chronic bifascicular block

1. Advanced second degree or intermittent third degree AV block
2. Type II second degree AV block
3. Alternating bundle branch block
4. Unexplained syncope, when other likely causes have been excluded

Pacing during an AMI

1. Persistent and symptomatic second or third degree AV block
2. Persistent second degree AV block with alternating bundle branch block
3. Transient second or third degree AV block associated with a bundle branch block

PACING FOR SINUS NODE DYSFUNCTION

SND is the most common indication for pacemaker implantation in the US. SND is also referred to as sick sinus syndrome (SSS) or tachycardia-bradycardia syndrome. SND is characterized by a constellation of symptoms and arrhythmias. The more common symptoms include syncope, presyncope, fatigue, decreased exercise tolerance, and palpitations. Syncope is the most important presenting symptom of SND in elderly patients. Episodes are often unheralded. In elderly patients who present with repeated falls, syncope should be considered a potential precipitating factor. Typical arrhythmias include sinus bradycardia, sinus pauses (usually at AF termination), paroxysmal or permanent AF, atrial flutter, or atrial tachycardias.

Sinus bradycardia can be physiologic, due to high vagal tone or pathologic, due to SND. Even resting heart rates of 40 or 50 bpm while awake or as low as 30 bpm while asleep may be normal for some patients, especially those with excellent cardiovascular fitness. The incidental finding of sinus bradycardia alone is not an indication for pacemaker implantation. However, if a patient gives a history of recurrent unexplained syncope or easy fatigability and is found to have resting extreme bradycardia, permanent pacemaker implantation should be considered.

Symptomatic sinus bradycardia may be iatrogenic due to medical therapy such as beta-blockers or calcium channel blockers. Pacemaker implantation is indicated in this situation if no suitable alternative to these medications is advisable. For example, a patient with chronic stable angina or prior myocardial infarction should, in most cases, receive beta-blockers. A pacemaker may be needed to support the use of beta-blockers. High-grade AV block develops with an annual incidence of up to 1.8% per year in patients with a normal QRS duration and with a higher incidence in patients with preexisting bundle branch block is present. Therefore, in the US, dual chamber pacemakers are almost invariably implanted for SND.

Bradycardia may also be an unavoidable consequence of the medications used to prevent a rapid ventricular response associated with AF. Beta-blockers, calcium channel blockers, and digoxin are used to control rapid ventricular rates during AF, but the use of these can result in intermittent symptomatic bradycardia or long pauses that can lead to syncope or presyncope. Of note, pauses of up to 3 to 4 s during sleep are not unusual and are not solely an indication for pacing. Rather, bradycardia may be a reflection of the relatively high vagal tone present during sleep. Adjustment of medication dose or the use of beta-blockers with intrinsic sympathomimetic activity can sometimes mitigate the bradycardia or pauses but can also result in suboptimal rate control when a patient is active and awake. A pacemaker is indicated to facilitate the use of medications that are considered essential and for which there are no other suitable alternatives. Patients with paroxysmal AF and intermittent symptomatic bradycardia or long offset pauses at the terminations of AF should receive a dual chamber pacemaker. Patients with chronic AF and intermittent symptomatic pauses should receive a single chamber ventricular pacemaker. In addition to pharmacologic therapy to control the tachycardia, AV junction ablation may be needed for adequate rate control.

The guidelines for pacing emphasize the importance of symptoms attributable to bradycardia. Asymptomatic resting bradycardia, even with heart rates less than 40 bpm while awake, is not an indication for permanent pacing. In the absence of reversible causes, symptomatic bradycardia, regardless of the mechanism, is generally a universally accepted indication for pacing. The clinical challenge in some cases is to establish the correlation between symptoms and bradycardia. This may require the use of monitors such as Holter monitors, event monitors, or ILRs. A formal exercise treadmill test, although not required, may be needed to diagnose chronotropic incompetence. An EP study to evaluate sinus node function is typically of limited benefit. However, in a patient with syncope of unknown origin, it is reasonable to implant a pacemaker if prolonged sinus node recovery times are provoked during an EP study. Occasionally, an upright tilt table test can reveal SND in the form of carotid sinus hypersensitivity in patients presenting with unexplained syncope. Despite these diagnostic studies, a correlation between symptoms and rhythm cannot be established. Therefore, it is reasonable to implant a pacemaker for patients with heart rates less than 40 bpm who have symptoms consistent with bradycardia (class IIa) such as syncope, even if a direct relationship cannot be proven clinically.

Paroxysmal AF is the most common tachyarrhythmia seen in many patients with SND. In appropriate patients with AF, pacemaker implantation and AV junction ablation provide clinical benefit. It should be considered in any patient with suboptimal rate control and in any patient who is at risk of developing or has developed a tachycardia mediated cardiomyopathy. Although this procedure is most often done in patients with chronic AF, it is also appropriate for some patients with paroxysmal AF. The benefits of pacing in patients with a cardiac resynchronization therapy (CRT) device may be maximized in those patients with AF who have undergone AV junction ablation. In patients with chronic AF who are receiving a CRT device, AV junction ablation can be recommended if adequate rate control to allow LV pacing cannot be achieved by medical therapy. This issue is unresolved in patients with paroxysmal AF who receive a CRT device. Pacing algorithms that attempt to promote biventricular pacing even during AF are not effective, and pacing algorithms that attempt to prevent AF have limited value. In patients without a bradycardia indication, permanent pacemaker implantation is not currently recommended solely for the purpose of implementation of AF prevention algorithms. Multisite and novel site (Bachmann bundle) pacing strategies do not have broad clinical applications at this time. An exception is the use of short-term multisite pacing in the immediate postoperative period following cardiac surgery.

PACING FOR ACQUIRED OR CHRONIC ATRIOVENTRICULAR BLOCK

AV block is the other major cause of bradycardia resulting in the need for pacemaker implantation. First degree, second degree (types I and II), and third degree AV blocks may have indications for permanent pacing. The definitions of each of these conduction abnormalities should be known. Advanced second degree AV block refers to the block of two or more consecutive P waves with some conducted beats, which indicates some preservation of AV conduction. In the setting of AF, a prolonged pause (e.g., >5 s) should be considered to be due to advanced second degree AV block. As in SND, the presence of symptoms attributable to bradycardia establishes a class I indication for pacing regardless of the anatomic level of block. Symptoms of AV block not only include fatigue, syncope, and presyncope but also CHF and exercise intolerance. Unlike in patients with SND, there are some types of heart block for which there are class I and IIa indications for pacing even in the absence of symptoms. Bradycardia-dependent torsade de pointes or VT associated with complete or advanced AV block is a class I indication for pacing even without associated symptoms. Complete or advanced AV block with asystole greater than 3 s or escape rates less than 40 bpm is an indication for pacing in symptom-free, awake patients.

First degree AV block is rarely an indication for permanent pacing. However, occasionally patients may experience symptoms due to an extremely long PR interval (>300 ms) even without progression to second or third degree AV block. A very long PR interval can lead to symptoms of "pacemaker syndrome" such as palpitations, chest pain, and fatigue. A dual chamber pacemaker programmed with shorter AV delays may relieve these symptoms, although there is no data to suggest a mortality benefit.

Type I second degree AV block is usually due to block at the AV node and does not usually progress to complete heart block. PM implantation is indicated if Type I AV block is associated with symptoms. Type II AV block due to intra-hisian or infra-hisian block is associated with unpredictable progression to more advanced AV block or third degree AV block. Type II second degree AV block with a wide QRS typically indicates diffuse conduction system disease and constitutes an indication for pacing even in the absence of symptoms. Type II second degree AV block with a narrow QRS complex may not be due to intra-hisian or infra-hisian block. If asymptomatic, these patients may need a diagnostic EP study to determine the site of block.

Another type of AV block requiring permanent pacing occurs after cardiac surgery. Aortic valve, mitral valve, and tricuspid valve surgery are all associated with the need for postoperative permanent pacing. Complete heart block or advanced AV block at any level can be seen. The reported incidence varies from 1% to 5%. Predictors of need for permanent pacing following cardiac surgery include multiple valve surgery, reoperation, prolonged pump time, preexisting bundle branch block, and preoperative rhythm other than sinus. It is appropriate to wait 3 to 5 postoperative days before implantation of a pacemaker. Despite this conservative observation period, later recovery of AV conduction has been observed, especially in patients with stable junctional rhythms at the time of implantation.

AV block or long sinus pauses during sleep in a patient with sleep disordered breathing is not an indication for PM implantation. These bradyarrhythmias should resolve after treatment of the sleep apnea. AV block during exercise is due to infra-nodal block and if it is not due to ischemia, a PM is indicated. Infiltrative diseases such as sarcoidosis or amyloidosis are progressive and even transient asymptomatic AV block should alert the clinician to the need for PM implantation or at the very least, close clinical follow-up.

Chronic bifascicular block (i.e., RBBB with left anterior fascicular block) reflects significant conduction system disease below the AV node. Unexplained syncope or symptoms suggestive of bradycardia justify pacemaker implantation. Incidental findings during EP study such as infra-hisian AV block during decremental pacing or HV interval greater than 100 ms are class IIa indications, irrespective of symptoms. An EP study is reasonable in patients with chronic bifascicular block and second degree type I AV block to further characterize the site of AV conduction delay. The incidental finding of asymptomatic "trifascicular block" (RBBB with left anterior fascicular block and prolonged PR interval) is not an indication for pacing.

The need for permanent PM implantation in the recovery phase of an acute myocardial infarction (AMI) is not necessarily related to the presence or absence of symptoms attributable to AV block. Furthermore, the requirement for temporary pacing in AMI does not by itself constitute an indication for permanent pacing. Alternating bundle branch block or second degree AV block associated with bundle branch block, with or without symptoms, is an ominous prognostic sign and permanent pacing is indicated. Consideration should be given to the location of the AMI. Heart block associated with an inferior wall MI is typically transient and does not usually require permanent pacing. Heart block associated with an anterior wall MI suggests extensive damage to the conduction system and permanent pacing is usually indicated.

INDICATIONS FOR PACING NOT RELATED TO SND OR AV BLOCK

There are several other conditions for which a permanent PM may be indicated. However, collectively these diagnoses represent a small fraction of the total number of pacemaker implants in the US. These diagnoses include neurocardiogenic syndrome, sleep apnea, carotid sinus hypersensitivity syndrome, neuromuscular disorders, and bradycardia in the transplanted heart.

Neuromuscular disorders such as myotonic dystrophy and Emery-Dreifuss muscular dystrophy are associated with an unpredictable progression to complete heart block. While second and third degree AV blocks are clear indications for pacing, pacemaker implantation may be considered in patients with first degree AV block, irrespective of the symptoms.

Sleep apnea syndrome is a very common respiratory disturbance occurring during sleep, especially in patients with CHF. Atrial overdrive pacing above the average baseline nocturnal heart rate has not consistently been shown to improve sleep apnea. Overdrive pacing as a treatment modality for sleep apnea is not an accepted indication for permanent pacing. However, both the obstructive and central forms are associated with significant bradyarrhythmias (sinus bradycardia, sinus arrest, and AV block) during sleep. There is a high degree of intrapatient and interpatient variability in the severity of nocturnal bradyarrhythmia. The main objective in the management of these patients is to treat the sleep apnea. If patients have persistent extreme (i.e., 10 s) asystole during sleep despite treatment with nasal continuous positive airway pressure, many clinicians would recommend permanent pacing.

Initial hemodynamic studies of pacing in patients with hypertrophic obstructive cardiomyopathy suggested a decrease in outflow gradient. Larger randomized clinical trials have failed to show improvement in quality of life or survival. Therefore, pacing to relieve the outflow gradient in medically refractory hypertrophic obstructive cardiomyopathy is a class IIb indication. Permanent pacing is indicated in these patients if it is needed only for standard bradycardia indications. The reader is referred to the guidelines for specific details.

INDICATIONS FOR INTERNAL CARDIOVERTER-DEFIBRILLATOR IMPLANTATION

Sudden cardiac death (SCD) is defined as death attributable to a cardiac cause that occurs soon after the onset of symptoms. This definition is more selective for arrhythmia related death when the time course is restricted to one hour from the onset of symptoms. Of course, other processes can lead to sudden death within less than an hour, including pulmonary embolism and AMI. Despite efforts to determine the cause of death, it cannot always be determined with certainty. Therefore, clinical trials have used total mortality as endpoints for evaluating the benefits of ICD therapy.

Indications for ICD implantation are divided into secondary prevention of cardiac arrest (or sustained VT) and primary prevention of SCD. Secondary and primary prevention indications are summarized in Table 10-4. A secondary prevention indication exists when a patient has survived an episode of sudden cardiac arrest or sustained VT. Primary prevention of SCD refers to the use of ICDs in individuals who are at risk for but have not yet had an episode of sustained VT, VF, or resuscitated cardiac arrest.

The results of the major secondary prevention trials (cardiac arrest or spontaneous sustained VT) are summarized in Table 10-5. Patients who have unexplained syncope and inducible sustained VT during EP study are likely to have had a significant ventricular arrhythmia leading to syncope (aborted cardiac arrest). Therefore, patients who have inducible VT during an EP study may be grouped with those patients with secondary prevention indication because they risk stratify to a higher risk group than those without

TABLE 10-4 Primary and Secondary Prevention Indications for ICD

Class I

1. Resuscitated cardiac arrest due to VF or hemodynamically unstable VT
2. Sustained VT and structural heart disease
3. Unexplained syncope and sustained VT or VF induced during EP study
4. Prior MI (at least 40 days prior) EF < 35%, and NYHA class II and III CHF or prior MI, EF < 30% and NHYA class I CHF
5. Nonischemic dilated CMP, EF ≤ 35%, and NYHA class II and III CHF
6. NSVT, prior MI, EF < 40%, inducible VT or VF during EP study

Class IIa

1. Unexplained syncope, dilated cardiomyopathy, and significant LV dysfunction
2. Sustained VT, normal or near-normal LV function
3. Hypertrophic cardiomyopathy and one or more major risk factors for SCD
4. Arrhythmogenic right ventricular dysplasia/cardiomyopathy (ARVD/C) and one or more risks factors for SCD
5. LQTS or CPVT associated with syncope or VT while receiving beta-blockers
6. Brugada syndrome associated with syncope or documented VT
7. Nonhospitalized patients awaiting cardiac transplantation
8. Patients with cardiac sarcoidosis, giant cell myocarditis, or Chagas disease

Class IIb

1. Nonischemic CMP, EF ≤ 35%, and NYHA Class I CHF
2. Unexplained syncope and advanced structural heart disease, when no cause of syncope can be determined
3. LQTS and risk factors for SCD but no history of syncope or VT
4. Familial cardiomyopathy associated with sudden death
5. Patients with LV noncompaction

Class III: see text

CMP, cardiomyopathy; LQTS, Long QT syndrome.

TABLE 10-5 Secondary Prevention ICD Trials

Trial (year)	Patients (*n*)	Inclusion Criteria	Design	Results
Multicenter Automatic Defibrillator Implantation Trial (MADIT). *N Engl J Med.* 1996;335(26):1933–1940.	196	**EF ≤ 0.35**, NYHA class I–III, spontaneous NSVT and **inducible VT**	All-cause mortality comparing ICD vs. medical therapy	56% relative risk reduction with ICD
Multicenter Unsustained Tachycardia Trial (MUSTT). *N Engl J Med.* 1999 Dec 16; 341(25):1882–1890.	704	**EF < 0.40**, NYHA class I–III, nonrecent MI, spontaneous NSVT and **inducible VT**	Cardiac arrest or death from arrhythmia comparing ICD vs. antiarrhythmic drug (AAD)	76% relative reduction with ICD in primary endpoint
Cardiac Arrest Study Hamburg (CASH). *Am Heart J.* 1994 Apr;127 (4 Pt 2):1139–1144.	191	Cardiac arrest due to VF or VT, no reversible cause	All-cause mortality comparing ICD vs. medical therapy	23% relative risk reduction with ICD in primary endpoint
Canadian Implantable Defibrillator Study (CIDS). *Circulation.* 2000 Mar 21;101(11):1297–1302.	659	VF, sustained VT and syncope, sustained VT and **EF ≤ 0.35**, syncope with inducible VT, no reversible causes	All-cause mortality comparing ICD vs. amiodarone	20% relative risk reduction with ICD in primary endpoint
Antiarrhthymics vs. Implantable Defibrillators (AVID). *N Engl J Med.* 1997 Nov 27; 337(22):1576–1583.	1,016	VF, sustained VT and syncope, sustained VT with **EF ≤ 0.40** and severe symptoms, no reversible causes	All-cause mortality comparing ICD vs. AAD	31% relative risk reduction with ICD in primary endpoint

inducible VT. Overall, secondary prevention trials demonstrate significant (as much as 50%) and consistent relative risk reduction with ICD therapy over medical management.

When considering a secondary prevention indication, reversible causes of cardiac arrest or VF should be evaluated. Careful clinical judgment is needed before attributing a cardiac arrest to a reversible cause and thus withholding ICD therapy. Electrolyte abnormalities are occasionally seen in patients who survive a cardiac arrest. Unless these abnormalities are exceptional in magnitude (i.e., severe hyperkalemia) and are the sole reason for cardiac arrest, these patients should be treated as patients with VT or VF who do not have electrolyte abnormalities. Likewise, patients who have VT or VF and who are coincidently on antiarrhythmic drugs should receive an ICD unless the arrest is clearly directly due to a toxicity of that antiarrhythmic medication (i.e., flecainide toxicity). Sustained monomorphic VT in patients with prior MI is rarely due to an acute ischemic event. Rather, it is typically due to reentry related to prior myocardial scar. Minor elevations in cardiac biomarkers should not be interpreted as an acute coronary syndrome that caused the VT or VF. Clinically, such patients often undergo cardiac catheterization and percutaneous coronary intervention (PCI) to vessels with significant but noncritical lesions. ICD implantation should not be delayed if these patients had preexisting myocardial infarctions or LV dysfunction. Patients who are resuscitated from VF in the context of an acute ischemic event and undergo emergent revascularization represent a unique challenge. Data suggest that revascularization alone may be adequate therapy in patients with a normal EF and no prior myocardial infarction. Finally, decompensated CHF may present with VT or VF and elevated biomarkers. An ICD should be implanted after management of the heart failure.

Patients with no prior cardiac history who present with VT or VF should undergo a standard cardiovascular workup as well as other relevant medical evaluation. Workup should include a complete 2D echocardiogram and an ischemic evaluation including cardiac catheterization in appropriate cases. In select patients, it may be appropriate to perform a diagnostic EP study or cardiac MRI or both. Genetic testing is not necessary to establish the diagnosis of a suspected channelopathy. An ICD should be implanted for these patients if a secondary prevention indication exists.

The clinical trials for primary prevention ICD implantation are summarized in Table 10-6. Left ventricular ejection fraction (LVEF) is the primary means to risk stratify patients to determine who should receive an ICD. It is noteworthy that the specific degree of LV dysfunction needed to qualify for an ICD (30% vs. 35%) varies based on clinical heart failure class. Given that there is no "gold standard" for determining LVEF, it is important to use all the data available. A given patient may have more than one assessment of LVEF during the course of an evaluation. Undue emphasis should not be placed on a single measurement, especially if it is not consistent with other available studies. Although the relative risk reduction is less than secondary prevention indications, a significant benefit exists to justify recommendation of an ICD to this relatively large patient population group. In total, the number of patients that need to receive an ICD to save one life is between 13 and 17 patients over a time of 3 years. This means that a large number of patients will receive no mortality benefit from an ICD.

When considering a patient for a primary prevention indication, it is important to define the nature of the structural heart disease as well as associated comorbid conditions. A comprehensive but targeted evaluation should be performed to identify treatable causes of a cardiomyopathy. Some form of ischemic workup is needed in all patients with risk factors for coronary artery disease. A cardiac MRI or right ventriculogram may be needed to diagnose arrhythmogenic RV cardiomyopathy. Genetic testing is available for the diagnosis of channelopathies such as long QT syndrome, Brugada syndrome, or catecholeminergic polymorphic VT (CPVT). Genetic testing is expensive and a negative test does not exclude a channelopathy. Therefore, these tests are not widely utilized. A diagnostic EP study with procainamide infusion can be helpful in suspected cases of Brugada Syndrome. Patients with coronary disease and prior MI are the largest subgroup who

TABLE 10-6 Primary Prevention ICD Trials

Trial (year)	Patients (*n*)	Inclusion Criteria	Design	Results
Second Multicenter Automatic Defibrillator Implantation Trial (MADIT-II). Prophylactic implantation of a defibrillator in patients with myocardial infarction and reduced ejection fraction. *N Engl J Med.* 2002;346:877–883.	1232	Remote MI, **EF < 0.30**, NYHA class I–III	All-cause mortality ICD vs. best medical therapy	31% relative reduction in primary endpoint
Amiodarone vs. Implantable Cardioverter Defibrillator Trial (AMIOVIRT). *J Am Coll Cardiol.* 2003;41(10):1707–1712.	103	Dilated cardiomyopathy, **EF ≤ 0.35**, NYHA class I–IV, NSVT	All-cause mortality ICD vs. medical therapy	No significant benefit to ICD
Cardiomyopathy Trial (CAT). *Circulation.* 2002;105(12):1453–1458.	104	Dilated cardiomyopathy, recent onset heart failure (<9 months), **EF ≤ 0.30**, NYHA class II and III	All-cause mortality ICD vs. medical therapy	No significant benefit to ICD
Sudden Cardiac Death Heart Failure Trial (SCD-HeFT). *N Engl J Med.* 2005;352(*3*):225–237.	1676	NYHA class II and III, **EF ≤ 0.35**, nonrecent MI, not recent onset heart failure	All-cause mortality, ICD vs. amiodarone	23% relative risk reduction with ICD
Defibrillators in nonischemic Cardiomyopathy Treatment Evaluation (DEFINITE). *N Engl J Med.* 2004;350(21):2151–2158.	458	NYHA class I–III, **EF ≤ 0.35**, dilated cardiomyopathy, NSVT, or ≥10 PVCs/h	All-cause mortality, ICD vs. medical therapy	35% relative reduction with ICD
Defibrillator in Acute Myocardial Infarction Trial (DINAMIT). *N Engl J Med.* 2004;351:2481–2488.	674	NYHA class I–III, **EF ≤ 0.35**, MI with 6–40 days, impaired heart rate variability	All-cause mortality, ICD vs. medical therapy	No difference in all-cause mortality, lower risk of arrhythmic death in ICD group

may have an indication for an ICD. Patients should be on stable and optimal medical therapy prior to ICD implantation. Medical therapy, including beta-blockers and ACE inhibitors (assuming no contraindications), should be titrated appropriate doses and LV function should be reevaluated after a reasonable period of time (90 days). The requisite duration of this therapy prior to ICD implantation is no longer specified in the guidelines. However, the early implantation of prophylactic ICD within 6 to 40 days of an MI, even in high-risk patients is not recommended. The DINAMIT (Defibrillator in Acute Myocardial Infarction Trial) study is a randomized trial that compared patients that received an ICD within 6 to 40 days of an MI to those receiving optimal medical management only. Both groups received excellent medical therapy. As expected, the risk of arrhythmia related death was significantly lower in the ICD group compared to the medical therapy group. However, the ICD group had a higher risk of nonarrhythmia related death. Overall mortality between the two groups was the same. Therefore, a prophylactic ICD should be delayed at least 40 days post-MI in patients who otherwise meet the guidelines. Except in the case of a recent MI, the duration of waiting ("blanking") periods are not specified in the current guidelines. However, the timing of a prophylactic ICD relative to revascularization is still an important consideration. It is still common practice to wait at least 40 days post-PCI and 90 days post-CABG before implantation of an ICD. A repeat assessment of LV function may be indicated if an improvement is expected after revascularization.

Previous versions of the guidelines recommended a waiting period of 9 months before implantation of a prophylactic ICD in patients with dilated, nonischemic cardiomyopathy. Patients with nonischemic DCM experience equivalent rates of life-threatening arrhythmias regardless of the diagnosis duration. In fact, data from the DEFINITE study showed that patients with a recent diagnosis of DCM benefited equally from an ICD as those with a remote diagnosis. The requisite duration of optimal medical therapy to determine its impact on LV function is unknown. Even though there is no "blanking" period specified by the current guidelines in terms of prophylactic ICD placement in DCM patients, it is also reasonable to wait 3 months. This is the same waiting period recommended before placement of a CRT device (see below). The clinician should exercise caution when delaying the recommendation of a prophylactic ICD, especially in patients who develop heart failure and LV dysfunction despite already receiving appropriate medical therapy.

The potential population eligible for a primary prevention ICD is very large. This is particularly important when the impact of inappropriate shocks is considered. There is a 10% to 24% chance of receiving an inappropriate shock. This includes shocks for non–life-threatening arrhythmias such as AF with a rapid ventricular response, shocks related to electromagnetic interference, or shocks due to myopotential oversensing. ICD shocks have been shown to have an adverse effect on the quality of life. Although rare, the triggering to fatal VF from an inappropriate shock has been reported. Patients with severe psychiatric illness or advanced dementia that prevents them from understanding the nature of ICD therapy are not candidates for ICD therapy.

It is also important to recognize when a primary prevention ICD is unlikely to improve mortality or when an ICD should not be implanted. The challenge to the clinician is to identify and consider the impact of comorbid conditions (end-stage kidney disease, severe COPD, pulmonary hypertension, NYHA IV heart failure, malignancy, etc.) and advanced age on the potential mortality benefit of an ICD. Patients with comorbid conditions associated with expected survival less than 1 year are not likely to benefit from a primary prevention ICD. Patients with class IV inotrope dependent CHF who are not candidates for transplantation should probably not receive an ICD. However, patients who have ambulatory class IV heart failure and are receiving a chronic ionotrope infusion as a bridge to transplant are suitable candidates for ICD implantations. Incessant VT or VF should first be controlled with antiarrhythmic drugs prior to ICD implantation. An electrical storm (clustering of hemodynamically destabilizing VT or VF, requiring multiple cardioversions or defibrillations within 24 to 48 h) is a contraindication to ICD implantation. VT may occur in the complete absence of structural heart disease or channelopathy and is referred to as idiopathic VT. These forms of VT include RV outflow tract VT, LV outflow tract VT (including noncoronary cusp VT), and fascicular VT (Belhassen VT) and are more appropriately treated pharmacologically or with catheter or surgical ablation, rather than an ICD. VF associated with rapidly conducted AF in a patient with Wolff-Parkinson-White syndrome is not an indication for ICD implantation. Catheter ablation of the accessory pathway is indicated.

CARDIAC RESYNCHRONIZATION THERAPY

As mortality rates for ischemic and nonischemic cardiomyopathy have declined, there is large and expanding population of patients with chronic CHF. An estimated 800,000 patients have advanced symptomatic heart failure (NYHA III or IV). Dilated cardiomyopathy, and to a lesser extent, ischemic cardiomyopathy, is associated with a disruption of electromechanical events. The most important electromechanical events of the cardiac cycle are characterized by the following: interatrial synchrony, AV synchrony, intraventricular synchrony, and interventricular synchrony. To varying degrees, each of these parameters is impaired in patients with cardiomyopathy. The term synchrony should not be taken to mean simultaneous, but rather, sequential. For example, LV mechanical events normally precede RV events. In the presence of a left bundle branch block (LBBB), the RV is preexcited relative to the LV, contributing to the reduction of global cardiac output. LBBB is also associated with dyssychronous contraction of the LV. It is this LV dyssynchrony that usually has the largest impact on cardiac output in patients with systolic dysfunction. There is no universally accepted definition of dyssynchrony and there is no single, universally accepted marker to identify or quantify dyssynchrony. Given that mechanical dyssynchrony measures have not proven useful, we now rely on electrical dyssynchrony measured by QRS duration as a surrogate for mechanical dyssynchrony.

CRT, also termed titrated pacing, has emerged as an important treatment modality in select patients with advanced CHF and LV dyssynchrony. Extensive clinical trial data shows that CRT improves acute and chronic hemodynamic function, quality of life, heart failure class, exercise tolerance, heart failure hospitalization, and mortality. In addition to clinical outcomes, CRT has been shown to result in remodeling of the ventricle, reducing mitral regurgitation, reducing chamber sizes, and improving LVEF.

Patients with a LVEF of less than 35%, QRS duration of more than 120 ms, and NYHA class III heart failure should be considered for a CRT device. Because CRT is an adjunctive therapy for the management of select patients with symptomatic heart failure, patients should be on stable medical therapy for at least 90 days. Optimal medical therapy may vary from patient to patient but should include ACE inhibitors and beta-blockers. In patients with the first presentation of decompensated heart failure, clinical heart failure class should be reassessed when a euvolemic state has been reached. Although the CARE-HF Trial demonstrated a significant reduction in mortality with CRT-P without the backup of a defibrillator, most patients who receive a CRT device receive a CRT-D.

The benefits of CRT are primarily affected through LV preexcitation and optimization of AV timing. With careful patient selection, the response rate to CRT is about 70%. To date, the presence of a LBBB seems to be the most practical means of identifying patients with LV dyssynchrony. Not all patients with a LBBB have significant LV dyssynchrony. Although baseline QRS duration is only moderately predictive of response, a QRS duration more than 150 ms is associated with a better response rate. Echocardiographic markers of dyssynchrony have proven difficult to reproducibly apply to identify those likely to have clinical response to CRT.

The current indications for a CRT device apply to a relatively select subgroup within the larger population of patients with moderate to severe heart failure. Many patients have class III CHF but not a LBBB. In patients with a relatively narrow QRS duration, the use of echocardiographic parameters to identify LV dyssynchrony in order to predict clinical response has been disappointing. There are also a large number of patients with class I or II CHF and LBBB whose progression to more severe stages of heart failure may be delayed with the use of CRT. Clinical trials testing this hypothesis are underway. The guidelines specify QRS duration but not the form of intraventricular conduction delay. However, the response rate to CRT in patients with a right bundle branch block (RBBB) or nonspecific IVCD is less than in patients with a LBBB. The presence of a left anterior fascicular block with a RBBB is associated with a better response rate than RBBB alone. The presence of AF or atrial flutter is associated with a lower response rate.

SUMMARY

Device therapy for the management of patients with cardiac rhythm disorders can have a major impact on morbidity and mortality. Just as with pharmacologic therapies, careful patient selection and device selection are needed to prevent the potentially adverse effects of these devices. In patient receiving a pacemaker, thoughtful programming and follow-up is needed to minimize ventricular pacing. In patients receiving ICDs, the greatest challenge is to minimize inappropriate shocks. Ongoing clinical research seeks to more specifically identify patients that should receive primary prevention ICDs. Similarly, clinical research in the area of CRT seeks to identify predictors for the nonresponder. Indications for device therapy are likely to expand. The challenge for the clinician is to identify the appropriate patients to receive these devices.

KEY POINTS

1. Indications for pacing are based primarily by presence of symptomatic bradycardia. It is therefore important to establish a correlation between symptoms such as fatigue, exercise intolerance and syncope, and rhythm. Symptomatic bradycardia is a class I indication for pacing in both sinus node dysfunction and acquired AV block.
2. Pacing to facilitate medical management of atrial fibrillation or to support the use of essential medications is an important indication for permanent pacemaker implantation.
3. Optimal pacemaker or ICD programming should promote intrinsic ventricular conduction and minimize right ventricular pacing.
4. An ICD is indicated (secondary prevention) when a patient has sustained VT or a ventricular fibrillation arrest in the absence of reversible causes. A "reversible cause" should be carefully distinguished from incidental abnormal findings such as electrolyte abnormalities or elevated cardiac biomarkers not associated with a critical coronary lesion.
5. Co-morbid conditions that limit prognosis to less than 1 year are a contraindication to ICD implantation for either primary or secondary prevention indications.
6. The current guidelines define relatively small fraction of heart failure patients who are likely to benefit from CRT devices. Markers of dyssynchrony other than QRS > 130 have yet not proven to useful for indentifying potential responders.

SUGGESTED READINGS

Guidelines

ACC/AHA/ESC 2006 Guidelines for the management of patient with ventricular arrhythmias and the prevention of sudden cardiac death. *J Am Coll Cardiol.* 2006;48:e247–e346.

ACC/AHA/HRS 2008 Guidelines for device-based therapy of cardiac rhythm abnormalities. *J Am Coll Cardiol.* 2008;51:e1–e62.

ESC Guidelines: Guidelines for cardiac pacing and cardiac resynchronization therapy. *Europace.* 2007;9: 959–998.

Clinical trials and review articles: Pacing

DAVID: Dual-chamber pacing or ventricular backup pacing in patients with an implantable defibrillator: The Dual Chamber and VVI Implantable Defibrillator (DAVID) Trial. *JAMA.* 2002;288(24):3115–3123.

MOST: Adverse effect of ventricular pacing on heart failure and atrial fibrillation among patients with normal baseline QRS duration in a clinical trial of pacemaker therapy for sinus node dysfunction. *Circulation.* 2003;107:2932–2937.

Review: Device-based therapies for atrial fibrillation. *Curr Treat Options Cardiovasc Med.* 2005;7:359–370.

SAVEPACe: Minimizing ventricular pacing to reduce Atrial Fibrillation in Sinus-Node Disease: The Search AV Extension and Managed Ventricular Pacing for Promoting Atrioventricular Conduction (SAVE PACe) Trial. *N Engl J Med.* 2007;357(10):1000–1008.

UKPACE: The United Kingdom Pacing and Cardiovascular Events Trial [UK Pacing Clin Electrophysiol]. *Heart.* 1997;78:221–223.

Clinical trials: ICD therapy

AVID: A comparison of antiarrhythmic-drug therapy with implantable defibrillators in patients resuscitated from near-fatal ventricular arrhythmias. The Antiarrhythmics versus Implantable Defibrillators (AVID) Investigators. *N Engl J Med.* 1997;337(22):1576–1583.

DEFINITE: Prophylactic defibrillator implantation in patients with nonischemic dilated cardiomyopathy. *N Engl J Med.* 2004;350(21):2151–2158.

DINAMIT: Prophylactic use of an implantable cardioverter-defibrillator after acute myocardial infarction. *N Engl J Med.* 2004;351:2481–2488.

MADIT: Improved survival with an implanted defibrillator in patients with coronary disease at high risk for ventricular arrhythmia. Multicenter Automatic Defibrillator Implantation Trial Investigators. *N Engl J Med.* 1996;335(26):1933–1940.

MADIT II: Prophylactic implantation of a defibrillator in patients with myocardial infarction and reduced ejection fraction. *N Engl J Med.* 2002;346:877–883.

Review: Implantable cardioverter-defibrillators after myocardial infarction. *N Engl J Med.* 2008;359: 2245–2253.

SCD-HeFT: Amiodarone or an implantable cardioverter-defibrillator for congestive heart failure. *N Engl J Med.* 2005;352(3):225–237.

Clinical trials and review articles: CRT

CARE-HF: The effect of cardiac resynchronization on morbidity and mortality in heart failure. *N Engl J Med.* 2005;352:1539–1549.

Cardiac resynchronization therapy and death from progressive heart failure: A metaanalysis of randomized control trials. *JAMA.* 2003;289:730–740.

PROSPECT: Results of the predictors of response to CRT trial. *Circulation.* 2008;117:2608–2616.

ReTHINQ: Cardiac-resynchronization therapy in heart failure with narrow QRS complexes. *N Engl J Med.* 2007;357(24):2461–2471.

Review: Cardiac resynchronization therapy: Past, present and future. *Rev Cardiovasc Med.* 2007;89(2):69–77.

CHAPTER 11

Miscellaneous Procedures

Aysha Arshad and Suneet Mittal

Various noninvasive monitoring tools are available to the cardiologist for the evaluation of patients with symptoms suggestive of an arrhythmia. These include ambulatory ECG recording systems designed to "capture" arrhythmias and various tools for the risk stratification of patients possibly at risk for sudden death. In addition, all trainees in Cardiology need to be familiar with commonly performed procedures such as electrical cardioversion, tilt table tests, and temporary venous pacemaker insertion. In fact, the most recent ACCF COCATS training statement stipulates the need to perform at least ten temporary pacemaker insertions and ten electrical cardioversions during the course of training. The aim of this chapter is to review the appropriate indications and techniques for these "miscellaneous" procedures.

NONINVASIVE MONITORING TOOLS

Several tools are now available for the outpatient evaluation of patients with intermittent symptoms (e.g., palpitations, dizziness, and syncope) suggestive of an arrhythmia and to gauge the efficacy of therapeutic interventions, such as institution of antiarrhythmic drug therapy and catheter ablation. In this chapter, we will explore some of these tools in greater detail. In the end, the clinical indication, frequency and duration of symptoms, underlying substrate, the patient's ability to participate in either transmitting or recording events, and cost are important considerations toward making a final choice (Table 11-1).

HOLTER MONITORING

The Holter monitor is the prototypical continuous electrocardiographic monitor and the one most commonly utilized in clinical practice. The device is battery operated, is connected to bipolar electrodes that allow the recording of two and up to five different leads (although some current systems allow for recording of all 12 leads), and provides continuous electrocardiographic data for 24 to 48 h. Data are recorded onto a microcassette, magnetic tape cassette, or compact disc, converted to a digital format, and analyzed using software that helps identify abnormalities in heart rhythm, including trends in heart rate. Recorders use patient-activated event markers and time markers to allow for a symptom-rhythm correlation. Holters are simple to place and use and require minimal patient participation. They are excellent for assessing heart rate trend and for quantifying the burden of atrial and ventricular ectopy. However, the short recording period usually precludes making a definitive diagnosis in patients in whom symptoms occur only intermittently.

TRANSTELEPHONIC ELECTROCARDIOGRAPHIC MONITORING

Transtelephonic electrocardiographic monitoring is useful when more than 1 to 2 days of monitoring are necessary in a given patient. Acquired data are transmitted to a central monitoring system from where they can be made available to the physician via either

TABLE 11-1 Options for Remote Monitoring: A Continuum

Holter Monitoring	Event Monitoring	Outpatient Telemetry	Implantable Loop Recorder	Hospital Inpatient Telemetry
Patients are likely to experience frequent (daily) events When real-time, heartbeat by heartbeat analysis is not required When results reporting within 3–5 days is acceptable	Patients are likely to experience infrequent, symptomatic events Patients are able to detect, transmit, and report events When stat MD reporting may be required	Patients are likely to experience infrequent, symptomatic or asymptomatic events When patients may have difficulty activating devices When real-time heartbeat by heartbeat analysis may be required When stat MD reporting may be required	Patients are likely to experience very infrequent, symptomatic or asymptomatic events Patients are able to visit physician's office for analysis When stat MD reporting is not required	Patients who require acute care When real-time, heartbeat by heartbeat analysis may be required When stat MD reporting may be required

fax or Internet. There are two distinct types of monitors available. Postsymptom event monitors do not require the patient to wear chest electrodes. These devices can either be carried by the patient (and applied to the chest when a symptom occurs) or worn on the wrist. When a symptom occurs, the patient presses a button to trigger storage of an electrocardiographic recording. This type of system is most useful in a patient who has intermittent symptoms that are sustained (allowing the patient time to apply and activate the monitor) and not associated with loss of consciousness. In contrast, presymptom event monitors ("loop recorders") require the patient to wear chest electrodes, usually for up to 30 days. These devices store an electrocardiographic recording as part of an ongoing rolling buffer. When the device is activated by the patient, a 1- to 2-lead electrocardiographic tracing is "saved," usually consisting of a few minutes of data preactivation and about a minute postactivation. The major limitation of loop recorders is the ability to capture data only on symptomatic arrhythmias. As a result, loop monitors have largely been replaced by mobile cardiac outpatient telemetry monitoring systems.

MOBILE CARDIAC OUTPATIENT TELEMETRY MONITORING

Mobile cardiac outpatient telemetry monitoring systems utilize cardiac event monitors with extended memory, which provide continuous electrocardiographic data over several days to weeks. The data obtained is similar to that obtained with hospital-based in-patient telemetry systems. These systems couple an automatic arrhythmia detector with cellular telephone transmission technology so that all electrocardiographic data are automatically and continuously transmitted to a centralized monitoring center. The physician is notified immediately if the patient develops an arrhythmia that meets physician-defined notification criteria. A daily report is provided to the physician, even in the absence of an arrhythmia. A major strength of these systems is the ability to capture information on both symptomatic and asymptomatic arrhythmias, which makes them superior to standard loop recorders.

Another reason for noninvasive monitoring is to risk stratify patients deemed at potential high risk for sudden cardiac death. The most commonly used tests are the signal-averaged electrocardiogram (SAECG), heart rate variability (HRV), and T wave alternans (TWA) testing. Unfortunately, to date, none has been conclusively shown to be able to identify high-risk patients among a cohort with left ventricular dysfunction.

SIGNAL-AVERAGED ELECTROCARDIOGRAM

The SAECG detects "late potentials" which represent areas of delayed myocardial activation and represent a substrate for reentrant ventricular arrhythmias. During this test, an ECG is recorded using a standard bipolar X, Y, and Z lead system. The X lead is positioned at the fourth intercostal space in both midaxillary lines; the Y lead is positioned on the superior aspect of the manubrium and on the left iliac crest; the Z lead is positioned at the fourth intercostal space, with the second electrode directly posterior on the left side of the vertebral column.

Signal averaging to reduce noise allows high gain amplification and filtering to expose these late potentials on the surface ECG. More than 200 beats are typically averaged to obtain a noise level of less than 0.3 μV (mean, 0.22 μV) at 40 Hz. There are three forms of noise encountered in high-resolution electrocardiographic studies: the noise inherent within electronic instrumentation, power line interference, and physiologic noise originating from chest wall muscles (electromyographic noise). Averaging high number beats mitigates the influence of noise on the test results, because noise has a nonconsistent relationship to the physiologic cardiac signal.

The SAECG is most commonly interpreted using time-domain analysis, which is performed using a high-pass bidirectional (Butterworth) filter (most commonly at 40 Hz)

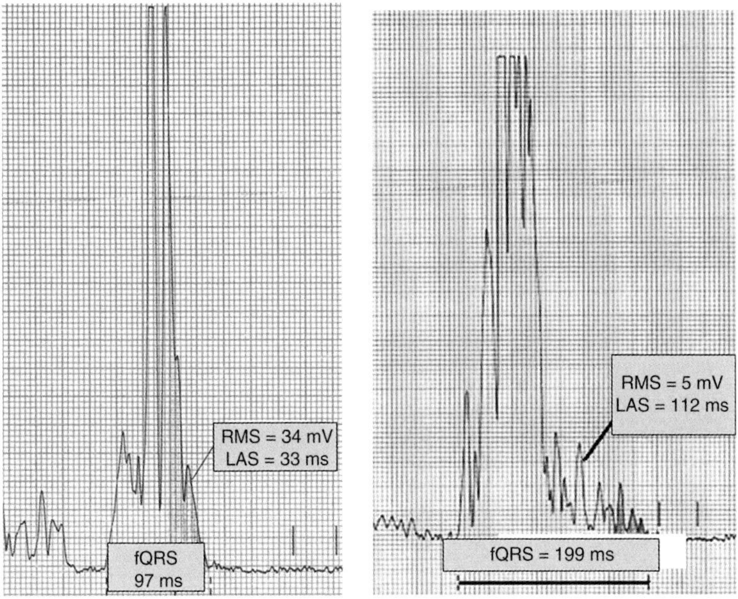

FIGURE 11-1. Signal-averaged ECG (SAECG). **Left:** Normal SAECG. **Right:** Abnormal SAECG. See text for discussion.

and a low-pass frequency of 250 Hz. Three standardized indexes are computed: the duration of the total filtered QRS (fQRS) complex, the duration of the low-amplitude signal (LAS) after the voltage decreases to ≤40 μV, and the root-mean-square (RMS) of the amplitude of signals in the last 40 ms of the fQRS complex. Late potentials are considered to be present if any two of the following three criteria are met: (i) fQRS greater than 114 ms, (ii) LAS greater than 38 ms, or (iii) RMS less than 20 μV (Fig. 11-1).

Not surprisingly, the data for using SAECG are strongest for patients with underlying ischemic heart disease who have previously suffered a myocardial infarction. Nonetheless, this is an infrequently used test as current practice guidelines do not recommend incorporating the test results in the decision to pursue either electrophysiologic testing or implantation of a cardioverter-defibrillator (ICD). However, the test is currently a diagnostic component of the Task Force criteria on arrhythmogenic right ventricular dysplasia/cardiomyopathy.

HEART RATE VARIABILITY

HRV refers to the beat-to-beat alterations in heart rate. Under resting conditions, healthy individuals exhibit periodic variation in RR intervals. This rhythmic phenomenon, known as respiratory sinus arrhythmia (RSA), fluctuates with the phase of respiration—cardioacceleration during inspiration and cardiodeceleration during expiration. RSA is predominantly mediated by respiratory gating of parasympathetic efferent activity to the heart. Reduced HRV has been used as a marker of reduced vagal activity. To date, over 26 different types of arithmetic manipulations of RR intervals have been used in the literature to represent HRV. Over half a dozen prospective studies have shown that reduced HRV predicts sudden arrhythmic death in patients postmyocardial infraction, independent of other prognostic indicators including ejection fraction. Additionally, a small number of studies also suggest that reduced HRV also predicts survival in patients without ischemic heart disease, especially in patients with congestive heart failure.

HRV can be analyzed using either time-domain or frequency-domain methods. A commonly used measurement of HRV, termed the SDNN, is the standard deviation of all normal RR intervals (those measured between consecutive sinus beats). The SDNN may be easily calculated from a 24-h Holter monitor. In calculating SDNN, any RR interval that begins or ends with a PAC or PVC is simply deleted from the calculation. SDNN is typically measured over 24 h and reported in units of milliseconds. Two variants of the SDNN, created by dividing the 24-h monitoring period into 5-min segments, are the *SDNN index* and the *SDANN index*. The SDNN index is the mean of all the 5-min standard deviations of NN (normal RR) intervals during the 24-h period (i.e., the mean of 288 NN standard deviations), while the SDANN index is the standard deviation of all the 5-min NN interval means (i.e., the standard deviation of 288 NN means). Other noteworthy time-domain indices are the *r-MSSD* and the *pNN50*. The r-MSSD, or the RMS successive difference, calculates the square root of the mean of the squared differences between successive NN intervals over 24 h. The pNN50 calculates the percentage of differences between successive NN intervals over 24 h that are greater than 50 ms. Both of these indices measure short-term variation in the NN interval because they are entirely based on comparisons between successive beats. All these HRV indices are time-domain measures because they are based on a time series of normal RR intervals.

On the other hand, frequency-domain analysis is performed by taking a series of numbers along a time axis and computing the fast Fourier transform. This yields a set of frequency-domain indices by partitioning the heart rate variance into spectral components and quantifying their power. The following indices are calculated: ultra low frequency ($1.15 \times 10 - 5$ to 0.00335 Hz), which reflects circadian and other long-term variations in heart rhythm; very low frequency power (0.0033 to 0.04 Hz), which in addition to sympathetic and parasympathetic inputs, may be influenced by the thermoregulatory, peripheral vasomotor, and renin-angiotensin systems; low-frequency power (0.04 to 0.15 Hz), which reflects largely sympathetic tone; and high-frequency power (0.15 to 0.45 Hz), which is modulated by respiration and in healthy subjects primarily reflects vagal tone.

The UK-Heart study prospectively assessed a cohort of patients with chronic heart failure. This prospective study followed up 433 outpatients (62 ± 10 years of age) with NYHA class I to III congestive heart failure, and an ejection fraction of 41% ± 17%. Time-domain indices of HRV and conventional prognostic indicators were related to death by multivariate analysis. During 482 ± 161 days of follow-up, the risk ratio for a 41.2-ms decrease in SDNN was 1.62 (95% CI: 1.16 to 2.44). The annual mortality rate for the study population was 5.5% for a SDNN greater than 100 ms, 12.7% for a SDNN 50 to 100 ms, and 51.4% for a SDNN less than 50 ms. The SDNN, serum creatinine, and serum sodium were related to progressive heart failure and death. The cardiothoracic ratio, left ventricular end-diastolic diameter, the presence of nonsustained ventricular tachycardia, and serum potassium were related to sudden cardiac death. A reduction in SDNN was the most powerful predictor of the risk of death due to progressive heart failure (Fig. 11-2). Similarly, the Autonomic Tone and Reflexes After MI (ATRAMI) study assessed the impact of HRV in post-MI patients and found a 3.2-fold higher mortality in patients with reduced HRV.

It has been shown that smoking cessation, beta-blockers, angiotensin converting enzyme (ACE) inhibitors, and cardiac resynchronization devices all improve HRV. In fact, many ICDs now report information on HRV. Unfortunately, there are no data on the use of HRV to identify candidates for ICD implantation. The DINAMIT study enrolled 675 patients within 40 days of myocardial infraction if they had an EF ≤ 35% and low HRV (or elevated heart rate). Patients were randomized to receive an ICD or no ICD in conjunction with optimal medical therapy. No improvement in overall survival

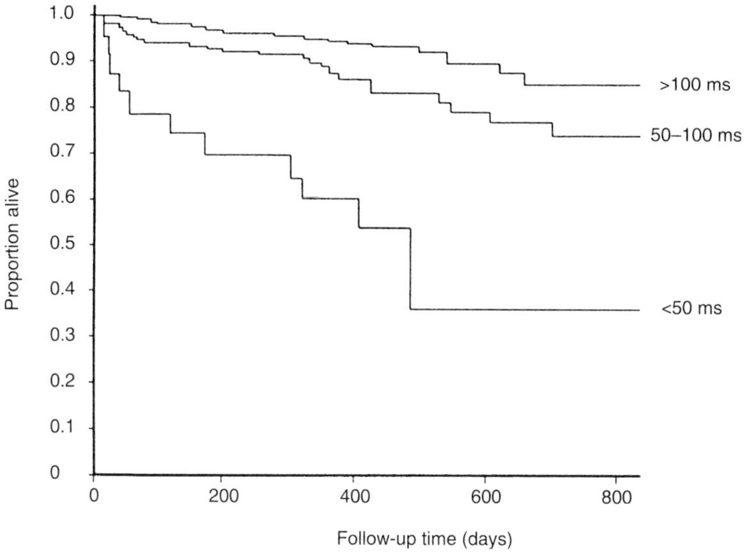

FIGURE 11-2. HRV and mortality in chronic heart failure (UK-Heart). Kaplan-Meier survival curves in patients categorized into SDNN subgroups. $p < 0.0001$ for difference in survival. (Reproduced from Nolan J, et al. Prospective study of heart rate variability and morality in chronic heart failure: Results of the United Kingdom heart failure evaluation and assessment of risk (UK-Heart). *Circulation.* 1998;98:1510–1516, with permission.)

was associated with ICD implantation. Therefore, there are limited reasons to incorporate HRV into routine clinical decision making.

T WAVE ALTERNANS TESTING

TWA refers to the beat-to-beat variability in the T wave amplitude. Macroscopic TWA, which is observed rarely, has long been associated with very high short-term arrhythmic mortality. More recently, there has been considerable interest in the detection of microvolt T wave alternans (MTWA) and its utility as a noninvasive marker to identify patients at high risk of sudden death. MTWA testing is performed by placing high-resolution electrodes, designed to reduce electrical interference, on a patient's chest prior to a period of controlled exercise. These electrodes detect tiny beat-to-beat changes, on the order of one-millionth of a volt, in the amplitude of the T wave (Fig. 11-3). Two methods currently exist to perform MTWA testing—the spectral analytic and the modified moving average methods. All available clinical data have been derived from studies using the spectral analytic method (Table 11-2). Currently available data do not support the use of TWA for risk stratification in patients with an ischemic cardiomyopathy. It may be useful in patients with nonischemic cardiomyopathy by identifying patients at extremely low risk for ventricular arrhythmias; however, more data are needed in this patient population.

HEART RATE TURBULENCE

The term heart rate turbulence (HRT) describes short-term fluctuations in sinus cycle length that follow spontaneous ventricular premature complexes (VPCs). In normal subjects, the sinus rate initially briefly accelerates and subsequently decelerates compared with the pre-VPC

TABLE 11-2 Prospective Trials of MTWA Testing

Study	Year	Study Cohort	Patients (*n*)	Mean follow-up	Primary endpoint	MTWA non-negative	MTWA negative	HR	*p*-Value
ABCD (AHA, 2006)	Nov 2006	• Prior MI • NSVT • EF ≤ 40% • EPS	566	24 months	Ventricular arrhythmia events	71%	29%	Event rates • EP/TWA (–): 2.3% • EP/TWA (+): 12.6%	0.016
ALPHA (ACC, 2007)	April 2007	• NICMP • NYHA Classes II–III • EF ≤ 40%	446	18 months *No patient received an ICD*	Cardiac death and life-threatening arrhythmias	292 (65%)	154 (35%)	4.01 *NPV* 98.7% @ 12 months	0.002
SCD-HeFT substudy	Nov 2008 *Circulation.* 2008:118: 2022–2028	• NYHA Classes II–III • EF ≤ 35%	490	30 months	SCD, sustained VT/VF, appropriate ICD therapy	355 (72%)	135 (28%)	1.28 (95% CI: 0.65–2.53)	0.46
MASTER	Nov 2008 *JACC.* 2008; 52:1607–1615	• Prior MI • EF ≤ 30%	575	2.1 years	Appropriate VT/VF (All pts were implanted with an ICD)	361 (63%)	214 (37%)	1.26 (95% CI: 0.76–2.09)	0.37

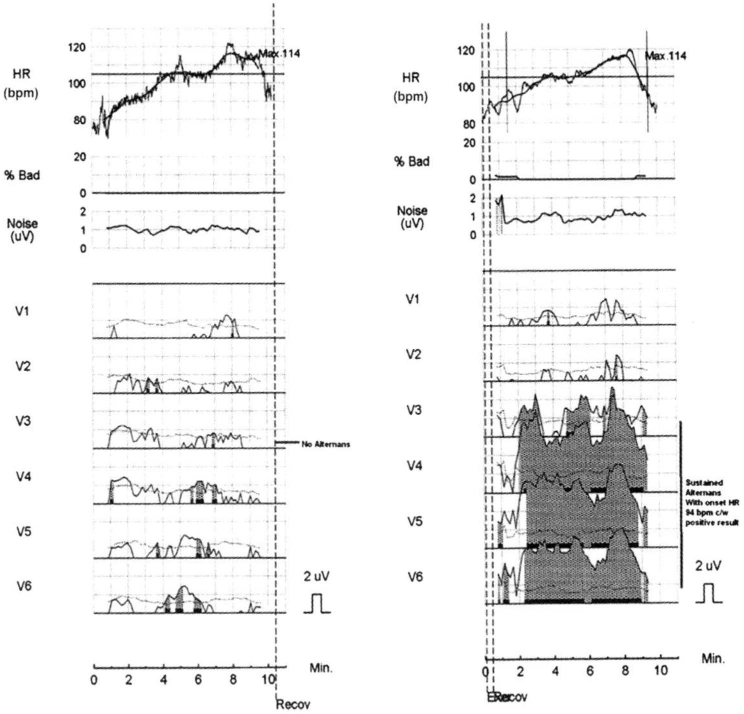

FIGURE 11-3. Exercise MTWA testing. Shown are (from **top** to **bottom**) heart rate trend, percentage of bad beats, noise level, and MTWA amplitudes in ECG leads V1 to V6. (The amplitudes in vector magnitude lead VM and the orthogonal leads X, Y, and Z are not shown but they demonstrated similar results.) **Left:** Absence of MTWA during exercise-induced elevation of the heart rate to a maximum heart rate of 114 bpm. **Right:** Exercise-induced sustained MTWA (shaded gray area), which starts at an onset rate of 94 bpm.

rate, before returning to baseline. The HRT is usually assessed from 24-h Holter recordings as an average response to VPCs. From such recordings, a VPC tachogram is constructed by aligning and averaging the RR interval sequences surrounding isolated VPCs (Fig. 11-4). Two phases of HRT, the early sinus rate acceleration and late deceleration, are quantified by two parameters termed turbulence onset and turbulence slope, respectively. Overall, HRT is an indirect measure of baroreflex function. Future studies will likely evaluate the role of HRT in risk stratification of patients post-MI and/or chronic congestive heart failure.

ELECTRICAL CARDIOVERSION

Patients with atrial fibrillation, the most commonly encountered sustained clinical arrhythmia, are often managed using electrical cardioversion. Introduced 45 years ago, electrical cardioversion initially typically utilized a damped sine wave monophasic waveform (Fig. 11-5). However, using such an approach, up to 20% of patients failed to convert to sinus rhythm. This was defined as the inability to restore sinus rhythm as opposed to an early recurrence of atrial fibrillation, in which the cardioversion was successful, although only transiently. Initially, patients who failed to cardiovert were subject to either internal cardioversion or left in atrial fibrillation permanently.

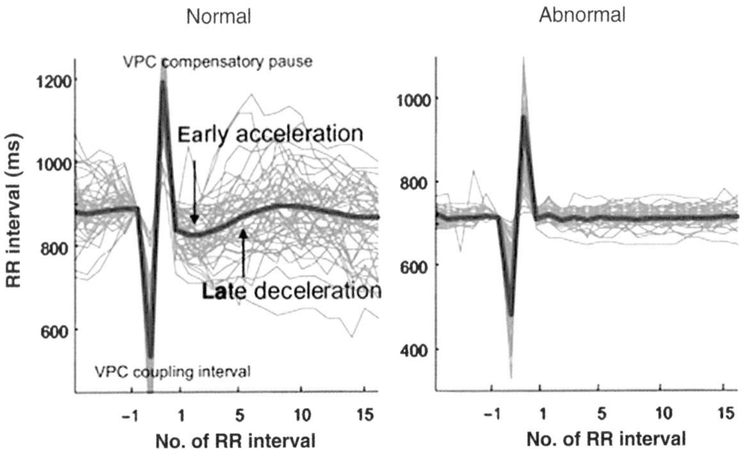

FIGURE 11-4. Heart rate turbulence. VPC tachograms showing normal **(left)** and abnormal **(right)** HRT. HRT is composed of the transient acceleration phase of heart rate (RR interval shortening) immediately after the compensatory pause followed by a subsequent and gradual deceleration phase (RR interval prolongation). *Orange curves* show single VPC tachograms. *Bold brown curves* show the averaged VPC tachogram over 24 h. (Reproduced from Bauer A, Malik M, Schmidt G, et al. Heart rate turbulence: Standards of measurement, physiological interpretation, and clinical use-International society for Holter and noninvasive electrophysiology consensus. *J Am Coll Cardiol.* 2008;52:1353–1365, with permission.) (See color insert.)

When using monophasic shocks, there are several possible methods to increase the overall efficacy of transthoracic cardioversion for atrial fibrillation. First, although current American Heart Association Advanced Cardiac Life Support Practice Guidelines recommend an initial 100-J shock, followed by sequential shocks of escalating energy if necessary, it has recently been demonstrated in a relatively small group of patients that delivery of an *initial* 360-J damped sine wave shock is associated with a higher success rate and requires less total shocks and cumulative energy than the conventional strategy of sequential shocks of increasing strength.

There are two additional options in patients who remain refractory to cardioversion. The first is to proceed to a 720-J shock, which is accomplished by using two defibrillators, with each delivering simultaneously a 360-J damped sine wave shock using an orthogonal electrode configuration. A pair of electrodes is applied in an anteroposterior position on the patient's chest and a second pair of electrodes is applied in an antero-apical position. This approach delivers greater current (due to the higher cumulative energy output) and reduces the transthoracic impedance (due to increased electrode surface area). A second option is administration of the class III antiarrhythmic agent, ibutilide (1 mg intravenously), prior to cardioversion. This strategy is reported to lower the atrial defibrillation threshold, which facilitates successful cardioversion.

Today, all of the above have been supplanted by the routine use of biphasic waveforms for cardioversion of atrial fibrillation. Two types of biphasic waveforms are commercially available; these include a truncated exponential (BTE) and a rectilinear waveform (Fig. 11-6). Several prospective randomized clinical trials have compared each of these biphasic waveforms to a damped sine wave waveform for the cardioversion of atrial fibrillation.

The initial study by Mittal et al. evaluated a rectilinear biphasic waveform, which consists of a constant-current 6-ms first phase and a truncated exponential 4-ms second phase. Unlike monophasic waveforms, this waveform is impedance compensated.

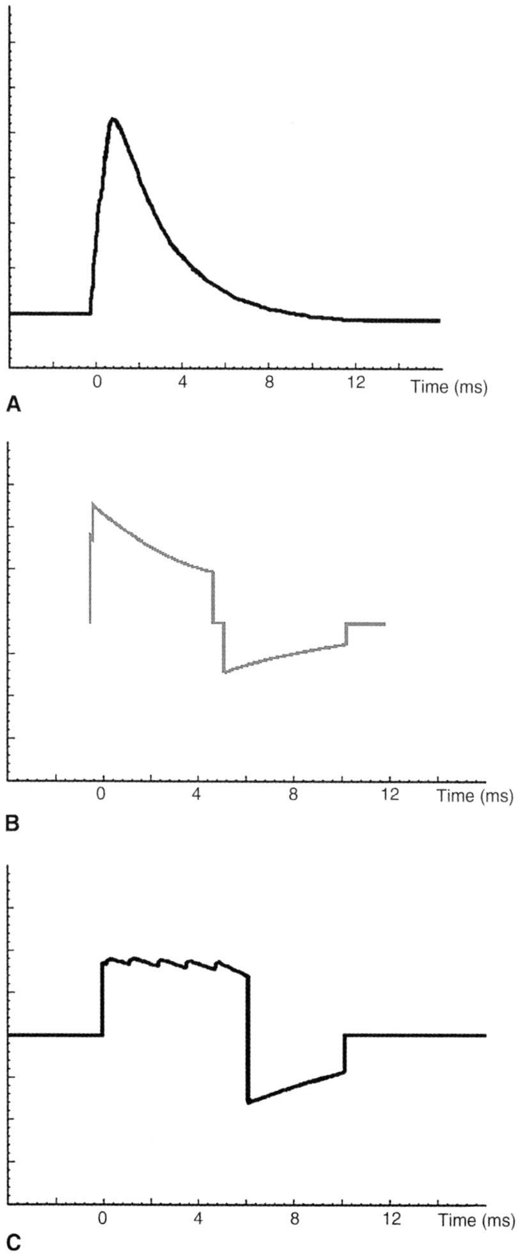

FIGURE 11-5. Shock waveforms. **A:** Damped sine wave waveform. **B:** Truncated exponential biphasic waveform. **C:** Rectilinear biphasic waveform.

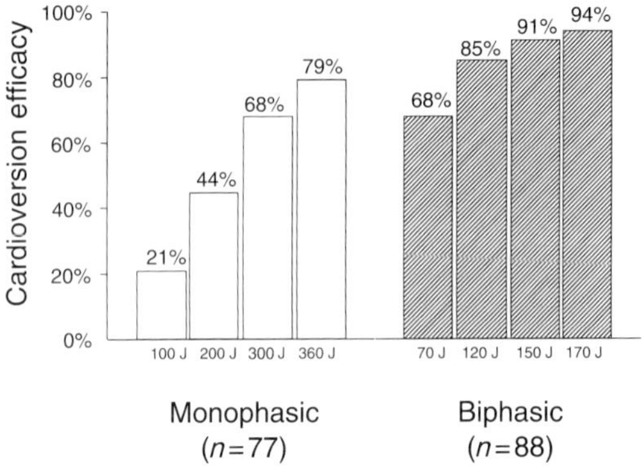

FIGURE 11-6. Cumulative cardioversion efficacy of damped sine wave monophasic and rectilinear biphasic shocks. The first-shock cardioversion efficacy with the 70-J biphasic waveform (60/88 patients, 68%) was significantly greater than that with the 100-J monophasic waveform (16/77 patients, 21%, $p < 0.0001$). Similarly, the cumulative cardioversion efficacy with the biphasic waveform (83/88 patients, 94%) was significantly greater than that with the monophasic waveform (61/77 patients, 79%, $p = 0.005$). (Reproduced from Mittal S, Ayati S, Stein KM, et al. Transthoracic cardioversion of atrial fibrillation: Comparison of rectilinear biphasic versus damped sine wave monophasic shocks. *Circulation.* 2000;101:1282–1287, with permission.)

A constant-current first phase is maintained by automatically adjusting the internal resistance of the defibrillator circuit based on the patient's transthoracic impedance, which is automatically determined at the onset of shock delivery. The first shock as well as cumulative shock efficacy with the rectilinear biphasic waveform was significantly greater than that with the damped sine wave waveform (Fig. 11-5). Approximately 70% of patients were successfully cardioverted with only a 70-J rectilinear biphasic shock and nearly 95% of patients who were randomized to receive biphasic shocks were successfully cardioverted. In contrast, only 21% of patients were successfully cardioverted with a 100-J monophasic shock and the cumulative success rate was only approximately 80%. In clinical practice, based on the observed difference in cardioversion efficacy between the two waveforms, for every seven patients who undergo cardioversion of atrial fibrillation, one additional patient will be successfully cardioverted with the rectilinear biphasic waveform. Similar results have been observed with use of the truncated exponential biphasic waveform. These data have heralded an era where biphasic shocks are routinely used for the transthoracic cardioversion of atrial fibrillation, which results in a near 100% efficacy of the procedure for the immediate restoration of sinus rhythm.

TEMPORARY VENOUS PACING

Transvenous pacing provides the most consistent and reliable means of temporary pacing in clinical practice. When required (Table 11-3), a decision needs to be made regarding the site of vascular access, the need for single or dual chamber pacing, and selection of the appropriate pacing catheter(s). Observation of proper sterile surgical technique is *critical*, as these systems are highly prone to infection.

Common venous access routes include the internal and external jugular, subclavian, femoral, or brachial veins. The right internal jugular venous route has been recommended for its direct route to the right ventricle, potential for the highest success rate, and lowest complication rate. Femoral venous access may be considered in the event of a bleeding diathesis or coagulopathy because pressure may be more easily applied to this site in the

TABLE 11-3 Indications for Temporary Transvenous Pacing.

Bradycardia associated with an acute myocardial infarction

1. Asystole
2. Symptomatic bradycardia (sinus bradycardia or Mobitz I second-degree AV block associated with hypotension [not responsive to atropine])
3. Bilateral bundle branch block (alternating LBBB and RBBB or RBBB with alternating LAHB/LPHB)
4. New or indeterminate age bifascicular block with first-degree AV block
5. Mobitz II second degree AV block

Bradycardia not associated with an acute myocardial infarction

1. Asystole
2. Second- or third-degree AV block associated with hemodynamic compromise
3. Ventricular tachyarrhythmias secondary to bradycardia (e.g., torsade de pointes)

event of hemorrhage. However, this site carries the greatest potential risk of infection and requires absolute immobility of the patient.

Catheter packaging will provide recommendations for the appropriate introducer size, most often between 4 and 7 Fr (1.5 to 2.3 mm). Providers credentialed for temporary venous pacemaker insertion and bedside nurses must be familiar with the particular equipment available at their institution. A pacing catheter is introduced into the selected access site through an introducer, advanced into the right atrium for atrial pacing or the right ventricular apex for ventricular pacing and finally, positioned to lodge against the endocardium. Once a stable position has been attained, pacing should be attempted and if capture is not obtained, the lead should be repositioned. Anchor sites should be used to tie the lead once positioned to prevent dislodgement, one at the site where the lead exits the skin and a second where a loop is formed with the lead.

There are many types of temporary pacing catheters. Fluoroscopy is needed for placement of stiff, nonfloating catheters while flow-directed catheters can be advanced with electrocardiographic or fluoroscopic guidance. Balloon catheters may decrease procedure time and improve lead positioning. The balloon should be deflated once in the ventricle to avoid displacement into the pulmonary artery. ECG guidance may be used when fluoroscopy is unavailable; however, a balloon-tipped, flow-directed catheter should be used in this setting. The use of echocardiography has also been described for placement of cardiac pacing leads. Four-chamber visualization of the heart may enhance lead positioning and may be especially useful when fluoroscopy is unavailable or undesirable, such as when treating pregnant women or patients in the emergency room setting.

When performing insertion using ECG guidance, standard limb leads are connected to the patient and V1, a precordial lead, is attached to the distal electrode of a balloon-tipped catheter. Continuous ECG monitoring is observed as the catheter is advanced into the heart. The location of the pacing catheter is deduced from the characteristics of the unipolar electrograms. A high right atrial location is usually indicated by an inverted P wave, a midatrial position by a biphasic P wave, and a low right atrial position by a positive P wave. Once the catheter crosses the tricuspid valve, the P wave amplitude decreases and QRS deflections are observed. Marked ST-segment elevation is an indicator of endocardial right ventricular contact. Simultaneous atrial and ventricular electrograms may be an indication of a coronary sinus position. A negative P wave is again noted as the electrode passes into the pulmonary artery as the catheter tip is above the level of the atrium.

TILT TABLE TESTING

Tilt testing is widely used to evaluate patients with suspected neurally mediated syncope. Current practice guidelines advocate that tilt testing be performed in a quiet

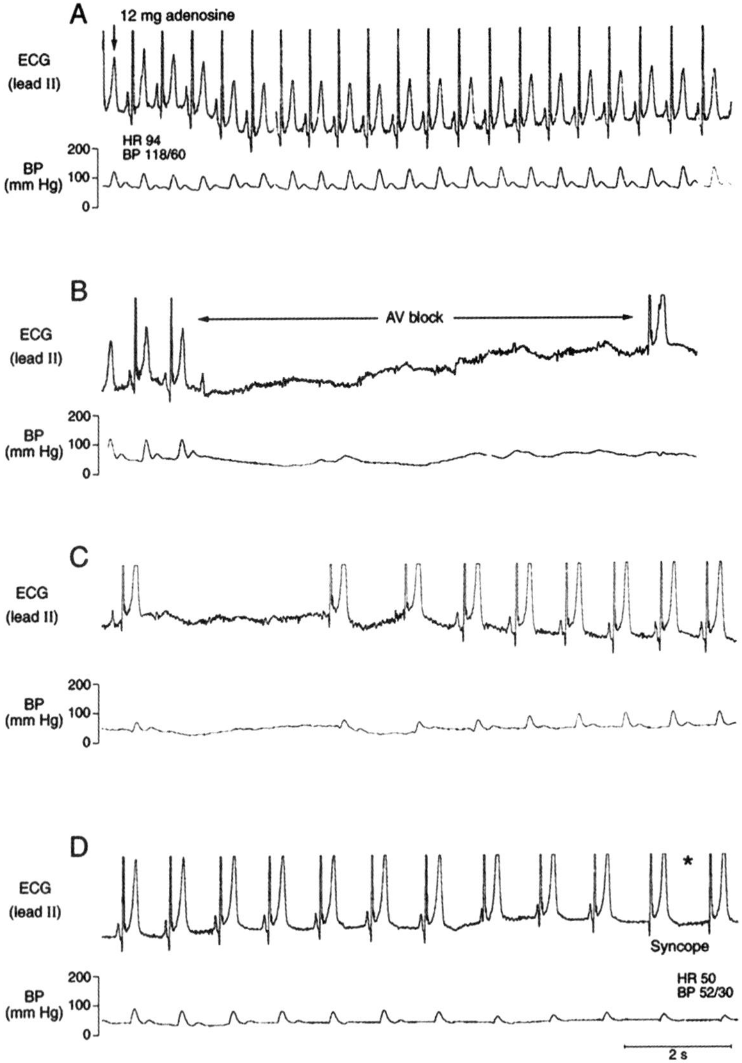

FIGURE 11-7. Adenosine-based tilt testing. **Panels A–D** represent a continuous recording from a patient referred for tilt testing to evaluate a history of recurrent syncope. Shown in each panel on top is a single-lead ECG recording (surface lead II). The bottom half of each panel shows a continuous tonometric blood pressure recording. **A:** At baseline, the blood pressure is 118/90 mm Hg and the rhythm is sinus at 94 bpm. While upright, the patient is administered 12 mg adenosine. **B:** The patient develops transient AV block, which is associated with hypotension. **C:** The AV block resolves and the patient's blood pressure returns to baseline. **D:** The patient then develops progressive sinus slowing and hypotension, which results in syncope (*). At the time of syncope, there is an underlying junctional rhythm at 50 bpm and the blood pressure is 52/30 mm Hg. (Reproduced from Mittal et al. A single-stage adenosine tilt test in patients with unexplained syncope. *J Cardiovasc Electrophysiol.* 2004;15:637–640, with permission.)

room with dim lighting. The patient should be fasting for at least 2 h prior to the test. Ideally, patients should be supine for 20 to 45 min (especially when venous cannulation is performed) prior to upright tilt; however, in practice this is quite difficult. Heart rate and blood pressure should be monitored continuously on a beat-to-beat basis. A tilt table with a footboard is essential. Finally, the patient should be tilted to 60 to 70 degrees; tilting to 80 degrees reduces the specificity of the test protocol.

Unfortunately, there is no standardized tilt test protocol. Currently used protocols usually consist of an initial drugfree tilt phase (usually at least 20 min and up to 40 min) followed by a phase using pharmacologic provocation, most commonly with isoproterenol, nitroglycerin, or adenosine. Isoproterenol is infused at a rate of 1 to 3 μg/min in order to increase the resting heart rate by 20% to 25%. Nitroglycerin is typically administered as a 400-μg sublingual spray. At our institution, we do not perform nitroglycerin tilt testing because of concerns over test specificity. Rather, we routinely use adenosine to facilitate the induction of neurally mediated syncope. Adenosine, like isoproterenol, has sympathomimetic effects, which are mediated through baroreflex and chemoreceptor activation. Single-stage adenosine tilt testing has a diagnostic yield comparable to a two-stage test protocol using drugfree and isoproterenol tilt stages. An attractive feature of adenosine tilt testing is that it takes only 3 min to complete (Fig. 11-7).

The major problem with tilt testing remains its poor sensitivity when using a protocol that maintains high specificity. This limitation is acknowledged in the recent AHA/ACC scientific statement on the evaluation of syncope. In patients without structural heart disease, the pretest probability that the diagnosis is neurally mediated syncope is high, irrespective of the tilt test result. Therefore, it is generally more important to exclude the possibility of serious bradyarrhythmia or tachyarrhythmia as the etiology for syncope. In addition, the sensitivity of tilt testing worsens significantly as the patient population being evaluated becomes older. Furthermore, prospective studies have demonstrated that in patients without structural heart disease who present with syncope, the clinical outcome is similar irrespective of the tilt test response (see Chapter 5). As a result, the clinical role for tilt testing remains controversial.

KEY POINTS

1. Mobile cardiac outpatient telemetry monitoring is being increasingly used to evaluate unexplained symptoms of palpitations and presyncope/syncope as well as for monitoring the burden of atrial fibrillation (to assess efficacy of antiarrhythmic drug therapy or catheter ablation).
2. A variety of tools for risk stratification of patients at high risk of sudden death are available. These include HRV, heart rate turbulence, signal-averaged electrocardiography, and microscopic TWA testing. Unfortunately, to date, none has proven effective in being able to identify patients most likely to benefit from ICD implantation.
3. Transthoracic shocks using biphasic waveforms have become standard practice in patients undergoing electrical cardioversion of atrial fibrillation.
4. All fellows should be familiar with the indications and techniques for temporary pacemaker insertion.
5. There is no accepted standardized protocol for tilt testing. All protocols that have acceptable specificity (low likelihood of a false-positive test result) are limited by a low positive yield. Adenosine-based tilt testing is attractive because it can be completed within 3 min.

SUGGESTED READINGS

Risk stratification

Bauer A, Malik M, Schmidt G, et al. Heart rate turbulence: Standards of measurement, physiological interpretation, and clinical use-International society for Holter and noninvasive electrophysiology consensus. *J Am Coll Cardiol.* 2008;52:1353–1365.

Goldberger JJ, Cain ME, Hohnloser SH, et al. American Heart Association/American College of Cardiology Foundation/Heart Rhythm Society scientific statement on non-invasive risk stratification techniques for identifying patients at risk for sudden cardiac death: A scientific statement from the American Heart Association Council on Clinical cardiology Committee on Electrocardiography and Arrhythmias and Council on Epidemiology and Prevention. *Circulation.* 2008;118:1497–1518.

Hohnloser SH, Kuck KH, Dorian P, et al. for the DINAMIT investigators. Prophylactic use of an implantable cardioverter-defibrillator after acute myocardial infarction. *N Engl J Med.* 2004;351:2481–2488.

Task Force of the European Society of Cardiology and the North American Society of Pacing and Electrophysiology. Heart rate variability: Standards of measurement, physiological interpretation and clinical use. *Circulation.* 1996;93:1043–1065.

Electrical cardioversion

Mittal S, Ayati S, Stein KM, et al. Transthoracic cardioversion of atrial fibrillation: Comparison of rectilinear biphasic versus damped sine wave monophasic shocks. *Circulation.* 2000;101:1282–1287.

Tilt table testing/syncope

Benditt DG, Ferguson DW, Grubb BP, et al. Tilt table testing for assessing syncope. *J Am Coll Cardiol.* 1996;28:263–275.

Brignole M, Alboni P, Benditt DG, et al. Guidelines on management (diagnosis and treatment) of syncope – Update 2004. The task force on syncope, European Society of Cardiology. *Europace.* 2004;6:467–537.

Mittal S, Stein KM, Markowitz SM, et al. Induction of neurally-mediated syncope with adenosine. *Circulation.* 1999;99:1318–1324.

Strickberger SA, Benson DW, Biaggioni I, et al. AHA/ACCF scientific statement on the evaluation of syncope: From the American Heart Association council on clinical cardiology, cardiovascular nursing, cardiovascular disease in the young, and stroke, and the quality of care and outcomes research interdisciplinary working group; and the American College of Cardiology Foundation in collaboration with the Heart Rhythm Society. *J Am Coll Cardiol.* 2006;47:473–484.

SECTION III

The Pacemaker and Defibrillator Clinic

CHAPTER 12

Device Interrogations and Utilization of Diagnostic Data

Charles J. Love

Implantable cardiac rhythm devices have progressed from fixed function, fixed rate, nonprogrammable pacemakers to the current generation of incredibly sophisticated, microprocessor-based, automated, implantable cardioverter-defibrillators (ICDs). A good friend of mine likes to compare device management 20 years ago to what we do today as flying a Cessna versus flying an F-16. The level of sophistication is several orders of magnitude greater for the latter, and the chance and consequences of making an error is much greater as well. On the other hand, the ability to provide phenomenal improvements in individual therapy and the opportunities to capture and manage critical information about patients and their rhythms has expanded markedly as well.

Learning how to manage and use the vast amount of data that can be retrieved from a device can be overwhelming, even for a "seasoned" device expert. Full interrogations of devices can produce dozens of sheets of paper with parameters, device information, diagnostics, and electrograms. The best way to approach this volume of data is to "divide and conquer," that is, to deal with each part of the functionality of the device one piece at a time. I prefer to look at the interrogations in the following manner:

(1) Device functional information
(2) Patient rhythm diagnostics
(3) Rhythm-specific information
(4) Appropriate programming values based on observed data
(5) Other monitored parameters

GETTING STARTED

The first step to analyzing the data from a device is to obtain the data from the device. In order to do this, one must first identify the manufacturer so that the proper programmer is utilized. Unfortunately, despite many years of requests from those of us doing device work, there is no "universal programmer," nor is there likely to be one in the

TABLE 12-1 Phone Numbers of Major Device Companies

Biotronik: 1-800 547-0394	Pacesetter: See St Jude Medical
Boston Scientific: 1-800-CARDIAC	Sorin (ELA): 1-763-519-9400
CPI: See Boston Scientific	St Jude Medical: 1-800-SHOCK VF
ELA: See Sorin	Telectronics: See St Jude Medical
Guidant: See Boston Scientific	Ventritex: See St Jude Medical
Intermedics: See Boston Scientific	Vitatron: See Medtronic
Medtronic: 1-800 MEDTRON(ic)	

foreseeable future. The manufacturer can be determined by one of several methods. First, most patients carry an identification card with them that will have the manufacturer, model, and serial number of the device. One word of caution is that if a patient has had more than one device, they may still have the card from the previous device which can lead to an erroneous identification. Should the patient not have an ID card, a chest radiograph can be inspected. Many devices have a radio-opaque identification tag that will have the company logo. If no logo is present, or getting a radiograph is not possible or convenient, each company has a toll-free phone number that can be called to obtain device registration information. One can call the number of each company until the one that has the information on the patient is reached. The phone numbers of the major device companies are listed in Table 12-1. As you can see, there has been a lot of consolidation in the industry!

Finally, if none of these options are available, one can try to interrogate a device using each programmer in turn until one "links up" with the device. This is generally frowned upon due to the (at least theoretical) possibility of an unintended effect on the implanted device. Note that on some occasions, the device may be nonfunctional or the battery will be so low that interrogation may not be possible.

Once the proper programmer is obtained, the programmer is turned on, and the wand is placed over the device; interrogation will begin automatically, or one simply presses the "Interrogate" button to initiate the process. It is always a good idea to print out everything you can at this point, so that if any of the counters are cleared (some do this automatically after each device interrogation), the data will not be lost, and your attending staff (or worse, the device clinic nurses) will not be upset with you. Other than the potential for some data to be cleared, as long as the "Program" or "Transmit" button is not pushed, you will not change anything regarding device function. Now that you have access to the information, it is possible to attempt to make some sense of it.

DEVICE FUNCTIONAL INFORMATION

My first attention is generally to the basics of device function. What are the current settings for mode and rate? Is the battery status OK? Is the lead integrity and function within normal limits? For an ICD, is the high-voltage circuit working properly?

BASIC PROGRAMMED DATA

In order to evaluate what a device is doing, and whether it is doing it correctly, there are many parameters that need to be evaluated (Fig. 12-1). However, for the novice, we will keep it simple and look at the two key parameters for pacing; pacing mode and pacing base rate. Obviously, the rate seen on an ECG should not be lower than the rate programmed into the device. There are some exceptions to this (such as rate hysteresis, sleep rate, and rate drop response), but we will stick to the most common methods of device setup. The mode will be expressed as a series of three or four letters denoting which chambers are paced, which are sensed, and the response to a sensed event. A fourth letter "R" may be present if rate modulation is activated (e.g., activity sensor). For ICDs, one will also need to evaluate whether the device is active or inactive/monitoring. This may be displayed in a number of ways as noted in Figure 12-2. One can also evaluate the rates at which ventricular tachycardia (VT) and ventricular fibrillation (VF) will be detected and treated. There may be occasion when the device will need to be disabled due to unnecessary shocks, or when the VT rate will need to be lowered due to a slow VT falling below the detection rate of the device.

BATTERY STATUS

Most devices now give an estimated longevity or a "gas gauge" to let one know the status of the battery. Examples of battery status indicators are shown in Figure 12-3. Some devices display a graph of battery voltage and/or remaining longevity, which is also useful to determine the presence of adequate power for the device.

Parameter Settings Report

Modes/Rates

Mode	DDDR
Mode Switch	On
A. Detect Rate	140 bpm
Lower Rate	70 ppm
Upper Tracking Rate	120 ppm
Upper Sensor Rate	120 ppm

A-V Intervals

Paced AV	300 ms
Sensed AV	300 ms
Rate Adaptive AV	On
Start Rate	90 bpm
Stop Rate	120 bpm
Minimum Paced AV	100 ms
Minimum Sensed AV	110 ms

Rate Therapy Features

Non-Competitive Atrial Pacing	On
Interval	300 ms
V. Rate Stabilization	Off

Atrial Lead

Amplitude	2 V
Pulse Width	0.4 ms
Sensitivity	0.3 mV
Pace Blanking	200 ms

Ventricular Lead

Amplitude	2 V
Pulse Width	0.6 ms
Sensitivity	0.3 mV
Pace Blanking	200 ms

Refractory

PVARP	310 ms
PVAB	150 ms

Rate Response

Rate Response	7
Activity Threshold	Medium Low
Activity Acceleration	30 sec
Activity Deceleration	5 min

FIGURE 12-1. A printout of basic device parameters from a pacemaker. The parameters are divided into groups representing basic mode, timing outputs, and other therapy features.

Parameter Settings Report **Page 1**

Detection

	Enable	Initial	Redetect	V Interval (Rate)
VF	On	18/24	12/16	330 ms (182 bpm)
FVT	via VF			270 ms (222 bpm)
VT	Monitor	16	12	370 ms (162 bpm)

PR Logic

AFib/AFlutter	On
Sinus Tach	On
Other 1:1 SVTs	On
SVT Limit	320 ms

Additional Settings

1:1 VT-ST Boundary	50 %
High Rate Timeout	Off

Other Enhancements

Stability	Off

Sensitivity

Atrial	0.3 mV
Ventricular	0.3 mV

A

FIGURE 12-2. A, B, C: Three different programmer printouts showing the status of tachycardia detection and therapies from different manufacturers. These all appear different, and one must be aware that careful inspection may be needed to determine if the device is active or not.

Tachy Zone Configuration

VT-1	VT-2	VF
400 ms 150 bpm 12 intervals	350 ms 171 bpm 12 intervals	**270 ms *** **222 bpm *** 12 intervals
SVT Discrimination		
Monitor Only	**ATP x2 *** **20.0 J / 619 V *** 36.0 J / 830 V 36.0 J / 830 V x2	25.0 J / 693 V 36.0 J / 830 V 36.0 J / 830 V x4

SVT Criteria

SVT Discrimination: .... Dual Chamber
VT-1: On VT-2: On
AF/AFL (V < A Rate Branch)
VT Diagnosis Criteria .... If Any
Morphology .... On (60 %, 5 of 8)
Interval Stability .... On (80 ms), 12 intervals
AV Association Delta .... Passive (60 ms)
Sinus Tach (V = A) Rate Branch
VT Diagnosis Criteria .... If Any
Morphology .... On (60 %, 5 of 8)
Sudden Onset .... On (100 ms)
Template .... Active Jun 6, 2007 12:17 pm (Update every 1 day)

B

Settings

Ventricular Tachy Settings

VF	200 bpm	ATP		41J, 41J, 41Jx6
VT	170 bpm	Burst	Ramp	6J, 41J, 41Jx4

Atrial Tachy Settings

ATR Mode Switch 170 bpm VDI

C

FIGURE 12-2. Cont'd.

HIGH VOLTAGE CHARGE CIRCUIT STATUS

ICDs have the ability to take a 3-V battery and deliver an 800-V discharge. In order to do this, one or more capacitors are required to charge, in a matter of seconds, to the energy required to defibrillate the heart (Fig. 12-4). An excessive charge time can indicate a problem with the capacitor(s), or a depleted battery. Charge times to the full output of the device are device specific, but any charge time in excess of 20 s is abnormal and should be addressed.

LEAD STATUS

There are three major components to the status of a pacing lead. Note that for most ICD systems, the shock lead is a multicomponent lead, and has the ability to sense, pace, and deliver the high energy shock.

Impedance (Resistance)

This is a core measure of the integrity of the lead and connection to the device. For pacing leads (or the pacing component of an ICD lead), the impedance can be anywhere from 300 to 1,000 Ω. For the shock component, the impedance is much lower, usually from 30 to 80 Ω. The steadiness of the number over time is more important than the

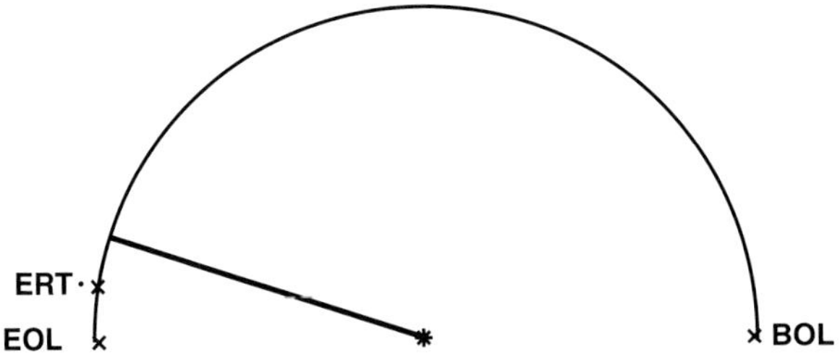

A

Battery OK

Approximate time to explant:	9 years
Charge Time	8.1 s
Last Capacitor Re-form	15 Oct 2008 08:37

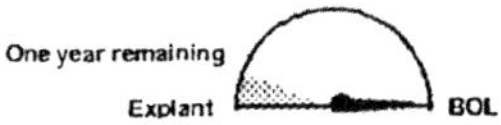

B

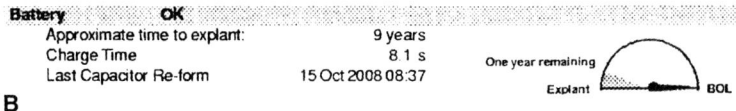

Estimated remaining longevity: 7 years, 5.5 - 8 years (Based on Past History)

Battery Status	OK
Voltage	2.76 V
Current	12.78 μA
Impedance	208 ohms

C

FIGURE 12-3. **A:** "Gas Gauge" from a device showing a device nearing the replacement time. This format does not estimate time remaining or give information about battery voltage or impedance. **B:** Another newer version of the "Gas Gauge," now showing a full battery reserve, and in this case an estimation of the longevity. **C:** Traditional form of data presentation showing battery voltage, battery impedance, and estimated longevity. Lead measurements are also shown. BOL, beginning of life; ERT, elective replacement time; EOL, end of life.

ICD Status

Battery Voltage (ERI=2.62 V)	2.99 V	Nov 24, 2008
Last Full Energy Charge	8.35 sec	Sep 23, 2008
Last Capacitor Formation (Interval = Auto)		Sep 23, 2008

Lead Performance	Atrial	Ventricular	
EGM Amplitude	3.4 mV	3.4 mV	Nov 24, 2008
Pacing Impedance	496 ohms	368 ohms	Nov 24, 2008
Defibrillation Impedance		37 ohms	Nov 24, 2008
SVC (HVX) Impedance 46 ohms			Nov 24, 2008

FIGURE 12-4. This data printout shows both the ICD status and lead data. The battery voltage is shown with the elective replacement indicator (ERI) referenced. Both the last full charge time and last capacitor reformation time (a test charge of the device) are shown. These may be the same. Generally, charge times to full output are in the range of 7 to 12 s. Times beyond 20 s are abnormal and should be addressed.

absolute value obtained. Many devices will store the values and display them as a graph upon interrogation (Fig. 12-5). A high impedance is associated with a fracture of the conductor coil or a poor connection to the device. A low impedance is associated with a short circuit, most commonly due to a failure of the insulation.

Sensing Threshold

The ability of a lead to sense the intrinsic activity of the chamber into which it has been placed is the second component of lead status. In most cases, sensing does not involve the shock coil; however, some leads utilize the shock coil as the pacing and/or sensing anode.

An abrupt or progressive change in the sensing threshold can indicate a failure of the lead, or it can simply be indicative of a change in the patient substrate. For example, if a patient has had a myocardial infarction, this could affect the sensing on the ventricular lead. Likewise, certain metabolic changes or pharmacologic interventions can affect sensing (these are usually reversible). As with impedance measurements, the absolute value of the P and R wave amplitudes are less important than the trend. Some devices maintain the sensing threshold history, while others do not (Fig. 12-5). In the latter case, the obtained values need be compared with those kept in the patient's device chart. This may not be available if the patient is followed up elsewhere.

Pacing Threshold

The last of the three components of lead evaluation is the amount of energy that it takes to pace the myocardium. This is known as the pacing threshold. As with sensing, some ICD leads may use the distal shock coil as part of the anode in the circuit. While low thresholds are uniformly good, a high threshold may be acceptable if it has been stable, or may indicate a lead problem if it is a new finding. Again, changes in substrate or certain metabolic changes and pharmacologic interventions may significantly affect the pacing threshold. Some devices have the capability of automatically testing the capture threshold on one or more of the leads. For many devices, these values must be determined manually (Fig. 12-6).

PATIENT RHYTHM DIAGNOSTICS

All modern devices keep information regarding the basic patient rhythm. The most basic data are the percent of time pacing and sensing occurs in each chamber. This can give a glimpse into the diagnosis for which the device was implanted. A device that is pacing

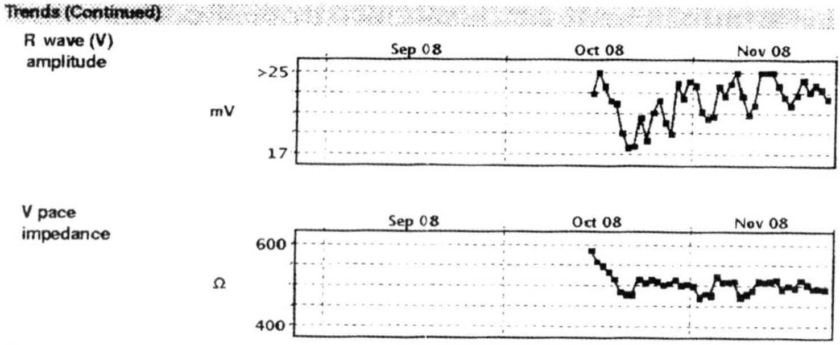

A

Leads Data	Implant 14 Oct 2008	Previous Session 15 Oct 2008	Most Recent 24 Nov 2008
Ventricular			
Intrinsic Amplitude	N/R mV	>25.0 mV	22.5 mV
Pace Impedance	N/R Ω	608 Ω	490 Ω
Pace Threshold	N/R V @ N/R ms	0.6 V @ 0.4 ms	
Shock Vector			
Shock Impedance	N/R Ω	47 Ω	49 Ω

B

FIGURE 12-5. A: Graph of lead sensing measurements ("R wave") and lead impedance measurements. After the early maturation phase, the lead impedance is very steady, indicating stable lead integrity. There is some variation of the R wave, but it is well within an excellent range. **B:** This device does not graph the impedance and R wave, but it does give a reference of the initial value and the last value for comparison.

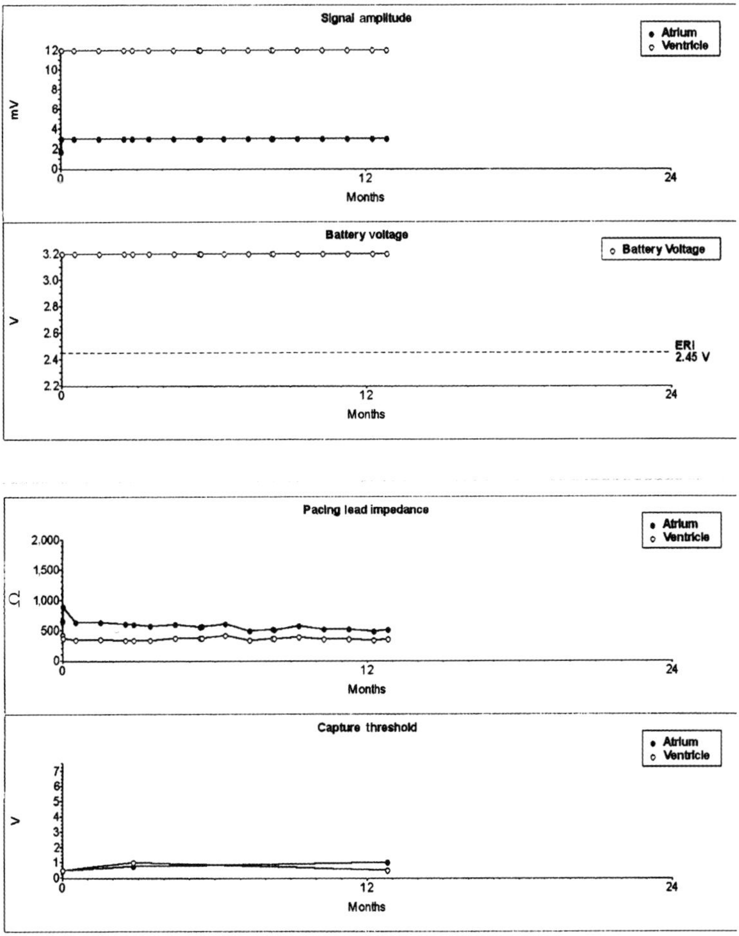

C

Pacemaker Status

Estimated remaining longevity: 3 years, 1.5 - 3.5 years (Based on Past History)
Battery Voltage/Impedance 2.71 V / 1,191 ohms

	Atrial	Ventricular
Amplitude/Pulse Width	2.57 V / 0.40 ms	5.37 V / 1.00 ms
Sensitivity	0.50 mV	2.80 mV
Measured Impedance	367 ohms	2,495 ohms

D

FIGURE 12-5. C: Multiple graph display showing measurements made at each clinic visit. They are not performed daily and automatically, but in this case, they are measured manually, stored, and graphed. **D:** This reading of lead status shows a very high impedance on the ventricular lead (2,495 Ω) consistent with a lead fracture.

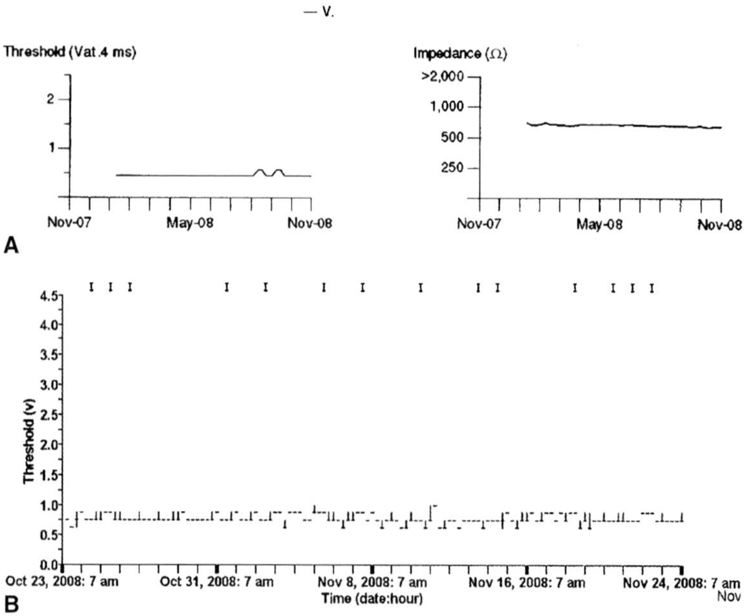

FIGURE 12-6. Pacing thresholds can be graphed by the device. **A:** This figure shows one manufacturer's device with the graph of capture threshold measured daily next to a graph of lead impedance. Both are steady, which is usually a good sign. **B:** This graph is from a different manufacturer that measures threshold every 8 h. Again, this shows a consistent and low threshold.

the atrium a large percentage of the time would be consistent with sick sinus syndrome, while one that is pacing the ventricle most of the time would indicate AV block. In some cases (such as in resynchronization therapy) there might be a reason for a high percentage of ventricular pacing, even when the AV node function is normal. Given the attention being paid to reduction of unnecessary ventricular pacing in non-CRT devices, these histograms can be used to guide programming therapy to achieve this goal.

The devices also provide histograms of heart rate and the percentage of time within these rate ranges that pacing or sensing occurs. Evaluation of this histogram is useful to determine the presence of chronotropic incompetence (sick sinus syndrome) or AV block, and allows identification of arrhythmias (Fig. 12-7). For patients who have rate response enabled, the sensor indicated rate histogram provides information as to the appropriateness of sensor response. This histogram depicts what the heart rate range would be if the sensor was controlling pacing at all times. Generally, the heart rate will be at the intrinsic rate or the sensor indicated rate, whichever is higher.

Histograms are useful, but provide only a "bird's-eye view" of the patient's heart rate and rhythms. Trend graphs provide up to beat-to-beat pacing, heart rate, and heart rhythm information, but over a much shorter period of time than histograms. These can be continuously recorded, such that only data from the time immediately prior to interrogation is available, or these can be "fixed," such that specific time frames are saved or specific triggers (e.g., high heart rate) cause a "snapshot" to be saved (Fig. 12-8). Many newer devices also save intracardiac electrograms that can be retrieved and reviewed as well (see text below).

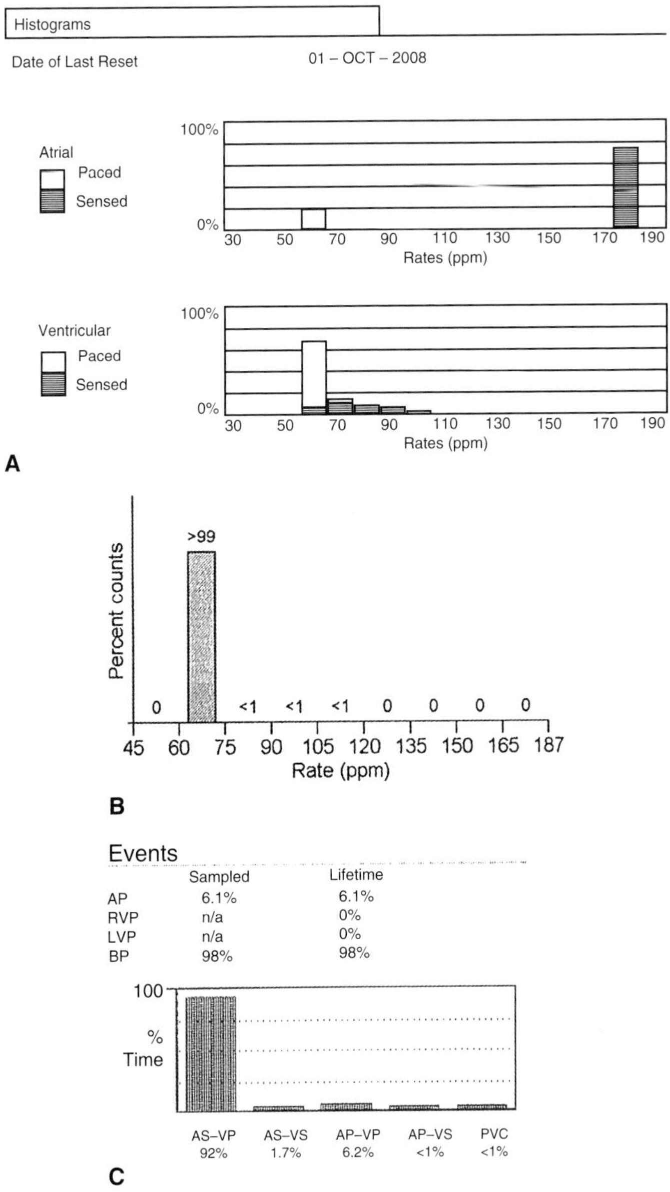

FIGURE 12-7. A: Atrial and ventricular histograms showing an 80% atrial fibrillation burden with a controlled ventricular response. **B:** Heart rate histogram showing all counts in the 60 to 75 bpm range. This patient has chronotropic incompetence. **C:** Pacing histogram showing the percent of time the device is pacing each chamber relative to the other chamber. This patient is mostly atrial sensed and ventricular paced (AS/VP) indicating the likely diagnosis of AV node disease.

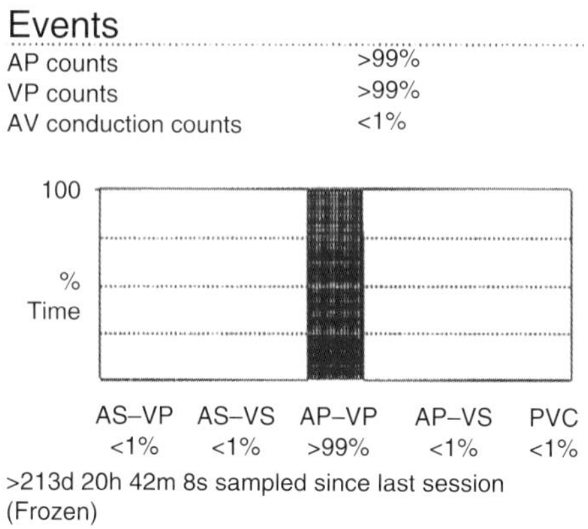

D

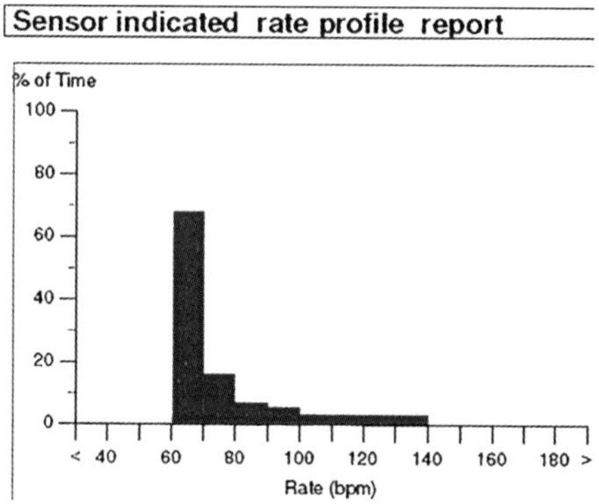

E

FIGURE 12-7. **D:** Pacing histogram showing virtually 100% pacing in both chambers, suggesting combined sinus and AV node disease. **E:** Sensor-indicated rate histogram. This histogram shows what the heart rate range would have been if the patient was 100% paced in the atrium (atrial or dual chamber devices,) or ventricle (single chamber ventricular devices or modes). It is useful to determine if the activity sensor is programmed appropriately for the patient's level of activity. This histogram shows a nice spread of projected heart rates.

RHYTHM-SPECIFIC INFORMATION

Specialized rhythm diagnostics are becoming increasingly common. For pacemakers, these can depict the frequency and duration of atrial and ventricular arrhythmias (Fig. 12-9). These data are very valuable to assist in determining the need for and effectiveness of medical or interventional therapy.

All implantable defibrillators now have the ability to store and retrieve information and electrograms from detected and treated arrhythmias. Most devices provide some level of overview as to how many arrhythmic events have occurred. The first level of diagnostic beyond this overview is the event log (Fig. 12-10). The log provides a

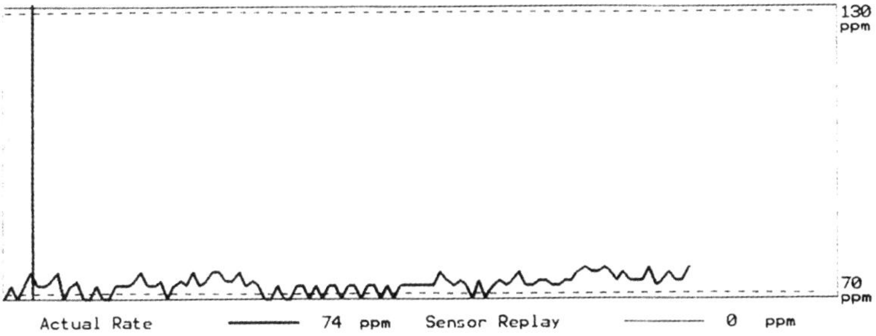

A

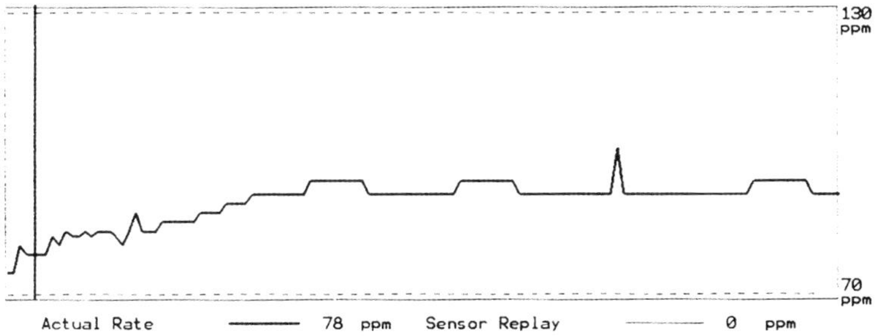

B

FIGURE 12-8. Trend graphs of the heart rate during an in-office exercise test to evaluate the reaction of the activity sensor. **A:** Graph of the heart rate at the original setting of the device shows minimal heart rate response with exercise. **B:** Graph of the heart rate after the activity sensor was made more responsive.

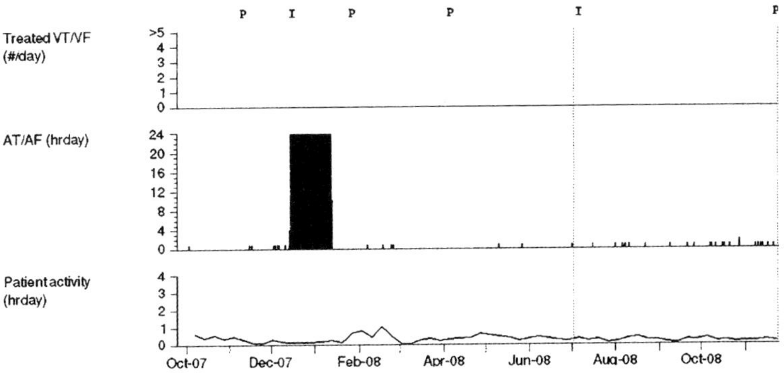

A

FIGURE 12-9. Specialized heart rhythm diagnostics. **A:** An example of the "Cardiac Compass" showing an episode of atrial fibrillation from December 2007 to January 2008. Note that there appear to be many brief nonsustained episodes during the recorded period as well. **B:** Another example, this time showing sustained atrial fibrillation. Note the bottom graph that shows the heart rate range during the atrial fibrillation. This is useful to assess rate control as well. **C:** Log of arrhythmias that met the trigger criteria programmed into the device. The time and date reference as well as the rhythm identified can be very useful to correlate events with patient symptoms.

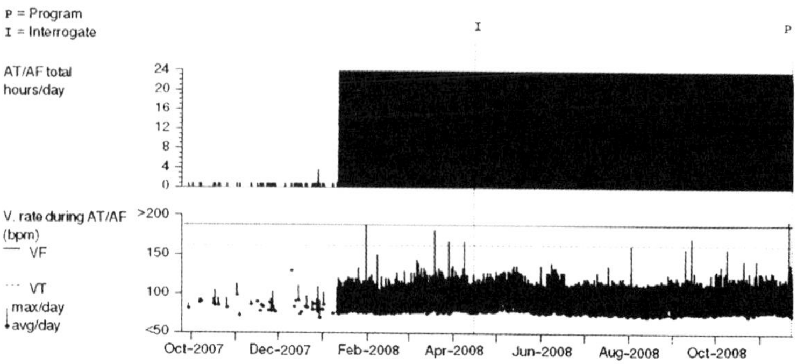

B

Trigger counts

Trigger	Count	EGMs
AT/AF detection	2	1
160 bpm		
High ventricular rate	10	7
150 bpm		
5 consecutive cycles		

Episode directory

	Date	Time	Type
⚠	Aug 21, 2008	6:45am	High ventricular rate
⚠	Aug 17, 2008	12:59am	High ventricular rate
⚠	Aug 7, 2008	3:59pm	High ventricular rate
⚠	Jul 24, 2008	10:34am	High ventricular rate
⚠	Jul 16, 2008	11:32pm	High ventricular rate
⚠	Jul 2, 2008	5:26am	High ventricular rate
	Jun 19, 2008	12:03pm	AT/AF Detection
⚠	Jun 7, 2008	9:44pm	High ventricular rate

C

FIGURE 12-9. Cont'd.

Episode Query Selections

Show All Episodes

Episode	Date/Time	Type	Zone	Rate bpm A	Rate bpm V	Therapy/ Duration	V:A	Stab	AFib	Ons	A&V
8	OCT-2008 04 10:30	V Spon				Nonsustained	-	N/R	-	44%	
7	MAY-2008 11 03:48	V Spon	VT		200	ATPx1	>	23	F	53%	
6	JUN-2007 28 09:40	V Spon				Nonsustained	-	N/R	-	19%	
5	MAY-2007 07 00:29	V Spon			182	Nonsustained	≤	5	F	6%	
4	07 00:28	V Spon	VT		175	ATPx1	≤	9	F	N/R	
3	07 00:28	V Spon			197	Nonsustained	≤	22	F	19%	
2	APR-2006 15 06:12	V Spon			76	Nonsustained	≤	N/R	F	56%	
1	MAR-2005 25 17:12	V Ind	VF		276	21J	>	12	F	N/R	

A

FIGURE 12-10. Event logs. **A:** This log is from the same patient shown in Figure 12-12. Note the five nonsustained events and the two VT events. These are time and date referenced. There is also a VF event, but this was "induced" at the time of device implant. It does not show on the overview in Figure 12-12 as the counters were cleared after the implant session. **B:** This log is from a different patient and shows numerous arrhythmic events in the atrium and the ventricle. Again, the time and date references are highly useful to correlate any patient symptoms to the presence or absence of arrhythmic events.

Episode	Date/Time	Type	Zone	Rate bpm	Therapy/ Duration
109	17-NOV-2008 11:55	ATR		141	00:04 m:s
108	16-NOV-2008 15:16	ATR		161	00:05 m:s
107	06-NOV-2008 20:55	Spont		82	Nonsustained
106	11-OCT-2008 21:43	ATR		68	00:04 m:s
105	16-SEP-2008 18:19	ATR		159	00:08 m:s
104	11-SEP-2008 01:42	PMT		120	
103	27-AUG-2008 19:31	ATR		77	00:00 m:s
102	12-AUG-2008 20:20	ATR		68	00:01 m:s
101	06-AUG-2008 22:39	PMT		120	
100	24-JUL-2008 01:02	PMT		120	
99	18-JUL-2008 16:55	PMT		120	
98	10-JUL-2008 15:03	PMT		120	
97	08-JUL-2008 07:17	ATR		87	00:01 m:s
96	24-JUN-2008 17:52	Spont			Nonsustained
95	24-JUN-2008 14:51	ATR		82	00:02 m:s
94	22-JUN-2008 05:44	PMT		120	
93	21-JUN-2008 01:54	ATR		120	00:01 m:s
92	11-JUN-2008 14:16	ATR		69	00:03 m:s
91	31-MAY-2008 06:46	PMT		120	
90	22-MAY-2008 21:56	PMT		120	
89	13-MAY-2008 13:05	ATR		94	00:00 m:s
88	13-MAY-2008 12:58	Spont		87	Nonsustained
87	10-MAY-2008 23:48	Spont		83	Nonsustained
86	06-MAY-2008 14:49	ATR		152	00:04 m:s
85	06-MAY-2008 14:28	ATR		155	00:10 m:s
84	21-APR-2008 10:26	ATR		86	00:02 m:s
83	18-APR-2008 19:28	ATR		80	00:01 m:s
82	01-APR-2008 20:05	ATR		63	00:02 m:s
81	25-MAR-2008 08:45	Spont			Nonsustained
80	24-MAR-2008 10:43	ATR		142	00:05 m:s
79	08-FEB-2008 09:06	ATR		75	00:01 m:s
78	15-JAN-2008 17:05	Spont		80	Nonsustained
77	07-JAN-2008 18:18	ATR		77	00:02 m:s
76	02-JAN-2008 13:16	ATR		164	00:08 m:s
75	14-NOV-2007 02:48	ATR		62	00:03 m:s
74	07-NOV-2007 08:05	ATR		90	00:02 m:s
73	20-OCT-2007 19:28	PMT		120	
72	20-OCT-2007 11:24	ATR		88	00:03 m:s
71	15-OCT-2007 21:19	ATR		61	00:02 m:s
70	09-OCT-2007 10:00	ATR		77	00:00 m:s
69	21-SEP-2007 17:37	ATR		104	00:04 m:s
68	19-SEP-2007 18:35	ATR		76	00:02 m:s

B

FIGURE 12-10. Cont'd.

listing of the most recent events, how they are classified, and how they were managed. Through the log, one is then able to retrieve in-depth information about the specific event. The ability to retrieve and evaluate intracardiac electrograms has been the greatest tool provided to the clinician. We are now able to play back the actual events as seen by the device. This is critical to determine the true cause of the arrhythmia. By evaluating the onset of the arrhythmia, the relationship between atrial and ventricular events, and how the rhythm was terminated, one is able to make a far more accurate diagnosis as compared to using heart rate information alone. Examples of some arrhythmias with the intracardiac recordings are shown in Figure 12-11.

APPROPRIATE PROGRAMMING BASED ON OBSERVED DATA

A comprehensive overview of device programming is beyond the scope of this chapter. However, it is useful for the novice to have a basic understanding of programming to deal with urgent or emergent situations related to the data obtained by a device interrogation. The following are four common clinical situations that would require urgent reprogramming of a device. Recognize that the suggested programming changes noted in this section are for *temporary* resolution of urgent/emergent problems. In all situations, it is essential that properly trained personnel be called in to fully evaluate and manage the device. It may also be necessary to place a temporary transvenous pacing lead as well.

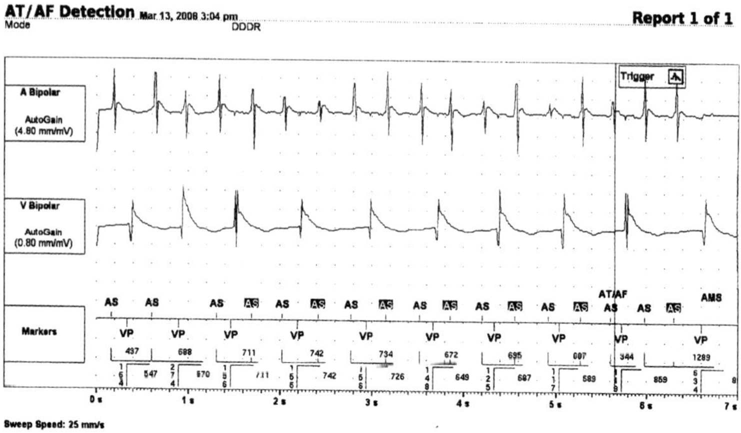

A

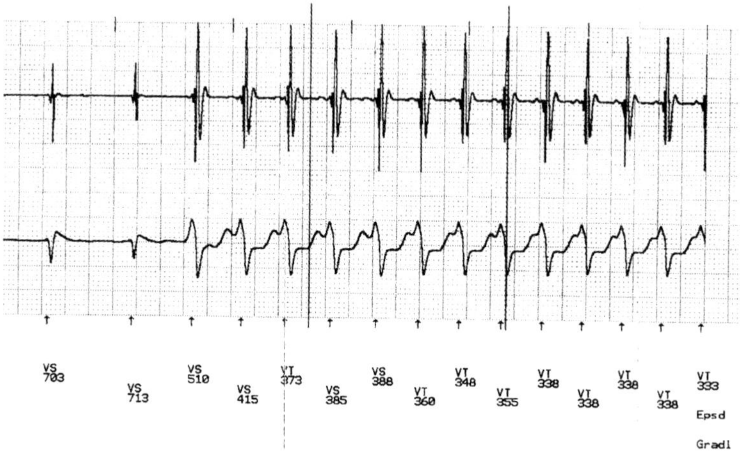

B

FIGURE 12-11. Intracardiac recordings automatically recorded during arrhythmias. **A:** The top tracing is of the atrial rhythm (atrial bipolar), and the middle is of the ventricular rhythm (ventricular bipolar). It can clearly be seen that the atrial rate is faster than the ventricular rate, and that the atrial rate is fairly regular, suggesting a form of atrial flutter. **B:** This tracing is from a single lead ICD. The top tracing is of the sensing bipole in the right ventricle. The bottom tracing is from the "far-field" RV coil to ICD can. The latter gives something close to a surface ECG recording. From this bottom tracing, the onset of ventricular tachycardia as suggested by the presence of a wide complex tachycardia can be easily seen.

ATRIAL FIBRILLATION WITH FAST PACING RATE

A common misperception of patients and some health care providers is that the pacemaker can be programmed to slow the fast ventricular response conducted down the AV node. In general, this is not true. However, there are situations where a dual chamber pacemaker or ICD has been programmed in such a way that it does not recognize or respond to pathologic atrial tachycardias (this is not an issue in ventricular single chamber devices). In such cases, the device may pace the ventricle at the programmed upper rate. Reprogramming the mode to a single chamber or nontracking mode (VVI or DDI) will immediately resolve the fast pacing rate. Note that pharmacologic agents that slow the AV node will have no effect on the conduction of the atrial fibrillation by the pacemaker.

LOSS OF CAPTURE

Pacing output with failure to capture can be an annoyance in a patient with a good intrinsic rhythm, or it can be life threatening in a patient who is pacemaker dependent. The two most common conditions that cause this problem are lead failure and elevated capture threshold. The latter is often due to an acute metabolic issue such as hyperkalemia, acidemia, or hypoxemia. In this situation, one needs to increase the programmed output (voltage and pulse width) in order to immediately restore capture and thus heart function. In an urgent or emergent situation, changing to the highest available voltage and longest available pulse width is simple and prudent. If a capture management algorithm is enabled (such as Autocapture), this should be turned off or disabled. In addition, if increasing the output alone does not result in capture, reprogramming the polarity to unipolar will allow capture if the problem is due to failure of the anode conductor. Note that polarity programmability for the right ventricular lead is not programmable on ICDs. A full evaluation of the leads and device can then be performed by qualified personnel in a more elective manner.

FAILURE TO PACE

Failure to output a pacing pulse can be due to many factors. There is generally not much that can be done for this unless the failure is due to oversensing or failure of the anode conductor (the latter can also cause the former). To diagnose an oversensing situation for a pacemaker (not ICD), placing a magnet over the device is a simple and helpful maneuver. If the device begins to pace, there is oversensing present or some algorithm is withholding pace output. Programming the device to an asynchronous mode (VOO or DOO) will force pacing without regard to any sensing events. Finally, all programmers have an "Emergency" or "STAT" button to automatically program a high output VVI mode. In many devices, the polarity is made unipolar as well. These program changes can be made as well in situations where rapid pacing occurs due to atrial fibrillation with tracking of the arrhythmia by the pacemaker.

INAPPROPRIATE SHOCKS

One of the most psychologically devastating situations for a patient is being shocked repeatedly by an ICD. This is most often caused by atrial fibrillation with a rapid ventricular response or a ventricular lead failure causing oversensing. Emergently, placing a magnet over the device will suspend device therapy, but only as long as the magnet remains over the device. Interrogating the device and turning off arrhythmia detection is the definitive way of preventing further shocks. In the case of atrial fibrillation, one can rate control the patient with the usual pharmacologic agents or cardiovert the patient.

OTHER MONITORED PARAMETERS

Implanted devices are rapidly evolving into devices that are capable of monitoring not only heart rhythms, but also other physiologic parameters. These now include "lung wetness," right ventricular pressure, and even left atrial pressure. The purpose of monitoring these parameters is to help identify the onset of congestive heart failure so that the patient can be managed prior to the need for hospitalization. An example of this is shown in Figure 12-12

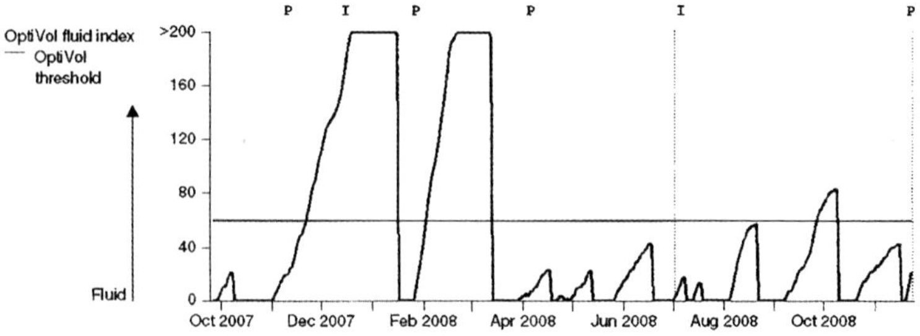

FIGURE 12-12. "Lung wetness" monitoring. This tracing is from an OpitVol enabled device that measures the chest resistance. By doing so, it is able to approximate the amount of fluid in the lungs. The episodes in late 2007 and early 2008 on the graph coincided with hospital admissions for congestive heart failure and pulmonary edema.

from a device with the OptiVol system. This method utilized chest wall plethysmography to monitor the electrical resistance of the lungs. As the "wetness" of the lung tissue increases, the electrical resistance will fall. It is hoped that by monitoring this parameter, and by intervening early in the process of developing congestive heart failure, hospitalization might be avoided. The same is true for monitoring right ventricular pressure (currently investigational). Utilizing this parameter, an estimated pulmonary artery diastolic pressure (ePAD) can be obtained. The ePAD will usually increase parallel to the left ventricular filling pressure, again allowing intervention to hopefully manage heart failure earlier. Left atrial pressure monitoring (also investigational) works in the same way, but measures left atrial pressures directly. Devices capable of monitoring other parameters to identify myocardial ischemia, blood glucose, and oxygen saturation are also being developed.

CONCLUSION

Complete evaluation and proper programming of implantable heart rhythm devices require significant training and experience. However, it is possible for one of minimal training to interrogate a device, and to gain basic knowledge of the device function and the presence or absence of significant arrhythmias. There are occasions when it is appropriate and necessary for one to interrogate a device, and to even make urgent or emergent changes to the programming. However, it is equally important that any time such circumstances exist, collaboration with and eventual evaluation by a trained expert occur as well.

KEY POINTS

1. Identify the device with regard to type (pacemaker, ICD, and Implantable Loop Recorder) and manufacturer so that the appropriate programmer and/or technical support staff can be utilized.
2. Interrogate the device and print all of the current settings at the beginning and end of your evaluation, so that you have a reference should there be a need to go back to the original settings or to evaluate what was changed.
3. Utilize the diagnostic data and graphs to look for changes in device, lead, or patient status.
4. Utilize the rhythm diagnostics to correlate patient symptoms with heart rhythms recorded by the device.
5. Make changes to the device only as needed to resolve a critical issue and then seek guidance from a qualified clinician for further evaluation and programming.

SUGGESTED READINGS

Barold SS, Stroobrandt RX. *Cardiac Pacemakers Step by Step: An Illustrated Guide*. Austin, TX: Futura; 2004. (A good text for those that learn by visual aid. This book is heavily illustrated to help the reader understand the timing cycles of pacemakers.)

Ellenbogen KA, Kay NE, Lau CP, et al. *Clinical Cardiac Pacing, Defibrillation and Resynchronnization Therapy*. 3rd Ed. Philadelphia, PA: W.B. Saunders; 2006. (This is a comprehensive resource that can serve as a complete reference for those in need of a core resource text.)

Ellenbogen KA, Wood MA. *Cardiac Pacing and ICDs*. 5th Ed. Cambridge, MA: Blackwell Science; 2008. (A somewhat more advanced text with an emphasis on ICDs and CRT devices.)

Kenny T. The *Nuts and Bolts of Cardiac Pacing*. Cambridge, MA: Blackwell Science; 2008. (A good starter text for non-cardiologists to understand the basics of pacing.)

Love CJ. *Cardiac Pacing and Defibrillators*. 2nd Ed. Austin, TX: Landes Bioscience; 2006. (This is an excellent basic resource for a novice to gain a good working understanding of device therapy and trouble shooting.)

Stroobrandt RX, Barold SS. *Implantable Cardioverter-Defibrillators Step by Step: An Illustrated Guide*. Malden, MA: Futura; 2009. (This is an excellent companion book to the pacing book by the same authors.)

SECTION IV
Miscellaneous Topics

CHAPTER 13

Approach to the Patient with Wide Complex Tachycardia

John M. Miller, Deepak Bhakta, John A. Scherschel, and Anil V. Yadav

Arriving at the correct diagnosis of wide complex tachycardia (WCT) can be one of the most anxiety-provoking tasks facing most cardiologists and trainees. Although many algorithms have been developed to assist in this process, these are often not easily recalled or applied. The purposes of this chapter are to try to simplify the methods used to make the correct diagnosis, as well as provide a guide to initial patient management. For the following discussion, WCT is defined as heart rate more than 100/min with QRS duration more than 120 ms. WCT may be uniform morphology (all QRS complexes identical) or polymorphic (PM) (varying QRS configuration). Left bundle branch block (LBBB) pattern is characterized by terminal negative vector in V1, whereas right bundle branch block (RBBB) pattern has a positive terminal vector in V1.

UNIFORM-MORPHOLOGY WIDE COMPLEX TACHYCARDIA—DIAGNOSTIC POSSIBILITIES

In order to establish the correct diagnosis of WCT, one must know what the possible diagnoses are. These include

(1) Ventricular tachycardia (VT)
(2) Supraventricular tachycardia (SVT) with
  (a) Aberrant (AB) interventricular conduction
    (i) Fixed (present during baseline rhythm)
    (ii) Functional (present only during WCT)
  (b) Atrioventricular (AV) conduction over accessory pathway (Wolff-Parkinson-White syndrome)
  (c) Abnormal QRS configuration not due to aberration or preexcitation
    (i) Present at baseline—hypertrophy, cardiomyopathy, and congenital heart disease
    (ii) Situational—drug toxicity and electrolyte disorders
(3) Ventricular pacing
(4) Electrocardiographic artifact

TABLE 13-1 Relative Frequency and Clinical Settings of WCTs

Cause of WCT	Relative Frequency[a]	Typical Clinical Setting
VT	+++++	Older patient; SHD; no prior episodes
SVT with aberration	++	Younger patient; no SHD; history of prior tachycardia episodes
SVT with abnormal baseline QRS	++	History of cardiomyopathy, heart surgery
Preexcited SVT	+	Younger patient; Wolff-Parkinson-White syndrome
SVT and pronounced antiarrhythmic drug effect	+	History of use of antiarrhythmic drug ± change in dose or metabolism
SVT with hyperkalemia	Rare	Acute renal failure, rhabdomyolysis
Ventricular paced rhythm	Rare	Pacing system present
ECG artifact	+	Asymptomatic; patient motion

[a]Number of + signs indicate relative frequency in a typical group of patients presenting with WCT.
SHD, structural heart disease.

All WCTs can be categorized as one of these causes; Table 13-1 gives their relative prevalence and typical clinical settings. Ventricular pacing and ECG artifact are rare causes, but their correct recognition is critical to prevent inappropriate testing and treatment for rhythm disturbances that are not present. In almost all published series, VT is the most common cause of WCT (in some series, 75%); therefore, if there is uncertainty as to the correct diagnosis, the WCT should be assumed to be VT. Although special populations have different proportions of the remaining diagnoses (e.g., pediatric centers with congenital heart disease patients), in most clinical situations the differential diagnosis of uniform-morphology WCT is between VT and SVT-AB. The following discussion deals with this distinction. Since the vast majority of both SVT-AB and VT are very regular, varying by no more than 30 ms in cycle length, they are generally readily distinguished from atrial fibrillation with either aberration or conduction over an accessory pathway (Wolff-Parkinson-White syndrome). The latter possibilities will thus not be considered further here.

VENTRICULAR TACHYCARDIA VERSUS SUPRAVENTRICULAR TACHYCARDIA WITH ABERRATION

The ECG appearance of VT can have immense variety, whereas that of SVT-AB has far fewer possible manifestations. Therefore, if one is familiar with all the configurations SVT-AB can have and the WCT being analyzed looks like one of those, most likely it is SVT; if not, it is probably VT. All of the published diagnostic algorithms take advantage of this distinction in one way or another. A brief summary of ECG distinctions follows; Table 13-2 summarizes many of these. The specificities of most criteria are tempered by whether or not the baseline QRS complex is fairly normal or not; if very distorted, such as in patients with cardiomyopathy or repaired congenital heart disease, ECG distinctions are blurred.

(1) QRS duration—The wider the QRS complex, the less likely it is SVT-AB (QRS ≤ 140 ms in over 70% of cases in older literature was SVT but only 40% in more recent studies). WCT with a QRS wider than 140 ms is thus more likely to be VT, and among WCT with QRS greater than 160 ms, 75% are VT.

(2) QRS axis—During SVT-AB, the frontal plane axis may be normal or either anterior or posterior fascicular block may occur; together, these encompass axis vectors from −90 degrees clockwise to 180 degrees, but the so-called northwest

TABLE 13-2 ECG Distinctions between VT and SVT

	SVT with aberration	VT
QRS duration	≤140 ms	>140 ms
QRS axis –90 to 180 degrees	Rare	Occasional (20%)
Precordial concordance	Rare	Occasional (20%)
QRS in V1 (LBBB type)		
Initial R wave duration	≤40 ms	>40 ms
QRS onset to S nadir	≤60 ms	>60 ms
QRS in V6 (RBBB type)		
R/S ratio	>1	<1
RS complex any precordial lead	Present	Absent (30%)
V_i/V_t in multiphasic lead	≥1	<1
QRS in aVR		
Narrow initial Q	Common	Rare
Tall R wave	Rare	Frequent (40%)
Wide/slurred Q	Rare	Occasional (20%)
AV relationship		
Dissociation	Extremely rare	Extremely rare
Non-1:1 relationship	Occasional (30%)	Frequent (40%)

axis (between 180 degrees and -90 degrees, with leads 1, 2, and 3 negative) is difficult to achieve with any type of aberration. Thus, if the axis is in this rightward superior quadrant, SVT is unlikely and VT is diagnosed. Though present in only 20% of VTs, its specificity is 95%.

(3) Precordial concordance—A pattern of all positive or all negative in the precordial leads ("concordance") has historically been unusual in SVT-AB and therefore when present, suggests VT as the WCT diagnosis. About 20% of all VTs have a concordant pattern, roughly evenly split between positive and negative. Recent evidence indicates that negative concordance is not as specific for VT, perhaps because of changes in patient characteristics (more patients with heart failure and very dilated hearts with delayed R wave development and LBBB in sinus rhythm will demonstrate negative concordance during SVT episodes).

(4) Specific QRS patterns in various leads—See Figure 13-1.

(a) Lead V1 and LBBB pattern—Normal septal depolarization causes a small, narrow R wave (≤40 ms) in V1 that is usually preserved with LBBB aberration. In addition, the descent to the nadir of the S wave is rapid (≤60 ms) in normal as well as LBBB aberration complexes. In VT with LBBB pattern, there is either no initial R wave or, if present, it is wider than 40 ms and the QRS onset to S wave nadir is more than 60 ms. These are subtle but readily measured differences.

(b) Lead V1 and RBBB pattern—The normal septal depolarization noted above is unaffected by RBBB aberration, so V1 in SVT with true RBBB shows an rSR′, rSr′, or rsR′. These patterns are unusual in VT, in which a tall, wide initial R wave, Rr′, or QR is more typically present.

(c) Lead V6 and RBBB pattern—Since the right ventricular (RV) muscle mass is small, delayed activation progressing away from V6 during true RBBB yields a qRs configuration (*R/S* ratio >1). Because RBBB-pattern VTs arise in the left ventricle (LV), all of the RV muscle mass as well as some from the LV contribute to the vector progressing away from V6. This yields rS or QS patterns in V6 (*R/S* ratio <1).

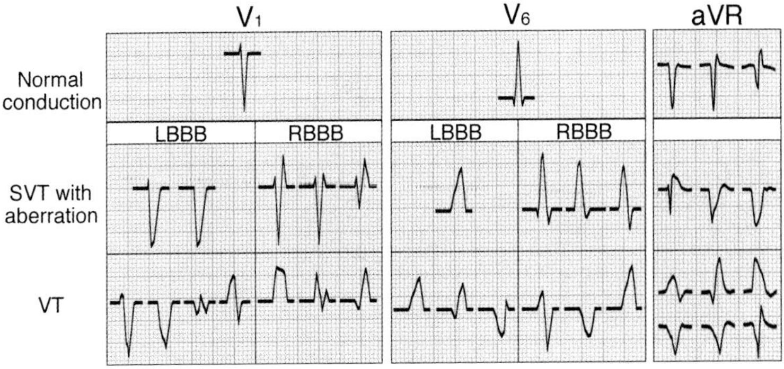

FIGURE 13-1. QRS configurations in SVT-AB and VT in several ECG leads. See text for discussion.

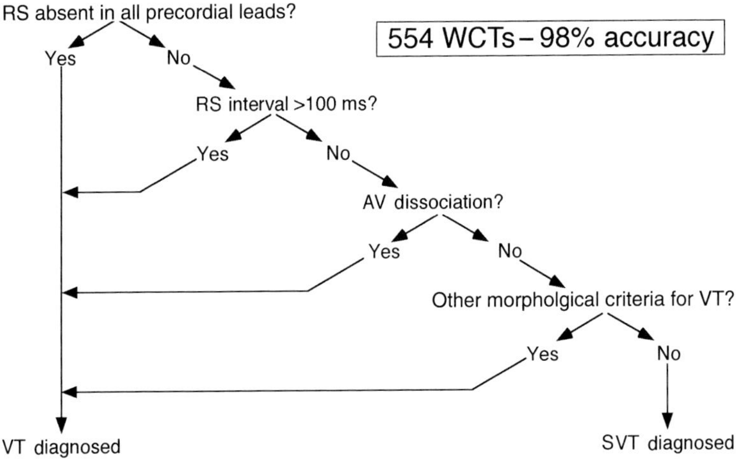

FIGURE 13-2. Brugada algorithm for diagnosis of WCT.

(d) RS complexes in precordial leads—Most cases of SVT-AB have at least one precordial lead showing an RS complex (usually mid-precordial). Brugada et al. (1991) showed that patients with VT often did not have any precordial lead with an RS complex, and thus, if a WCT lacks RS complexes in any precordial lead, VT should be diagnosed. The entire algorithm is shown in Figure 13-2.

(e) Initial versus terminal velocity vectors—As indicated above, in true BBB, the initial QRS vectors are relatively rapid, with conduction delay occurring later in the QRS complex. In VT, however, conduction velocity is relatively slow throughout the QRS. An index of the net voltage traversed in the initial 40 ms of a multiphasic QRS complex divided by the voltage traversed in the final 40 ms of the same QRS complex takes advantage of this disparity in conduction velocity. The resulting ratio, the V_i/V_t index, is ≥1 in the majority of SVT-AB cases and less than 1 in most VT cases. Figure 13-3 shows the algorithm for this criterion.

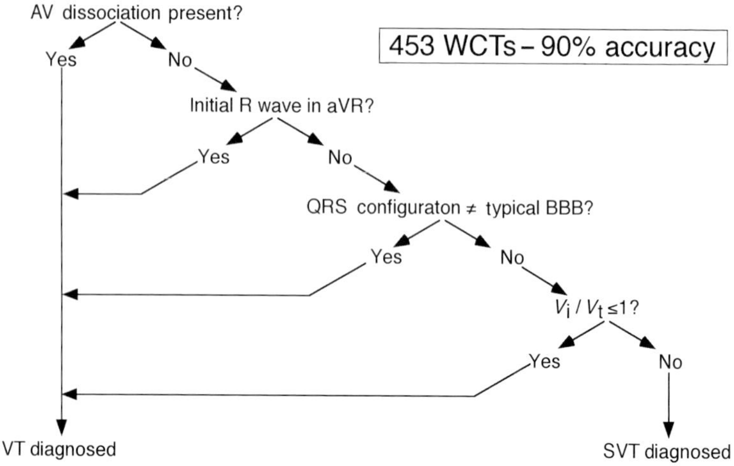

FIGURE 13-3. First Vereckei algorithm for diagnosis of WCT ("V_i/V_t algorithm").

(f) Pattern in aVR—Lead aVR usually shows a rapid QS, Qr, or QR configuration in normal QRS complexes as well as during SVT-AB. In VT, these patterns are rare and are replaced by R, Rs, or complexes starting with a Q but with slurred downstroke (>40 ms). The entire algorithm for this criterion is shown in Figure 13-4.

(5) AV relationship—In the vast majority of SVT-AB cases, there is at least one P wave for each QRS (sometimes more, as in atrial flutter with 2:1 conduction). In VT, this is not necessary; any AV ratio less than 1 is thus highly suggestive of VT. Though a highly specific criterion, it is not very sensitive: in only about 30% of VTs can AV dissociation be clearly seen, although 2:1 or Wenckebach

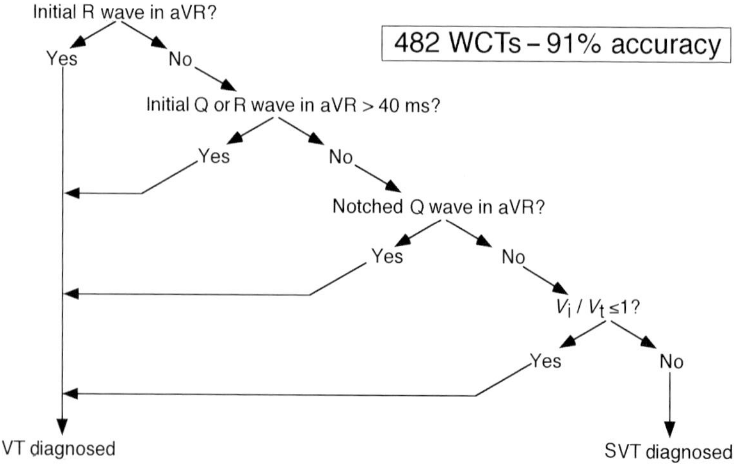

FIGURE 13-4. Second Vereckei algorithm for diagnosis of WCT ("aVR algorithm").

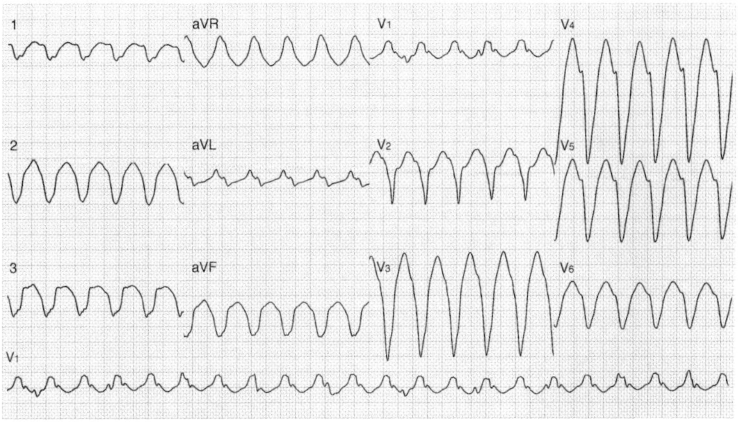

FIGURE 13-5. ECG of VT showing multiple criteria (QRS width 210 ms; axis—120 degree; Rr′ in V1; *R/S* ratio in V6 less than 1; AV dissociation (seen in V1 rhythm strip).

retrograde block can be seen in another almost 10% of VTs. Poor visualization of dissociated P waves due to obscuration by QRS complexes and T waves prevents more frequent diagnosis; in addition, some VT patients may have coexisting atrial flutter or fibrillation as the supraventricular rhythm, making determination of the presence and timing of P waves impossible.

Fusion complexes (a blend of VT and normally conducted complexes) and capture beats (complete supraventricular capture during VT) are the result of fortuitously timed atrial activity conducting to the ventricles to form a narrowed (partially or wholly normal) QRS complex during ongoing VT. These phenomena imply a non-1:1 AV relationship and thereby signify VT as the underlying rhythm in practically all cases. While highly specific, this is unfortunately a rare finding and is limited to relatively slow VTs (rate < 160/min) such that there is adequate time between QRS complexes for a P wave to conduct to some degree.

Figure 13-5 shows a WCT ECG (VT) in which many of the criteria are illustrated.

In patients with implanted cardiac devices (pacemakers and implantable cardioverter-defibrillators [ICD]), additional diagnostic and management options exist. For example, in a patient with a dual-chamber device of any type in whom the nature of WCT is uncertain, interrogation of the device showing "live" running electrograms will show clear atrial activity and generally enable definitive diagnosis. In addition, devices can be used to terminate arrhythmias with overdrive pacing (pacemakers or ICDs) or commanded shock (ICD only). These maneuvers can, however, result in initiation of less stable rhythms (e.g., ventricular fibrillation) and should only be attempted by a skilled electrophysiologist in a setting in which quick corrective action can be taken.

POLYMORPHIC WIDE COMPLEX TACHYCARDIA

PM WCT is not unusual but because the rate is usually very rapid, leading to hemodynamic instability and often death, it does not present the clinician with diagnostic challenges as often as uniform-morphology WCT. Possible causes of PM WCT include

(1) long-QT interval related arrhythmias (congenital vs. drug-related); see Figure 13-6
(2) myocardial ischemia (usually with obvious ST-T changes and normal QT interval; Fig. 13-7)

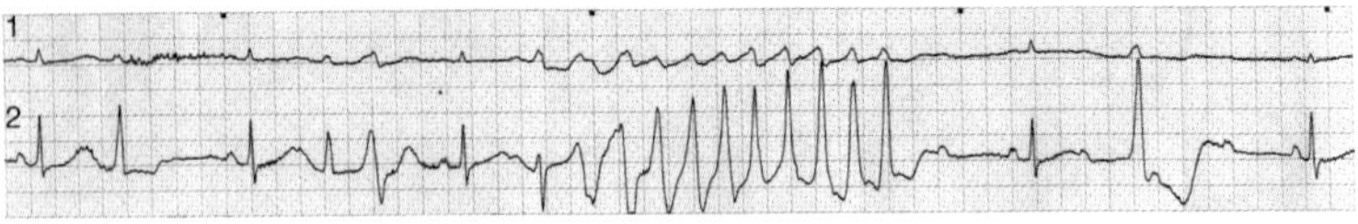

FIGURE 13-6. Rhythm strip of a long QT interval and high-grade AV block. Note constantly changing QRS configuration and prolonged QT before and after episode.

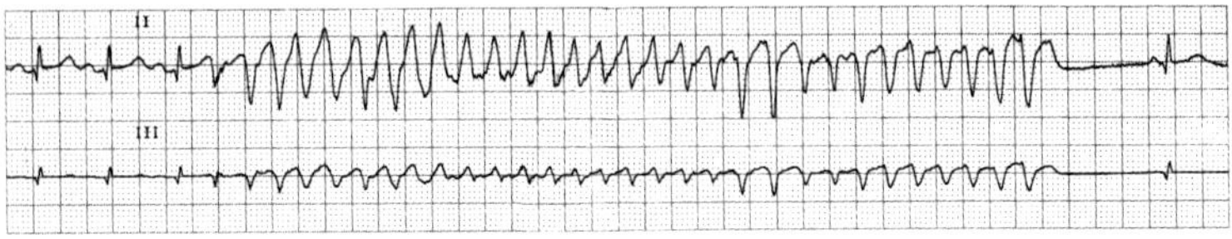

FIGURE 13-7. Rhythm strip of nonsustained PM VT occurring in the setting of myocardial ischemia. Note typical features of very rapid, constantly changing QRS during arrhythmia and mild ST elevation in lead 2.

(3) catecholaminergic PM VT
(4) short-coupled PM VT
(5) idiopathic ventricular fibrillation
(6) preexcited atrial fibrillation with multiple accessory pathways
(7) ECG artifact

ECG artifact is an important consideration in this diagnosis, but because the clinical status of the patient with PM WCT is generally very unstable, simply assessing the patient's status during the episode in question will allow distinction of real arrhythmia from artifact. The major differential in this category is between long-QT related arrhythmias and myocardial ischemia. By their nature, a large number of these cases have at least a potentially reversible cause, and thus, it is critical to make a correct analysis of the nature of the arrhythmia. In many or even most cases, these arrhythmias are either self-terminating after several seconds (with frequent recurrences) or require cardioversion due to hemodynamic instability. The ECG in sinus rhythm prior to onset of episodes will help in the diagnosis (long QT interval, ST segment shifts indicative of ischemia, etc.).

MANAGEMENT OF WIDE COMPLEX TACHYCARDIA

As noted earlier, optimal therapy of WCT hinges on correct diagnosis; conversely, disastrous results can ensue if the wrong diagnosis is made. For example, assuming SVT-AB as the cause of WCT since the patient "looks good" (rather than "sick" as VT patients should look) and administering either verapamil or esmolol can cause sudden hemodynamic collapse that can be difficult to reverse in patients with compromised LV function. Since the majority of WCT are VT, unless one is certain they are dealing with SVT-AB, treatment should be as though the patient had VT.

Initial evaluation of the patient with tachycardia is concerned with his or her overall clinical status—vital signs, assessment for chest pain, dyspnea, light-headedness followed by a search for potential reversible causes, and establishment of intravenous (IV) access (Fig. 13-8). If the patient is unstable (hypotension, loss of consciousness, severe chest pain, or dyspnea despite oxygen administration), urgent synchronized cardioversion is in order. Standard paddle/electrode positions should be used to deliver an initial 150 J biphasic shock. In most cases, lower energies will suffice but higher energies may also be required. This will almost always restore a stable rhythm (sinus, atrial fibrillation, etc.). If tachycardia recurs, repeated shocks may succeed but it is likely that an antiarrhythmic

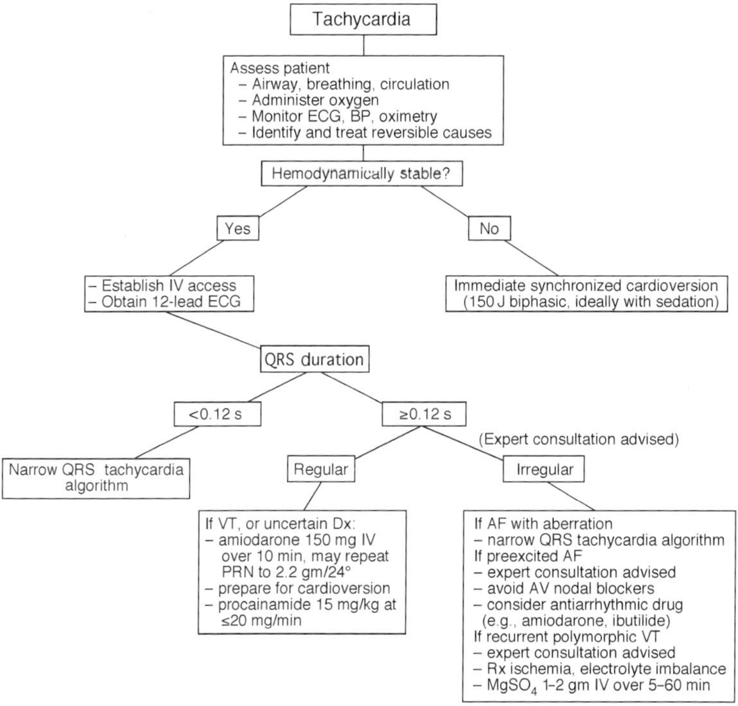

FIGURE 13-8. Algorithm for management of patients with WCT. (Modified from 2005 Advanced Cardiac Life Support Guidelines.)

drug will be needed to maintain a stable rhythm (usually amiodarone). If the patient is instead stable, a 12-lead ECG should be obtained and if the QRS is wide, a concerted attempt at applying one or more algorithms should be made to establish the correct diagnosis. It is always preferable to obtain a 12-lead ECG during an episode for subsequent analysis, even if the diagnosis seemed clear at the time, since ultimate therapy may be guided by ECG characteristics (especially catheter ablation). If VT is the cause or the cause is not clear, IV amiodarone 150 mg over 10 min should be administered. If this fails to convert the rhythm, IV procainamide 15 mg/kg at up to 20 mg/min (limited by hypotension) may be used. If this does not work or at any time the patient becomes unstable, cardioversion may be applied after adequate sedation.

Only very rare cases of PM WCT are due to atrial fibrillation transmitted to the ventricles over multiple accessory pathways; thus, most cases are PM VT and, further, due to a reversible cause (long QT from medications, ischemia, etc.). Discerning such a cause and treating this should proceed on a parallel track with treating the acute arrhythmia episode.

SUMMARY

The differential diagnosis of WCT remains challenging. The clinician has a wide variety of excellent tools at his/her disposal to make the correct diagnosis in the majority of cases, although no diagnostic system or algorithm is without fault. Establishing the correct diagnosis has critical implications for immediate correction of the rhythm disorder as well as subsequent evaluation and management.

KEY POINTS

1. Most cases of WCT are VT.
2. Patient appearance (conversant or comfortable) is an unreliable indicator of diagnosis.
3. A fundamental question in diagnosing WCT is whether it does or does not resemble a known pattern of aberration: if it does, it is probably aberration; if not, it is probably VT.
4. Recent changes in patient characteristics and disease patterns have blurred some ECG distinctions.
5. Existing algorithms can correctly categorize only about 90% of all cases of WCT.
6. Unless the diagnosis is clearly otherwise, WCT should be treated as VT.

SUGGESTED READINGS

Brugada P, Brugada J, Mont L, et al. A new approach to the differential diagnosis of a regular tachycardia with a wide QRS complex. *Circulation*. 1991;83(5):1649–1659.

Miller JM, Das MK, Yadav AV, et al. Value of the 12-lead ECG in wide QRS tachycardia. *Cardiol Clin*. 2006;24(3):439–451.

Vereckei A, Duray G, Szenasi G, et al. Application of a new algorithm in the differential diagnosis of wide QRS complex tachycardia. *Eur Heart J*. 2007;28(5):589–600.

Vereckei A, Duray G, Szenasi G, et al. New algorithm using only lead aVR for differential diagnosis of wide QRS complex tachycardia. *Heart Rhythm*. 2008;5(1):89–98.

Wellens HJJ, Bär FWHM, Lie KI. The value of the electrocardiogram in the differential diagnosis of a tachycardia with a widened QRS complex. *Am J Med*. 1978;64:27–33.

CHAPTER 14

Antiarrhythmic Medications

Katia Dyrda, Paul Khairy, Stanley Nattel, Mario Talajic, Peter G. Guerra, Bernard Thibault, Marc Dubuc, Laurent Macle, and Denis Roy

The ultimate purpose of antiarrhythmic drugs is to restore a normal rhythm and/or prevent the onset of recurrent, rapid, or more serious arrhythmias. All antiarrhythmic drugs alter cellular membrane conductances, either directly or indirectly. Their effectiveness is limited and side-effect profiles range from cardiovascular consequences such as hypotension, worsened heart failure, or conduction tissue impairment to central nervous system and gastrointestinal tract manifestations. Antiarrhythmic drugs should, therefore, be carefully selected, titrated, and monitored. As patients respond variably to individual antiarrhythmic drugs, management strategies are typically fraught with trial and error. Underlying structural heart disease involving the conduction tissue or myocardium must be considered when selecting a drug regimen, as well as the hemodynamic stability of the patient, type of arrhythmia, intended duration of therapy, and associated comorbid conditions.

ANTIARRHYTHMIC DRUG CLASSIFICATION

The most commonly used drug classification is based on electrophysiologic effects of antiarrhythmic drugs at the cellular level. This "action potential" classification was proposed by Singh and Vaughan Williams in 1970. However, antiarrhythmic drugs are complex and their action depends on various factors including tissue type, heart rate, membrane potential, acute or chronic damage to the myocardium, and patient age. They may also produce hemodynamic effects and may alter autonomic nervous system function or cardiac metabolism. The mechanism of action of a given antiarrhythmic drug may, therefore, extend beyond the predominant class to which it was assigned. For example, amiodarone is a class III agent, but also exerts class I, II, and IV actions. In addition, some drugs may not be categorized within this classification system, such as adenosine and digoxin. Table 14-1 summarizes the various drug class and the commonly used agents within each class. Table 14-2 provides standard doses and indicates the routes of elimination of these agents.

Class I drugs impede the rate of Na^+ entry via cardiomyocyte-membrane Na^+ channels across the cell membrane during the upstroke phase of cellular activation. They are, therefore, commonly referred to as Na^+-channel blockers. There are three subclasses, namely A, B, and C, based on the degree of modification of the upstroke velocity of the action potential during phase 0 and their effect on repolarization and conduction velocity. The mechanism or duration of action differs between the subgroups because of variable rates of drug binding to, and dissociation from, the channel receptor. Action potential duration (APD) is increased by class IA drugs, decreased by class IB drugs, and

TABLE 14-1 Classification of Antiarrhythmic Drugs

	Class			
	I	II	III	IV
A	Quinidine	Atenolol	Amiodarone[a]	Verapamil
	Procainamide	Bisoprolol	Sotalol[b]	Diltiazem
	Disopyramide	Carvedilol	Dofetilide	
B	Lidocaine	Esmolol	Ibutilide	
	Mexiletine	Labetolol	Bretylium	
	Phenytoin	Metoprolol	Azimilide	
	Tocainide	Nadolol		
C	Flecainide	Propranolol		
	Propafenone	Timolol		
	Moricizine			

[a]Amiodarone is a class III agent with classes I, II, and IV activity.
[b]l-sotalol has beta-blocking and class III activity while D-sotalol is a pure class III agent.
Source: Adapted from Bennett DH. *Cardiac Arrhythmias: Practical Notes on Interpretation and Treatment.* 7th Ed. London: Hodder Arnold Publishers; 2006.

mostly unaffected by class IC drugs. Class I drugs may also be subclassified on the basis of the type of cells primarily targeted. Class IA and IC affect both atria and ventricles, with intraventricular conduction being particularly slowed by IC drugs, while class IB drugs work particularly at the ventricular level.

Antiarrhythmic agents in this class typically exhibit use-dependence. During faster heart rates, less time is available for the drug to dissociate from the receptor, which results in an increased number of blocked channels and enhanced blockade. Such an effect may lead to a progressive decrease in impulse conduction velocity and widening of the QRS. This is rare with class IB agents since their effect is selective for depolarized tissue, but is more common with class IA and frequent with class IC agents.

Class II drugs interfere with cardiac effects of the sympathetic nervous system, as typified by beta-blockers (although drugs that decrease noradrenalin release, like amiodarone, also have class II actions). They reduce the slope of spontaneous depolarization (phase 4) of cells with pacemaker activity, particularly in SA and AV nodes. The pacemaker discharge rate is lowered as a result, explaining the heart-rate slowing typically seen with beta-blockers.

Class III drugs predominantly block potassium channels such as I_{Kr}, and thus prolong the duration of the action potential, length of the refractory period, and the QT interval. However, they do not modify phase 0.

Class IV drugs impede the slow inward movement of Ca^{2+} via L-type Ca^{2+} current (I_{CaL}) across cell membranes. They are thus referred to as Ca^{2+}-channel blockers. Cells in the sinus and AV nodes are particularly sensitive to their effect because of the prominent role of I_{CaL} in nodal depolarization. Verapamil, diltiazem, and dihydropyridines like nifedipine and felodipine all act on I_{CaL} but differ in the relative amount of cardiac versus vascular blockade at therapeutic doses. The dihydropyridines have little direct electrophysiologic effect on the heart but have strong vasodilator actions.

While the intent of drug therapy is to terminate or prevent arrhythmias, some agents can paradoxically increase the frequency of a preexisting arrhythmia, sustain a previously nonsustained arrhythmia, or cause new arrhythmias, a phenomenon called "proarrhythmia." Proarrhythmic effects are most often noted with class I and class III agents. Class III proarrhythmic events most commonly occur shortly after introduction

TABLE 14-2 Bolus and Maintenance Doses of Commonly Used Antiarrhythmics

Drug	Primary Route of Elimination	Bolus or Loading Dose		Maintenance Dose	
		IV	po	IV	po
Adenosine		6 mg over 2 s followed by saline flush; repeat doses of 12 and 18 mg at 1 min intervals if unsuccessful			
Digoxin	Kidney	0.5 mg followed by 0.25 mg q6h ×2	0.5–1.0 mg	0.0625–0.25 mg q24h	0.0625–0.25 mg q24h
Disopyramide	Kidney	1–2 mg/kg over >15 min		1 mg/kg/h	100–300 mg q6–8h
Procainamide	Kidney	6–13 mg/kg at 0.2–0.5 mg/kg/min	500–1,000 mg	2–6 mg/min	250–1,000 mg q4–6h
Quinidine	Liver	6–10 mg/kg at 0.3–0.5 mg/kg/min	800–1,000 mg		300–600 mg q6h
Lidocaine	Liver	1–3 mg/kg at 20–50 mg/min	Not applicable	1–4 mg/min	Not applicable
Phenytoin	Liver	100 mg q5 min (maximum 1,000 mg)	1,000 mg		100–400 mg q12–24h
Mexiletine	Liver	250 mg in 5–10 min then 250 mg over 1 h	400–600 mg	0.5–1.0 mg/min	150–300 mg q8–12h
Flecainide	Liver	1–2 mg/kg over >10 min	100–200 mg q12h		50–150 mg q12h
Propafenone	Liver	1–2 mg/kg	450–900 mg		150–300 mg po q8–12h
Dronedarone	Kidney				400 mg q12h
Amiodarone	Kidney	150 mg over 10 min (may be repeated over 10–30 min) then 1 mg/min for 8 h then 0.5 mg/min for 16 h	800–1200 mg/day until a total of 10 g		100–400 mg q24h
Sotalol	Kidney	10 mg over 2 min			40–160 mg q8–12h
Bretylium	Liver	5–10 mg/kg at 1–2 mg/kg/min		0.5–2 mg/min	4 mg/kg/day
Dofetilide	Kidney	2–5 µg/kg			0.125–0.5 mg q12h
Verapamil	Liver	5–10 mg over 30–60 s	0.005 mg/kg/min		120–360 mg q24h

or after altering the dose. Female sex, renal insufficiency, pretreatment QT interval, and the presence of heart failure significantly increase this risk in the case of sotalol. Class I proarrhythmia most typically occurs with acute ischemic events.

CLASS IA DRUGS—QUINIDINE, PROCAINAMIDE, AND DISOPYRAMIDE

Class IA agents moderately depress the phase 0 upstroke in non-nodal tissue, which is sometimes called "fast-channel" or "fast-response" tissue because of the rapidity of phase-0 upstroke and conduction caused by the large phase-0 Na^+ current. Reduced phase-0 Na^+ current causes a slowing of depolarization and conduction, and a corresponding prolongation of conduction time in fast-response cells of atrial muscle, ventricular muscle, His-Purkinje cells, and accessory pathways. Their kinetics of onset and offset is of intermediate rapidity (1 to 5 s). They also block K^+ channels, particularly I_{Kr}, and prolong APD. These effects are reflected by the surface ECG as an increase in QRS duration and prolongation of the QT interval.

Class IA agents have moderate potassium-channel blocking activity, which tends to slow the rate of repolarization and prolong APD. At slower heart rates, use-dependent blockade of the sodium current is not as manifest. This phenomenon, along with a tendency for APD prolongation due to potassium-channel blockade to increase at slow rates, produces increasing APD and QT prolongation with bradycardia, which is termed reverse use-dependence. In predisposed patients, excessive bradycardia-related repolarization-delaying actions of class IA drugs can lead to excess APD and QT prolongation, along with torsade de pointes arrhythmias.

While IA agents have little effect on the slow-response cells of the normal SA and AV nodes, interactions with the autonomous nervous system may exert indirect changes. In addition, the rate of SA node discharge may increase and AV nodal conduction may be enhanced by the anticholinergic effect of IA drugs.

The IA agents find their use in the treatment of reentry tachycardias, both at the level of the atria (atrial fibrillation [AF] and flutter) and of the ventricle (ventricular tachycardia), as well as with accessory pathways (WPW syndrome).

Intravenous procainamide continues to be used in centers in North America for conversion of AF with an efficacy that is probably less than that with Class IC agents. It can also be administered for acute termination of reentrant ventricular tachyarrhythmias in the setting of preserved left ventricular function with success rates reaching 80%. Its long-term oral use is limited by its restricted absorption, short half-life, and side effects including gastrointestinal symptoms, agranulocytosis, and lupuslike syndromes. Of note is that *N*-acetyl-procainamide, a metabolite of procainamide, acts as a class III agent, with little effect on inhibiting sodium current but preserved K^+-current blocking properties.

The use of *quinidine* has been largely abandoned because of a high incidence of gastrointestinal side effects and the proarrhythmic risk of torsade de pointes ventricular arrhythmia. Emerging evidence may support a role in minimizing ICD shocks in patients with the short QT syndrome. It has also been used to control arrhythmic storms in patients with the Brugada syndrome.

Disopyramide is an alternate agent that can be administered both parenterally and orally to treat supraventricular or ventricular tachyarrhythmias. In practice, it is used mainly in younger patients for the management of AF (in combination with an AV nodal blocking agent), for recurrent supraventricular arrhythmias, or in selected patients with PVCs. Dose adjustments are required if renal function is impaired, as the drug is partially excreted by the kidney. It is contraindicated in patients with QT prolongation as it can also cause torsade de pointes. Its use should be limited to patients with preserved left ventricular function because of its negative inotropic effects and the risk of precipitating heart failure. The intravenous loading dose should not exceed 0.5 mg/kg/min as severe hypotension may ensue. Its peripheral anticholinergic actions are responsible for the common side effects such as blurry vision, closed-angle glaucoma, dry mouth, constipation, and urinary retention and, more importantly, for the increased ventricular response to AF or flutter.

CLASS IB DRUGS—LIDOCAINE, MEXILETINE, AND PHENYTOIN

When administered in therapeutic doses, class IB agents cause a negligible decrease in the slope of phase 0 of normal fast-response action potentials. The surface ECG remains unaffected except possibly for a slight shortening of the QT interval. However, in the presence of cell damage, hyperkalemia, and acidosis, the effect is amplified. The refractory period and, to a lesser extent, the duration of the action potential, can shorten. Purkinje fibers and ventricular myocytes are particularly sensitive to these effects, which are far less notable in atrial tissue. Class IB agents do not influence slow-response cells of normal SA and AV nodes and have a trivial impact on autonomic tone. Fewer proarrhythmic events have been associated with IB agents. The kinetics of onset and offset of these agents is rapid (generally <500 ms).

Class IB agents are not indicated for the treatment of supraventricular arrhythmias. They are considered for the treatment of ventricular arrhythmias, especially those associated with acute myocardial infarction (MI) and a prolonged QT interval. They have limited efficacy for conversion of stable monomorphic ventricular tachycardia in the setting of chronic left ventricular dysfunction. Prophylactic *lidocaine* may worsen outcomes after MI and is thus no longer recommended for prophylaxis of ventricular arrhythmias in the setting of acute MI.

Lidocaine can only be administered intravenously, and as such, its use is limited to short-term therapy. Dose adjustments are required if liver function is impaired and in situations of low cardiac output, in which reduced liver blood flow slows lidocaine elimination. The bolus dose must be carefully selected as many dose-formulations are available on the market. A continuous infusion should follow if the bolus successfully terminated the arrhythmia. Titration of the drug may be difficult, given its narrow therapeutic range. A fall in plasma levels may permit a recurrence of the arrhythmia while supratherapeutic levels often affect the central nervous system. Confusion, light-headedness, paresthesias, and involuntary movements are the most common manifestations, with seizures and coma representing severe toxicity.

Mexiletine has a long elimination half-life, which allows for oral administration. It is a moderately effective agent for treating acute and chronic ventricular tachyarrhythmias, but not supraventricular tachycardias. It may also be considered for the treatment of patients with the LQT3 syndrome. It has a similar narrow therapeutic profile to lidocaine. Commonly experienced side effects include bradycardia and hypotension, nausea and vomiting, confusion, tremor, and ataxia. Dose adjustments are required if liver function is impaired and in low cardiac output states. Mexiletine may be useful in selected patients when combined with class I drugs or amiodarone.

Phenytoin may be administered via either route but is a weaker agent and is virtually never used as an antiarrhythmic drug at present.

CLASS IC DRUGS—PROPAFENONE AND FLECAINIDE

Class IC drugs do not affect autonomic tone but do cause a profound depression in the upstroke of phase 0 and a marked slowing of conduction in fast-response tissues. However, they have minimal impact on repolarization and APD. The refractory period is not typically prolonged, although the effective refractory period may be increased in the His-Purkinje system and accessory pathways. They are powerful inhibitors of abnormal automaticity and reentry within atrial and ventricular muscle, and accessory pathways. These drugs have slow onset and offset kinetics (10 to 20 s).

Characteristic ECG findings include a prolonged QRS resulting from slowing of intraventricular conduction and a secondarily lengthened QT interval with an unchanged T wave. The PR interval may be slightly prolonged.

Flecainide can be administered orally and intravenously. It is, however, unavailable intravenously in North America. It is effective in the treatment of paroxysmal AF, atrial flutter, AV reentrant tachycardias, pre-excitation syndromes, and idiopathic symptomatic ventricular ectopy. Typically this drug is used in patients with paroxysmal AF not associated with significant structural heart disease, where it is effective in preventing recurrences of AF in 50% of patients. It should be avoided in patients with heart failure because of its negative inotropic effects and in patients with coronary artery disease, even with preserved ventricular function. This drug has a narrow therapeutic range and a marked widening of the QRS is a sign of supratherapeutic levels. It can be proarrhythmic, especially in patients with a history of sustained ventricular tachycardia, with or without underlying heart failure. As a result of its potent atrial conduction slowing properties, it may transform AF into a slower atrial flutter, which may conduct 1:1 to the ventricles. Because of this potential atrial proarrhythmia, simultaneous beta-blocker or calcium-channel blocker therapy, intended to slow AV-nodal conduction, is recommended. Since it is metabolized by the liver and excreted by the kidney, dose adjustments are rarely required for end-organ impairment.

Propafenone is effective in treating supraventricular and ventricular arrhythmias. Proarrhythmic effects have been reported. It is contraindicated if left ventricular function is impaired. Similar to flecainide, propafenone can increase the ventricular response rate to atrial fibrillation and flutter. It is, therefore, often used in combination with an AV-nodal blocking agent in such patients, despite the fact that is has mild inherent beta-blocking properties.

Propafenone is metabolized by CYP2D6 and to a lesser extent by CYP1A2 and CYP3A4. Drugs that inhibit CYP2D6 (such as paroxetine, sertraline, and fluoxetine), CYP1A2 (such as amiodarone), and CYP3A4 (such as grapefruit juice and ketoconazole) will increase the plasma levels of propafenone. Propafenone itself is also an inhibitor of CYP2D6. Hence, coadministration of propafenone with drugs metabolized by CYP2D6 (such as quinidine, haloperidol, and venlafaxine) may lead to increased plasma levels of these drugs. In addition, concomitant use of propafenone and digoxin increases steady-state serum digoxin and decreases the clearance of digoxin. Plasma digoxin levels must thus be monitored in patients receiving propafenone and digoxin dose adjustments may be indicated.

CLASS II DRUGS—BETA-BLOCKERS

Beta-blockers exert their effect on cardiac arrhythmias through multiple and complex mechanisms. Competitive inhibition of catecholamine binding to cardiac beta-adrenoreceptors is the primary effect, resulting in a reduction of both normal and abnormal automaticity in nodal tissue, and slowing of AV-nodal conduction. Chronic therapy with high doses of certain agents like propranolol may also exert membrane effects such as prolongation of APD and effective refractory periods, in addition to increasing the ventricular fibrillation threshold.

Any arrhythmia that results from increased sympathetic nervous system activity on the heart may respond to beta-blockers. This includes exercise-related arrhythmias and those associated with pheochromocytoma, thyrotoxicosis, and ventricular arrhythmias in the setting of myocardial ischemia or long QT syndrome (particularly LQT1/5 and to a lesser extent LQT2). Catecholaminergic-mediated tachycardias due to abnormal automaticity or triggered activity at the atrial or ventricular levels may also respond favorably to beta-blocker therapy. Although generally less useful for reentrant tachycardias that do not involve the AV node, they may suppress premature beats that trigger reentry. When

TABLE 14-3 Characteristics and Usual Doses of Various Beta-blocking Agents

Drug Name	Alpha-blockade	Cardio selectivity	Dose		Route of Elimination	ISA
			po	IV		
Acebutolol	–	+	200–800 mg q24h	N/A	Renal and hepatic	+
Atenolol	–	++	50–200 mg q24h	N/A	Renal	–
Bisoprolol	–	+	2.5–20 mg q24h	N/A	Renal and hepatic	–
Carvedilol	+	–	3.125–25 mg q12h	N/A	Hepatic	–
Esmolol	–	++	N/A	5–10 mg/kg then 0.05–0.3 mg/kg/min	Blood esterases	–
Labetalol	+	–	100–400 mg q12h	20–300 mg q12h	Hepatic	–
Metoprolol	–	++	25–150 mg q12h	5–15 mg q6–8h	Renal	–
Nadolol	–	–	40–160 mg q24h	N/A	Renal	–
Propranolol	–	–	10–80 mg q6–8h	1–5 mg q6–8h	Hepatic	–

N/A, not applicable; ISA, intrinsic sympathomimetic activity.

used to treat supraventricular arrhythmias in which the AV node is a necessary part of the circuit, the therapeutic objective is to sufficiently depress the AV node so that conduction cannot be maintained during tachycardia. Beta-blockers must be given carefully in order to avoid significant bradycardia. This is particularly true if sick sinus syndrome is suspected, to prevent post-cardioversion pauses. In addition, beta-blockers can exert negative inotropic effects, which can precipitate or worsen heart failure. However, when beta-blockers are introduced under stable conditions and carefully titrated, they improve survival in patients with heart failure.

Nonselective beta-blockers affect cardiac Beta-1 and bronchial- and blood vessel-predominant Beta-2 receptors. Selective beta-blockers only affect B1 receptors. Selective B1-blockers are, therefore, often preferred since B2-blockade can aggravate reactive airway disease. Table 14-3 provides a summary of the various available beta-blockers, their target dose, and selectivity.

Several beta-blockers have been extensively studied in numerous clinical trials. For example, metoprolol, atenolol, and carvedilol (which also has alpha-adrenergic receptor blocking actions) decrease mortality and sudden death after MI. Although class effects common to all appropriately titrated beta-blockers confer benefit for arrhythmic indications, some exert unique pleiotropic actions. For example, *carvedilol* is a beta- and alpha-adrenergic blocker that inhibits calcium, potassium, and sodium currents, and prolongs APD. However, with chronic use of carvedilol, the number of channels increases.

CLASS III DRUGS—AMIODARONE, DRODENARONE, DOFETILIDE, IBUTILIDE, SOTALOL, BRETYLIUM, AND VERNAKALANT

Class III antiarrhythmic drugs prolong the action potential without affecting phase 0 and have a variable effect on the autonomic nervous system.

Amiodarone is the most potent antiarrhythmic available, with a unique pharmacokinetic and side-effect profile. It can block sodium channels in depolarized tissues and may inhibit calcium channels, potassium channels, and (nonspecifically) adrenergic receptors. It is generally used for life-threatening arrhythmias or arrhythmias refractory to other medical therapy. Although success rates vary according to the patient population and the type of arrhythmia targeted, 1 year arrhythmia-free rates of 60% to 80% for supraventricular arrhythmias and 40% to 60% for ventricular arrhythmias have been reported. It is considered to be the most effective antiarrhythmic drug to prevent recurrences of AF. Despite earlier trials suggesting an improvement in prognosis with amiodarone compared to placebo, amiodarone when compared to ICD therapy had no favorable effect on survival in patients with poor left ventricular function. In selected patients, amiodarone has resulted in a reduction in both appropriate and inappropriate ICD shocks as compared to beta-blocker therapy or sotalol.

The predominant electrical effect of amiodarone is prolongation of the APD and, hence, refractory period in fast-response cells of atrial and ventricular muscle, Purkinje fibers, and accessory pathways. Surface ECG changes include a decreased sinus rate, prolonged PR, mildly increased QRS duration, and prolonged QT. With significant QT prolongation, the risk of torsade de pointes may increase, although, notably, amiodarone can cause substantial QT prolongation without inducing torsade de pointes.

Amiodarone may be administered orally or intravenously. A central line is preferable for intravenous administration, given the risk of phlebitis. A loading period is required before a therapeutic effect can be fully appreciated, as the elimination half-life ranges from 20 to 100 days. With oral administration, the onset of action typically occurs 2 days to a week after the start of therapy, while peak levels are not reached for 1 to 2 months. These pharmacokinetic properties allow for stable serum levels over time but unfortunately render drug elimination very slow in cases of drug toxicity. Amiodarone is metabolized by the liver to desethylamiodarone, which maintains some antiarrhythmic effects. Amiodarone and its metabolites accumulate in the adipose tissue, cardiac muscle, lung tissue, and liver.

The lowest possible effective maintenance dose should be targeted in an attempt to minimize the risk of toxicity. In practice, this is usually 200 mg/day. However, the long-term risk of unwanted effects should not preclude therapy, particularly if the patient's prognosis is poor. Prior to initiation of chronic therapy, patients must be informed of the multiple potential extra-cardiac side effects including blue skin discoloration and photosensitive skin rash, corneal deposits, gastrointestinal disturbance, hypothyroidism or hyperthyroidism, hepatitis, peripheral neuropathy, pulmonary interstitial fibrosis, and adult respiratory distress syndrome. Adverse effects are noted in approximately 75% of patients treated for 5 years but only a third discontinue therapy.

Dronedarone is a novel antiarrhythmic drug with electrophysiologic properties similar to amiodarone but with a much shorter half life. Significant proarrhythmic effects have not been noted. Since it contains no iodine radical, it has a gentler side-effect profile, free of amiodarone's thyroid, pulmonary, hepatic, and dermatological toxicity. There is, however, concern about increased mortality in patients with moderate to severe heart failure. Serum creatinine levels have also been noted to rise due to reduced tubular excretion (without overt renal function impairment). In a recent very large trial (Athena), dronedarone was found to reduce cardiovascular hospitalizations and death in AF patients with cardiovascular risk factors. Dronedarone is currently under regulatory review for drug approval.

Sotalol is primarily a nonselective beta-blocker without intrinsic sympathomimetic activity at low doses, and exhibits class III properties at higher doses. Unlike pure beta-blockers, sotalol has a clear effect on the recovery period of atrial and ventricular myocardium and accessory pathways, particularly with higher doses. It has been used to treat supraventricular and ventricular tachyarrhythmias, including patients with defibrillators. Sotalol does have proarrhythmic potential, especially in the setting of hypokalemia or when associated with other QT-prolonging drugs. QT surveillance is thus mandatory. It is contraindicated in patients with prolonged QT or a family history of long QT syndrome. In addition, the risk of toxicity increases significantly in elderly, hypertensive females with low body weight taking diuretics and in the setting of impaired renal function.

Sotalol exhibits reverse use-dependence effects, manifested by prolongation of repolarization and the refractory period during slower heart rates. Effects are less pronounced at higher heart rates. This translates into a longer QT at lower heart rates, which shortens with an increase in heart rate.

Dofetilide is moderately successful in acutely converting and preventing atrial fibrillation and flutter. QT prolongation is expected, with torsade de pointes occurring in less than 5% of patients. Therapy must, therefore, be initiated under continuous cardiac monitoring for a minimum of 72 h. Dofetilide is contraindicated if the QTc exceeds 500 ms and the dose must be reduced if the QT increases by 15% after the first dose. Lower dosing is required in patients with renal dysfunction. Dofetilide does not have a negative inotropic effect and, in spite of its proarrhythmic potential, does not increase mortality in patients with impaired ventricular function. In fact, its use has been associated with fewer hospitalizations for heart failure. A careful review of the patient's drug profile is indicated prior to initiation of therapy as the concomitant administration of multiple other drugs may further increase the QT interval or raise serum levels. Dofetilide is commercially available only in the US.

Ibutilide is an intravenous class III agent, which converts atrial fibrillation and flutter to sinus rhythm in 30% to 50% of cases. It has been found to be more effective in converting atrial flutter. Torsade de pointes occurs in 3% of patients.

Bretylium has unique delayed-onset antiarrhythmic properties and autonomic effects. The cardiovascular response to the drug is biphasic, with an initial period of sinus tachycardia, increase in blood pressure, and possible worsening of the arrhythmia. These are due to the drug concentration at sympathetic nerve terminals, which results in an early phase of norepinephrine release. This initial response is followed by a decrease in blood pressure. Arrhythmias may subsequently terminate as norepinephrine release is eventually blocked. Bretylium is rarely used. It has little effect on sustained ventricular tachycardia but may prevent recurrence of ventricular fibrillation.

Vernakalant is an early-activating potassium-channel blocker and frequency-dependent sodium blocker with relative atrial selective effects. Phase 3 clinical trials of the intravenous formulation demonstrated vernakalant to be efficacious and safe in converting recent-onset AF to sinus rhythm. Common adverse effects included dysgeusia, sneezing, and paresthesia. Intravenous vernakalant is currently under regulatory review for drug approval for the acute conversion of AF.

CLASS IV DRUGS—VERAPAMIL AND DILTIAZEM

Calcium-channel blockers such as verapamil and diltiazem act predominantly on L-type Ca^{2+} currents in the cells of the SA and AV nodes, leading to a decreased phase 4 automaticity, a slowed phase 0 depolarization, and prolonged refractoriness and conduction time. The normal fast response action potential is largely unaffected in healthy myocardium. However, when injured, atrial and ventricular cells may demonstrate altered fast response action potential with exposure to calcium-channel blockers.

Few changes are noticeable on the surface ECG, namely, slight sinus slowing and PR interval prolongation, this without modification to the QRS or T wave.

Verapamil is often used intravenously for reentrant tachycardias that involve either SA or AV nodes as part of the circuit and may abruptly terminate the tachycardia. Examples include SA node reentry, AV node reentry, and macroreentry involving an accessory pathway with anterograde conduction through the AV node. Tachycardias arising from atrial muscle are much less likely to terminate but slowing of AV node conduction and refractoriness may permit better control of the ventricular response. In addition, right ventricular outflow tract tachycardia and fascicular tachycardia may be terminated with intravenous verapamil. Unfortunately, prevention of these arrhythmias with oral verapamil is uncommon.

Although verapamil is considered safe for acute termination of orthodromic reentry, it is not recommended for the acute treatment of atrial fibrillation or flutter in patients with WPW syndrome. The ventricular response to atrial fibrillation or flutter may significantly increase as conduction through the accessory pathway is enhanced, with potential degeneration into an unstable ventricular rhythm.

Verapamil may cause profound bradycardia and hypotension. Its intravenous administration is relatively contraindicated in patients already treated with beta-blockers Verapamil is also contraindicated in patients with impaired sinus or AV node activity. Finally, it has significant negative inotropic properties and is, therefore, contraindicated in patients with impaired ventricular function.

Diltiazem has a similar profile to that of verapamil but a less pronounced inhibitory effect. Diltiazem is generally better tolerated than verapamil for chronic oral therapy since it causes less hypotension and constipation.

UNCLASSIFIED DRUGS—ADENOSINE AND DIGOXIN

Adenosine is an endogenous nucleoside found in all cells in the body. In circulation, it has a half-life of only 10 s and is very quickly removed by erythrocytes and endothelial cells. If large doses are administered rapidly, adenosine can transiently block AV-nodal conduction and slow SA node automaticity by activating an adenosine-sensitive outward potassium current. It, therefore, has an attractive profile as an acute first-line agent for AV reentry tachycardias. Transient AV block may occur for a few seconds as the tachycardia terminates. Adenosine will also transiently slow the ventricular response to atrial flutter or fibrillation, unmasking the flutter or fibrillation waves. In patients with sick sinus syndrome, sinus function may transiently worsen when conversion to sinus rhythm occurs.

Adenosine may be helpful diagnostically, although a response or lack thereof is not an infallible indicator. For example, right ventricular outflow tract tachycardia may respond to adenosine while some supraventricular tachycardias will fail to terminate. In some instances, lack of response to adenosine is related to the rate of drug injection and travel time to the heart, which can be longer than its duration of action. In other cases, the administered dose may have been insufficient to break the tachycardia. Adenosine is generally not indicated for wide complex tachyarrhythmias unless there is a reasonable possibility that a supraventricular tachycardia is conducting aberrantly, in which case adenosine may confirm the diagnosis.

Contraindications to adenosine include a history of asthma with severe bronchospasm. Patients should be warned about the uncomfortable transient sensation of flushing, chest tightness, and/dyspnea that accompany adenosine administration.

Digoxin has a direct effect on cell membranes of atrial and ventricular muscle and on specialized conduction tissue, including accessory pathways. It causes a mild decrease in the duration of the action potential and refractory period. However, the predominant effect is an enhancement of vagal tone, which is demonstrated clinically by slowing of the SA node and depression of AV nodal conduction. It is, therefore, widely used for rate control in AF, although it does not have a significant effect on restoring sinus rhythm.

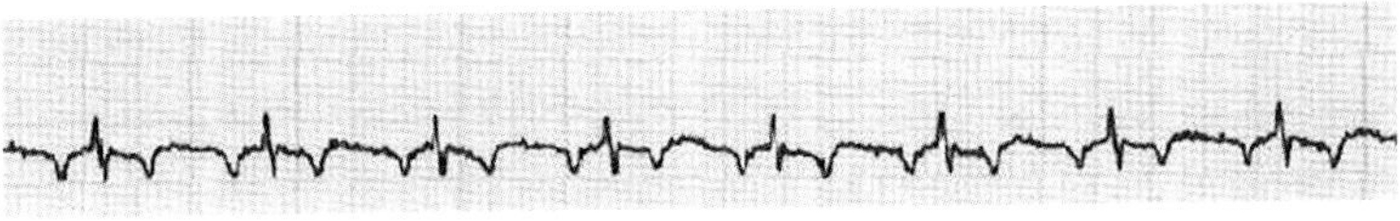

FIGURE 14-1. Atrial tachycardia with 2:1 AV block. (Source: Courtesy of Dr Marc Dubuc, Montreal Heart Institute.)

In situations of minimal vagal tone, such as when a patient is active, digoxin is often ineffective as monotherapy for rate control.

Typical ECG manifestations include sinus rate slowing, PR prolongation, and QT interval shortening. Depression of the ST segment with a scooped or hockey stick appearance and flattening of the T waves are characteristic.

Digoxin toxicity should be suspected if patients experience dizziness, nausea, vomiting, diarrhea, anorexia, blurry or yellow vision, confusion, weakness, or apathy. Predisposing factors include dehydration, renal impairment, hypokalemia, hypercalcemia, and combination therapy with amiodarone and other drugs. The serum digoxin level should be measured at least 6 h after the last dose and need not be elevated for toxicity to develop. Signs of toxicity can be noted on the ECG, such as sinoatrial block, sinus bradycardia, sinus or atrial tachycardia with AV block, AF with a junctional rhythm, slow response to AF, ventricular ectopic beats, or ventricular tachycardia. Figure 14-1 shows an ECG finding observed with digoxin toxicity.

The treatment of digoxin toxicity consists of stopping the drug, correcting electrolyte abnormalities, and providing supportive care including temporary pacing if indicated. In the absence of significant AV block, propranolol can be effective in treating digoxin-induced tachycardias. Otherwise, lidocaine and phenytoin are safer alternatives. Note that cardioversion is considered potentially dangerous in the setting of digoxin toxicity. If a shock is unavoidable, the lowest energy possible should be used and a lidocaine bolus administered.

In cases of life-threatening acute or chronic toxicity, digoxin-specific Fab fragments should be considered. Such indications include

- Arrhythmia causing hemodynamic instability (ventricular arrhythmia or severe bradyarrhythmia)
- Serum potassium level greater than 5 mmol/L
- Altered level of consciousness attributable only to digoxin toxicity
- Serum digoxin level greater than 12.8 nmol/L (or >3.6 nmol/L in case of renal impairment) measured 6 to 8 h after acute ingestion or as baseline level if chronic ingestion
- Acute ingestion of greater than 10 mg of digoxin

The antibody is given intravenously and binds circulating digoxin until it can be eliminated. It is important to note that once the antibody has been administered, measured total serum digoxin levels will not be interpretable for up to 7 days (while measured total serum levels will be increased, the bound fraction will be inactive). Management decisions must then be based solely on clinical judgment. Equations exist to calculate de dose of Digibind based on the amount ingested or on serum digoxin level. Unfortunately, these are difficult to remember in an emergency situation. A simple but safe rule of thumb is to administer 20 vials (standard dose of 38 mg/vial) in two separate doses for acute ingestions or 6 vials for chronic ingestions. The dose should be diluted in 50 mL of NS. Finally, anaphylactoid reactions have been reported and therefore, a cutaneous intradermal test should be performed in asthmatic patients or those who have previously been treated with Digibind.

Therapy with digoxin is not absolutely contraindicated once a diagnosis of digoxin toxicity is established, provided the factors which predispose to increased risk of toxicity can be alleviated and the dose reduced.

THE USE OF ANTIARRHYTHMIC DRUGS IN PREGNANCY

Several hemodynamic changes during pregnancy may predispose women to recurrent arrhythmias or development of new arrhythmias. While most tachyarrhythmias during pregnancy are benign and self-limited, the risk to mother and fetus is higher in the presence of underlying cardiac disease. To date, there is no strong evidence supporting the safety of antiarrhythmic medication in pregnancy, prompting a conservative approach to therapy in most. Table 14-4 summarizes the risk classification system for drug therapy in pregnancy.

The use of antiarrhythmics is further complicated by pharmacokinetic changes that occur in pregnancy, with difficulty maintaining therapeutic drug levels. Alterations in drug absorption can be attributed to changes in the gastric pH and decreased gastrointestinal motility. Intravascular volume increases, which may affect drug distribution and warrant increased dosages. A reduction in serum protein levels may increase the amount of free circulating drug. Enhanced drug elimination results from increased renal elimination and hepatic metabolism. As such, the use of antiarrhythmics should be restricted to those with severe symptoms and hemodynamic instability. In these extreme cases, a reasonable object is to limit the number of antiarrhythmic agents and target the lowest effective dose. Table 14-5 provides an overview of indications and possible adverse effects of antiarrhythmic drugs during pregnancy and lactation.

TABLE 14-4 Definition of FDA Pregnancy Risk Categories

Pregnancy Category	Definition
A	*Controlled studies show no risk*—adequate and well-controlled studies have failed to demonstrate a risk to the fetus in any trimester of pregnancy.
B	*No evidence of risk in humans*—animal reproduction studies have failed to demonstrate a risk to the fetus and there are no adequate and well-controlled studies in pregnant women or animal studies that have shown an adverse effect, but adequate and well-controlled studies in pregnant women have failed to demonstrate a risk to the fetus in any trimester. The chance of fetal harm is remote but remains a possibility.
C	*Risk cannot be ruled out*—animal reproduction studies have shown an adverse effect on the fetus and there are no adequate well-controlled studies in humans, but potential benefits warrant use of the drug in pregnant women despite potential risk.
D	*Positive evidence of risk*—there is positive evidence of human fetal risk but potential benefits may warrant the use of the drug in pregnant women despite potential risk.
X	*Contraindication in women who are or who may become pregnant*—studies in animals or humans have demonstrated fetal risk, and the risk involved in the use of the drug in pregnant women clearly outweighs the potential benefits.

Source: *Physicians Desk Reference*. 57th Ed. Montvale, NJ: Thomson PDR; 2004:3539.

TABLE 14-5 Indications and Potential Adverse Effects of Antiarrhythmic Drug Use in Pregnancy

Drug Name	Vaughan-Williams Class[a]	FDA Risk Class	Indication	Potential Adverse Effect in Pregnancy	Use During Lactation	Key Points
Adenosine	N/A	C	Acute termination of maternal SVT	Transient fetal bradycardia, maternal dyspnea	Unknown, probably safe	First line for acute treatment of SVT if failure of vagal maneuvers
Digitalis	N/A	C	Maternal and fetal SVT; AF rate control; CHF	Miscarriage (if digitalis toxicity in mother), premature labor; low birth weight	Compatible	Long record of safety
Quinidine	IA	C	Maternal and fetal arrhythmias including SVT with CBT; maternal malaria	Maternal and fetal thrombocytopenia; eighth nerve toxicity; torsade de pointes	Generally compatible but caution advised	Long record of safety
Procainamide	IA	C	Acute treatment of undiagnosed wide complex tachycardia	Lupuslike syndrome with long-term use; torsade de pointes	Compatible but long term therapy not recommended	Long record of safety; IV dosing; drug of choice for acute management of wide complex tachycardia
Disopyramide	IA	C	Variety of maternal and fetal arrhythmias but limited experience	Induction of labor; torsade de pointes	Compatible	Limited experience and alternatives available thus best avoided
Lidocaine	IB	B	Maternal VT; arrhythmias due to digoxin toxicity	CNS adverse effects; bradycardia	Compatible	Long record of safety but must be avoided in case of fetal distress
Mexiletine	IB	C	VT	CNS adverse effects; bradycardia; low APGAR scores; fetal hypoglycevmia	Compatible	Experience limited
Phenytoin	IB	D	Arrhythmias due to digoxin toxicity	Mental and growth retardation; fetal hydantoin syndrome; fetal hypoglycemia	Generally compatible but caution advised	Better alternatives available thus best avoided

(Continued)

TABLE 14-5 Indications and Potential Adverse Effects of Antiarrhythmic Drug Use in Pregnancy (Cont'd)

Drug Name	Vaughan-Williams Class[a]	FDA Risk Class	Indication	Potential Adverse Effect in Pregnancy	Use During Lactation	Key Points
Flecainide	IC	C	Maternal and fetal SVT and VT	Increased mortality in patients with prior MI but generally safe if structurally normal heart	Compatible	Best option for treatment of fetal SVT with hydrops
Propafenone	IC	C	Maternal and fetal SVT and VT	Similar concerns to flecainide; mild beta-blocking effect	Unknown	Experience limited
Beta-blocking agents	II	C (however D for atenolol)	Maternal and fetal SVT; AF/AFl rate control; idiopathic VT; HCM; maternal HTN; thyrotoxicosis	Intrauterine growth retardation; fetal bradycardia; fetal apnea; premature labor; hypoglycemia; hypocalcemia; hyperbilirubinemia	Avoid atenolol. Metoprolol and propranolol compatible	Generally considered safe, avoid during first trimester if possible, cardioselective agent preferable
Amiodarone	III	D	Life-threatening ventricular arrhythmias; fetal SVT	Fetal hyperthyroidism or hypothyroidism; prematurity; low birth weight; fetal bradycardia; congenital malformations; maternal and fetal QT prolongation	To be avoided since a large amount of drug is absorbed by the infant	Use only if no alternative exists; avoid especially in first trimester
Sotalol	III	B	Maternal and fetal SVT; maternal VT; hypertension in the past	torsade de pointes; beta-blocking effect	Generally compatible but caution advised	Experience limited but effective
Ibutilide	III	C	Acute termination of AF/AFl	Torsade de pointes	Unknown	No experience in pregnancy
Bretylium	III	C	Maternal ventricular arrhythmias	Unknown	Unknown	Very limited experience in pregnancy. Not recommended
Calcium antagonists	IV	C	Maternal and fetal SVT; AF/AFl rate control; idiopathic VT (verapamil); maternal HTN, premature labor	Fetal bradycardia and heart block; maternal hypotension; depression of cardiac contractility; maternal hepatitis; fetal distal digital defects	Compatible	Verapamil relatively safe but safer options available. Experience limited with diltiazem

[a] Vaughan Williams classification of antiarrhythmics.

AFl, atrial flutter; APGAR, appearance, pulse, grimace, activity, respiration; CBT, concealed bypass tract; CHF, congestive heart failure; CNS, central nervous system; HCM, hypertrophic cardiomyopathy; HTN, hypertension; IV, intravenous; N/A, not applicable; SVT, supraventricular tachycardia; VT, ventricular tachycardia.

Source: Adapted from Joglar JA, Page RL. Antiarrhythmic drugs in pregnancy. *Curr Opin Cardiol*. 2001;16:40–45, with permission.

KEY POINTS

1. Despite the fact that we presently live in an interventional era of electrophysiology, the vast majority of patients are still treated with drugs.
2. The ultimate purpose of antiarrhythmic drugs is to restore a normal rhythm and/or prevent the onset of recurrent, rapid, or more serious arrhythmias. Antiarrhythmic drugs are generally more effective at restoring sinus rhythm than at preventing the recurrence of an arrhythmia.
3. Antiarrhythmic drugs have side effects that may restrict long-term use.
4. The lowest effective dose should be sought.
5. ECG QTc measurements must be an integral part of titration protocols for any antiarrhythmic drug that potentially prolongs the QTc.
6. Antiarrhythmic drugs may exert proarrhythmic effects, especially in the setting of acute ischemia and ventricular dysfunction.
7. Electrical cardioversion in the setting of digoxin toxicity is considered dangerous and should be reserved for hemodynamic instability or life-threatening arrhythmia.
8. As patients respond variably to individual antiarrhythmic drugs, management strategies are typically fraught with trial and error.
9. Factors to consider when selecting a drug regimen include the nature of the arrhythmia, presence of underlying structural heart disease or hemodynamic instability, impairment of sinus or AV node function, and intended duration of therapy.
10. Beta-blockers are the first-line therapy to control the ventricular response to atrial fibrillation and flutter, and for arrhythmias initiated by exercise and emotions.
11. Sotalol, propafenone or flecainide are often used as first-line therapy for maintenance of sinus rhythm in patients with AF without underlying heart disease.
12. Adenosine remains the drug of choice to terminate reentrant tachyarrhythmias that involve the AV node as an obligatory part of the circuit.
13. Amiodarone remains the most effective antiarrhythmic drug but is also associated with the least favorable extracardiac side-effect profile. It is primarily used for arrhythmias that are life threatening or resistant to other drug therapy.
14. Many tachyarrhythmias can be conservatively managed during pregnancy. Digoxin and beta-blockers are considered first line agents. Antiarrhythmic medications should generally be avoided, particularly during the first trimester of pregnancy.

SUGGESTED READINGS

Bennett DH. *Cardiac Arrhythmias: Practical Notes on Interpretation and Treatment.* 7th Ed. London: Hodder Arnold Publishers; 2006.

Fogoros RN. *Electrophysiologic Testing.* 4th Ed. Oxford: Blackwell Publishing Ltd; 2006.

Kron J, Conti JB. Arrhythmias in the pregnant patient: Current concepts in evaluation and management. *J Interv Card Electrophysiol.* 2007;19:95.

Miller JM, Zipes DP. Therapy for cardiac arrhythmias. In: Libby P, Bonow RO, Mann DL, Zipes DP, eds. *Braunwald's Heart Disease: A Textbook of Cardiovascular Medicine.* 8th Ed. Philadelphia, PA: Saunders Elsevier; 2008, Chapter 33.

Qasqas SA, McPherson C, Frishman, et al. Cardiovascular pharmacotherapeutic considerations during lactation and pregnancy, *Cardiol Rev.* 2004;12:201–221.

Vaughan Williams EM. Classification of antiarrhythmic drugs, In: Sandoe E, Flensted-Jansen E, Olesen KH, eds. Symposium on Cardiac Arrhythmias. Sodetalje, Sweden: AB Astra; 1970:449–472.

Walsh EP, Saul JP. Cardiac arrhythmias. In: Keane JF, Lock JE, Fyler DC, eds. *Nadas' Pediatric Cardiology.* Philadelphia, PA: Saunders Elsevier; 2006:507–511.

CHAPTER 15

Channelopathies

Iwona Cygankiewicz and Wojciech Zareba

Last two decades witnessed a significant progress in our understanding of electrophysiology (EP) of myocardial cell and in appreciation of the role cardiac ion channels play in pathologies of the heart. Inherited arrhythmia disorders, starting with the long QT syndrome (LQTS), have served (and still serve) as a Rosetta Stone for elucidating how specific cardiac ion channel abnormalities might relate to arrhythmogenic conditions in myocardium. The duration and morphology of the action potential of myocardial cell is governed by a complex interplay of several membrane ion currents and by intracellular shifting of mostly calcium ions. As shown in Figure 15-1, activation of both atrial and ventricular myocardial cell depends on proper function of numerous ion channels. In this chapter, we will focus just on principal forms of channelopathies related to ventricular myocardial cells. Sodium and calcium inward currents and potassium outward currents maintain electrical balance of the myocardial ventricular cell. An overcharge of myocardial cell with positively charged ions during repolarization (excessive inflow of sodium or calcium ions or deficient removal of potassium ions) is arrhythmogenic. Such conditions could be caused by inherited arrhythmia disorders (i.e., LQTS, short QT syndrome [SQTS], and Brugada syndrome) or by acquired heart diseases (ischemic or nonischemic cardiomyopathies) where down-regulation of potassium currents and an overload of myocardial cells with calcium ions accompany the disease process. This chapter aims to provide an overview of the channelopathies (LQTS, SQTS, Brugada syndrome, and catecholaminergic polymorphic ventricular tachycardia [CPVT]) that should be considered when evaluating patients without apparent structural heart diseases who present with ventricular arrhythmia, unexplained syncope, cardiac arrest, or sudden death in family members.

LONG QT SYNDROME

The LQTS is a genetically determined disorder characterized by prolongation of QT interval and propensity to syncope, cardiac arrest or sudden death in association with torsade de pointes (TdP), and polymorphic ventricular tachycardia (VT) that might be self-terminating or deteriorate to ventricular fibrillation (VF) (Fig. 15-2). The prevalence of LQTS is estimated at 1:3,000 to 1:5,000 in the general population.

LQTS is caused by mutations of predominantly potassium and sodium ion channel genes or channel-related proteins leading to positive overcharge of myocardial cell with consequent heterogeneous prolongation of repolarization in various layers and regions of myocardium. Table 15-1 shows a list of genes and affected ion channels or related proteins associated with the LQTS. Among positively genotyped patients LQT1 and LQT2 account for about 90%, LQT3 accounts for about 5% to 8%, while the remaining types of LQTS are extremely rare. The most frequent LQTS forms are linked with gene mutations in KCNQ1 resulting in a reduction in I_{Ks} current (LQT1); KCNH2 resulting in a reduction in I_{Kr} current (LQT2); and SCN5A gene resulting in an increase in late INa current (LQT3).

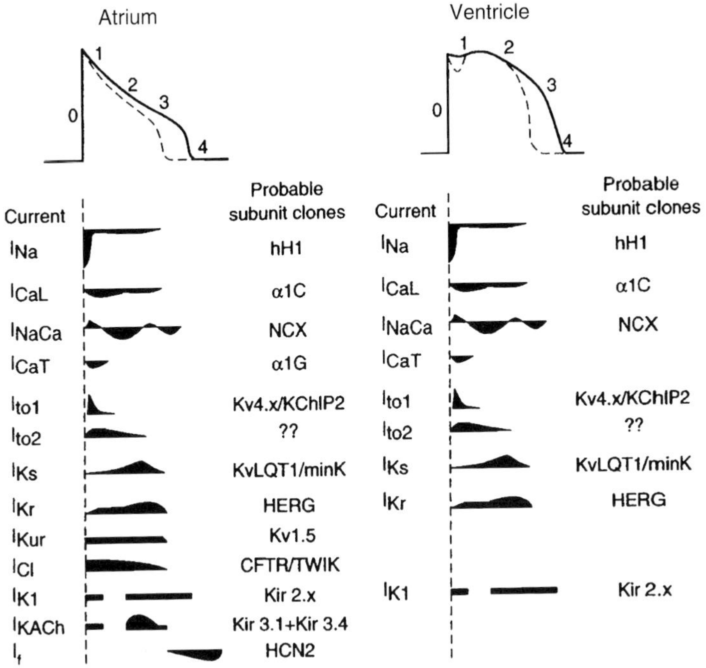

FIGURE 15-1. Action potential and membrane currents active during a ventricular action potential. (Reproduced from Tomaselli G, Roden DM. Molecular and cellular basis of cardiac electrophysiology. In: Saksena S, Camm AJ, eds. *Electrophysiological Disorders of the Heart.* Philadelphia, PA: Elsevier Inc., 2005, with permission.)

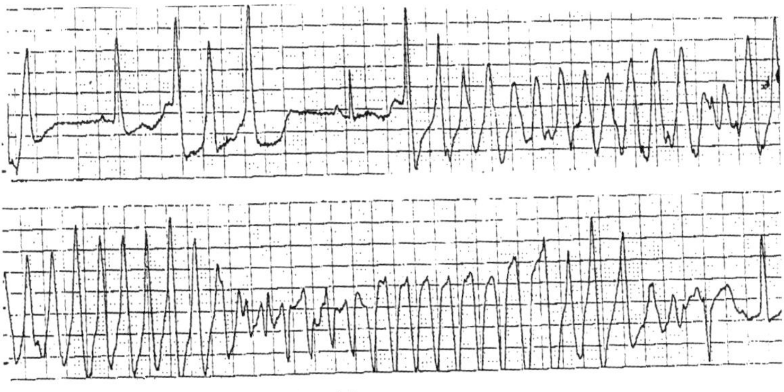

FIGURE 15-2. Exemplary *torsade de pointes* VT.

LQTS DIAGNOSIS

Diagnosis of LQTS is based on the ECG findings and clinical history. Symptoms including palpitations, syncope, an aborted cardiac arrest in evaluated individual, or sudden death/cardiac arrest in a relative are usually directing toward a suspicion of the LQTS.

TABLE 15-1 Genetic Types of the LQTS

Genotype	Chromosome	Affected Gene	Channel Protein	Ion-Channel Current	Frequency in Mutation-Identified LQTS Patients
LQT1	11	KCNQ1 (Kv7.1)	Four α-subunits each with six membrane spanning segments	$\downarrow I_{Ks}$	45%
LQT2	7	KCNH2 (hERG) (K_v11.1)	Four α-subunits each with six membrane spanning segments	$\downarrow I_{Kr}$	45%
LQT3	3	SCN5A (Na_v1.5)	One α-subunit with 24 membrane spanning segments	↑late I_{Na}	7%
LQT4	4	Ankyrin-B (ANK2)	Sodium pump and Na/Ca exchanger	I_{Na}[a]	<1%
LQT5	21	KCNE1 (MinK)	β-Subunit of KCNQ1 with one membrane spanning segment	$\downarrow I_{Ks}$	<1%
LQT6	21	KCNE2 (MiRP1)	β-Subunit of KCNH2 with one membrane spanning segment	$\downarrow I_{Kr}$	<1%
LQT7	17	KCNJ2 (Kir2.1)	Two membrane spanning segments	$\downarrow I_{K1}$	<1%
LQT8	6	CACNA1C (Ca_v1.2)	One α_1-subunit with 24 membrane spanning segments	$\uparrow I_{Ca}$	<1%
LQT9	3	CAV3 (Caveolin)	Altered gating kinetics of Na_v1.5	I_{Na}[a]	<1%
LQT10	11	SCN4B (Na_vB4)	β-Subunit of SCN5A with one membrane spanning segment	↑late I_{Na}	<1%
LQT11	7	AKAP9	A-kinaze anchor protein	$\downarrow I_K s$[a]	<1%
LQT12	20	SNTA1	Sodium current (SCN5A) regulator	$\uparrow I_{Na}$[a]	<1%

[a]Channel-related proteins, these are not proteins forming channels.

TABLE 15-2 Bazett-corrected QTc Values for Diagnosing QT Prolongation

Rating	1–15 years (ms)	Adult Male (ms)	Adult Female (ms)
Normal	<440	<430	<450
Borderline	440–460	430–450	450–470
Prolonged	>460	>450	>470

Source: Reprinted from Moss AJ, Robinson JL. Long QT syndrome. *Heart Dis Stroke*. 1992,1:309–314, with permission.

A standard surface 12-lead ECG is the baseline test used to recognize whether suspicious symptoms could be related to the LQTS or could be linked to other arrhythmogenic conditions like hypertrophic cardiomyopathy, arrhythmogenic right ventricular cardiomyopathy, or Brugada syndrome. An LQTS patient may present with a QTc interval duration that is prolonged, borderline, or normal, according to age and gender (Table 15-2). Patients with QTc > 500 ms usually do not pose a diagnostic problem as they present high likelihood of LQTS, while in symptomatic patients with QTc ranging from 440 to 500 ms, other confounding factors including underlying heart disease (e.g., cardiomyopathy), QT-prolonging drugs, or improper QT interval measurement should be ruled out.

Although the QT interval includes QRS complex, the entire QT interval is considered as a measure of repolarization since repolarization process starts during QRS complex for early activated regions of myocardium. The QT interval should be measured from the onset of QRS complex to the offset of T wave, defined as a deflection point terminating the descending arm of the T wave usually at the level of isoelectric line or as the nadir between T and U waves. Physiologically, QT interval duration should be considered from the earliest onset of QRS complex in any of the 12 leads to the latest offset of T wave in any lead. However, this approach is rarely used apart from some automatic algorithms. Limb lead II is the most frequently used to measure QT interval manually. When T and U waves are merged or when the T wave has a bifid pattern a careful inspection of repolarization duration in all 12 leads might be helpful in determining QT interval duration. In case of repolarization morphologies with the presence of a second component of T wave or U wave, some investigators suggest using the rule that U wave usually should be at least 150 ms behind the peak of the T wave, whereas closer deflections might be considered as the second component of T wave. Since QT duration changes with heart rate, QTc correction formulae were developed to compare given QT and given heart rate to QT at 60 beats/min. The most popular is Bazett formula ($QTc = QT/[RR^{1/2}]$), but Fridericia formula ($QTc = QT/[RR^{1/3}]$) is increasingly used especially in studies evaluating the effects of drugs on QT interval. Bazett QTc formula has limitations of overestimating repolarization duration at fast heart rates and underestimating it at slow heart rates. Fridericia formula causes less misjudgment.

In patients suspected for LQTS, analysis of T wave morphology might be of special values since QT prolongation is frequently accompanied by changes in T wave morphology. In addition to QT prolongation, abnormal T wave morphology including flattened, bifid, broad based, and biphasic T waves might be observed in 12-lead ECGs of LQTS patients. Figure 15-3 shows specific patterns associated with distinct LQTS genotypes: LQT1 is characterized by wide, broad-based T waves, LQT2 usually shows low-amplitude and frequently notched T waves, and LQT3 is characterized by a relatively long ST segment followed by a peaked, frequently tall, T wave.

Table 15-3 demonstrates a diagnostic score, based on ECG findings, clinical history, and family history proposed by Schwartz et al. (1993) to recognize the likelihood of LQTS. A high probability of LQTS diagnosis is present if score reaches a value of at

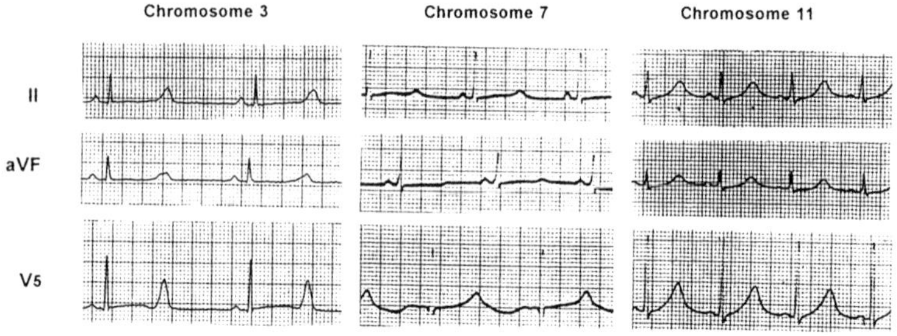

FIGURE 15-3. T wave morphology in ECG recordings from leads II, aVF, and V5 from patients with LQTS1, LQTS2, and LQTS3. (Reproduced from Moss AJ, et al. ECG T-wave patterns in genetically distinct forms of the hereditary long QT syndrome. *Circulation.* 1995;92:2929–2934, with permission.)

least 4, whereas in the case of score values of 2 to 3, the likelihood of diagnosis is lower. While facing patients suspected of LQTS, it is also necessary to pay attention to factors that triggered syncopal episodes or cardiac arrest. LQT1 patients are more likely to develop cardiac events during exercise and swimming, LQT2 patients have their episodes frequently associated with emotions, sudden noise, and LQT3 could develop events on awakening or during sleep.

Genetic testing of the LQTS is especially valuable in borderline cases and in early diagnosis of family members. The clinical course might be different by genotype, as well as the effectiveness of therapy with beta-blockers is different in LQT1 than LQT2 and LQT3 patients. Commercial genotyping covers the most frequent LQTS genes: LQT1, LQT2, LQT3, LQT5, and LQT6, whereas the remaining genes (LQT4, LQT7 to 10) are tested less frequently since mutations of these genes are very infrequent.

RISK STRATIFICATION AND MANAGEMENT OF LQTS PATIENTS

Risk stratification of LQTS patients should include the assessment of QT duration, history of prior syncope or cardiac arrest, gender, age, family history, and genotype. The QTc > 500 ms is associated with a twofold to threefold higher risk of cardiac events, defined as syncope, aborted cardiac arrest, or sudden death in comparison to individuals with shorter QTc. History of recent syncopal episodes that occurred less than 2 years before patient's seeking advice is associated with extremely high risk of aborted cardiac events. The risk of cardiac events in LQTS patients is modulated by a gender-age interaction. Males have higher risk of cardiac events than females till puberty and subsequently females tend to demonstrate higher risk of events. Carriers of LQT1 and LQT2 mutations have higher risk of cardiac events than LQT3 carriers. On the other hand, LQT3 patients were found to have higher lethality of cardiac events, meaning that their risk of dying during first cardiac event was few-fold higher than that of LQT1 or LQT2 patients.

Therapeutic approach to a LQTS patient should aim to decrease the risk of cardiac events and sudden death. LQTS patients have their arrhythmic events frequently triggered by stress, exercise, swimming, and sudden awakening. Patients and their family members should be advised to eliminate ringing clocks, phones, and other noise-making devices as much as possible. Circumstances where sudden noise (e.g., discotheque) and stress (e.g., rollercoaster rides) is likely to occur should be avoided. Patients should avoid getting involved in competitive sports and water sports since swimming or sudden immersion in water might trigger cardiac events. Patients should

TABLE 15-3 Diagnostic Criteria for LQTS

Findings	Score
Electrocardiographic[a]	
Corrected QT interval, ms	
≥480	3
460–470	2
450 (in males)	1
Torsade de pointes[b]	2
T wave alternans	1
Notched T wave in three leads	1
Low heart rate for age[c]	0.5
Clinical history	
Syncope[b]	
With stress	2
Without stress	1
Congenital deafness	0.5
Family history[d]	
Family members with definite LQTS	1

Scoring ≤1 point, low probability of LQTS; 2 to 3 points, intermediate probability of LQTS; and ≥4 points, high probability of LQTS.

[a]Findings in the absence of medications or disorders know to affect these electrocardiographic findings. The corrected QT interval (QTc) is calculated by Bazett formula: $QT/RR^{1/2}$.

[b]Torsade de pointes and syncope are mutually exclusive.

[c]Resting heart rate below the second percentile for age.

[d]The same family member cannot be counted in both categories.

Source: Reprinted from Schwartz PJ, Moss AJ, Vincent GM, et al. Diagnostic criteria for the long QT syndrome: An update. *Circulation*. 1993;88:782–784, with permission.

be informed about many cardiac and noncardiac drugs that might prolong QT interval and cause TdP VT. Protection with automatic external defibrillator, which could be located at home and could accompany patients during various activities, is another preventive option which is exercised in lower risk patients. Special emphasis should be put on the compliance of patients taking beta-blocker since gaps in beta-blocker treatment might contribute to sudden increase in propensity to develop life-threatening ventricular arrhythmias.

Antiadrenergic therapy consisting of beta-blockers is a mainstay of treatment in LQTS patients. In particular, LQT1 patients seem to well benefit from beta-blocker therapy and, if compliant, they rarely need implantable cardioverter-defibrillators (ICDs). In general, beta-blockers seem to be effective in LQT2 patients, but there are high-risk individuals who have recurrences of cardiac events despite beta-blocker treatment and these patients should qualify for ICD therapy (Table 15-4). There is a controversy regarding whether LQT3 patients benefit from beta-blocker therapy; however, no sufficient data exist justifying that LQT3 patients should not be treated with beta-blockers. In some high-risk LQTS patients, usually already with ICDs and on beta-blocker therapy, performing left cervicothoracic stellectomy (left cardiac sympathetic denervation) might lead to a significant improvement by further decreasing the probability of catecholaminergic response and risk of cardiac events.

High-risk LQTS patients qualify for prevention of sudden death with ICDs. The category of high-risk patients should include individuals after cardiac arrest, patients with recurrent syncope despite beta-blockers, individuals with QTc > 500 ms with syncopal episodes occurring during the past 2 years. There is no evidence that family history (sudden death cases in first-degree relatives) should drive decision making

TABLE 15-4 Indications for ICD Implantation in Patients with Channelopathies

	Primary Prevention	Secondary Prevention	
Channelopathy	**Class IA**[a]	**Class IIA**	**Class IIB**
LQTS	Past history of cardiac arrest	Syncope and/or VT on beta-blockers	High-risk LQTS patients[b] (QTc > 500 ms, syncope, LQT2, LQT3, and JLN)
SQTS[c]	Past history of cardiac arrest		
Brugada syndrome	Past history of cardiac arrest	Spontaneous type I ECG and syncope or asymptomatic with inducible VT/VF	Asymptomatic drug-induced ECG type I and family history of SD and positive EP study
		Drug-induced type I ECG and syncope	
CPVT	Past history of cardiac arrest	Syncope and/or VT on beta-blockers	

Note: According to ACC/AHA/ESC 2006 Guidelines for Management of Patients with Ventricular Arrhythmias and the Prevention of Sudden Death, ACC/AHA/HRS 2008 Guidelines for Device-based Therapy on Cardiac Rhythm Abnormalities, and Second Consensus on Brugada Syndrome HRS/EHRA.
[a]ICD therapy recommended in patients on optimal pharmacotherapy and life expectancy more than 1 year.
[b]For details refer to Table 15-3.
[c]Due to sporadic cases, SQTS risk stratification unknown, not included in guidelines.

regarding implantation of ICDs. High-risk LQT2 and LQT3 patients are those who might particularly benefit from ICD therapy, whereas in LQT1 patients, usually beta-blocker therapy is sufficient to protect the patient. It is worth stressing that implantation of ICD at a young age despite life-saving benefits carries a life-time consequences of device replacements, malfunction, inappropriate shocks and the decision regarding implanting device should be taken with understanding of risks and benefits of this therapy.

Shortening QTc with medication is a desired goal of therapy in the LQTS, but this concept is currently limited just to LQT3 patients who might benefit from administration of flecainide, the only sodium channel blocker evaluated to date in long-term studies. Late sodium channel blocker ranolazine might serve as an attractive alternative but a long-term use of this drug in LQT3 patients is not yet evaluated.

DRUG-INDUCED QT PROLONGATION AND THE RISK OF PROARRHYTHMIA

Drug-induced QT prolongation and TdP have been recognized as the side effects of several cardiac and noncardiac medications. The majority of these drugs act by blocking I_{Kr} current directly or through their metabolites, others demonstrate such action if administered together with a drug affecting function of the cytochrome P-450 enzymatic system. Not all medications that block I_{kr} current are associated with TdP, which means that QT prolongation induced by I_{Kr} blockade must be accompanied by a significant increase in transmural dispersion of repolarization to create conditions suitable for the development of TdP.

Transmural dispersion of repolarization seems to play the most important role in arrhythmogenesis in both drug-mediated and congenital forms of LQTS. The episodes of TdP usually start with a short-long-short pattern of RR cycles consisting of short-coupled premature ventricular beat followed by compensatory pause and another premature ventricular beat usually falling close to the peak of the T wave (R on T). This pattern increases heterogeneity of repolarization in the myocardium and promotes arrhythmogenic conditions. TdP episodes usually show a warm-up phenomenon with first few beats of VT presenting longer cycle lengths with subsequent shortening of the cycle lengths of tachycardia. TdP frequently terminates spontaneously with last two to three beats showing slowing of arrhythmia. However, in some cases TdP might degenerate into VF.

Susceptibility to drug-induced QT prolongation and TdP is multifactorial and a combination of several factors is needed for arrhythmia to occur. Genetic predisposition based on variations in genes encoding the function of ion channels is considered as a key factor underlying susceptibility to drug-induced QT prolongation and TdP. Polymorphisms in genes encoding ion channels may cause an increased sensitivity of these channels to drugs blocking I_{Kr}, while polymorphisms in genes encoding enzymes metabolizing drugs may increase serum levels of drugs to excessive levels blocking the channel.

Several clinical factors are known to be associated with an increased risk for drug-induced QT prolongation and TdP. Women account for 70% of cases of drug-induced QT prolongation and TdP indicating that sex-related differences in repolarization duration might predispose women to proarrhythmias. Older age, preexisting heart disease (especially heart failure with low ejection fraction), spontaneous or drug-induced bradycardia, or dyselectrolitemia (hypokalemia, hypomagnesemia) are additional factors increasing susceptibility to QT prolongation and proarrhythmia. It should be emphasized that it is unlikely that one of the above factors is sufficient to cause drug-induced QT prolongation. Usually, a combination of several above mentioned factors must coincide to precipitate drug-induced TdP.

There is no universal threshold for identifying significant drug-induced QTc prolongation, and each drug has to be analyzed on an individual basis. QTc prolongation by more than 30 ms should raise concerns, and with greater concern when the increase in QTc exceeds 60 ms, especially if the QTc prolongs beyond 500 ms. The analysis of the magnitude of QTc prolongation from baseline by a drug should be paralleled by evaluating the absolute value of the prolonged QTc. Almost all of the reported TdP occur in subjects with QTc > 500 ms.

To assess the probability of drug-induced QT prolongation and the risk of TdP one should first determine pretreatment probability of such incident based on known clinical factors. Secondly, a baseline ECG should be recorded to determine potential baseline QT prolongation, which could be related to genetic predisposition, underlying disease process, or drugs currently being taken. The QTc interval should be evaluated based on both automated and manual measurements. ECGs should be repeated in a period reflecting maximum plasma concentrations of the drug, and the QT should be measured using the same methodology as it was done for baseline ECGs. In case of significant QTc prolongation by 60 ms or above 500 ms, treatment should be stopped or the combination of drugs should be modified to diminish the risk of cardiac events. As an example, patients in whom dofetilide treatment is initiated should remain in the hospital ward for 3 consecutive days to assess potential QT prolongation. Drugs associated with an increased risk of QT prolongation and TdP are listed in Table 15-5 (the detailed list can be found on www.qtdrugs.org).

SHORT QT SYNDROME

The SQTS is characterized by persistently short QT interval (QTc ≤ 320 ms) associated with high incidence of atrial fibrillation, syncopal episodes, and/or sudden cardiac death in patients with no underlying structural heart disease. Up to date, only a few families and several sporadic cases have been diagnosed with SQTS.

TABLE 15-5 Drugs that Prolong the QT Interval

Category	Drugs
Antihistamines	Astemizole and terfenadine
Anti-infectives	Amantadine, clarithromycin, chloroquine, erythromycin, grepafloxacin, moxifloxacin, pentamidine, sparfloxacin, and trimethoprim-sulfamethoxazole
Antineoplastics	Tamoxifen
Antiarrhythmics	Quinidine, sotalol, procainamide, amiodarone,bretylium, disopyramide, flecainide, ibutilide, moricizine, tocainide, and dofetilide
Antilipemic agents	Probucol
Calcium channel blockers	Bepridil
Diuretics	Indapamide
Gastrointestinal agents	Cisapride
Hormones	Fludrocortisone and vasopressin
Antidepressants	Amiryptyline, amoxapine, clomipramine, imipramine, nortriptyline, and protriptyline
Antipsychotic	Chlorpromazine, haloperidol, perphenazine, quetiapine, risperidone, sertindole, thioridazine, ziprasidone, doxepin, and methadon

Note: For more complete listing please visit www.qtdrugs.org

Diagnosis of SQTS is based on clinical symptoms, typical ECG pattern, EP study, and genetic testing. In clinical setting, patients with SQTS may present as totally asymptomatic or may experience sudden cardiac arrest as the first symptom. In the largest to date database analyzed by Giustetto et al. (2006), cardiac arrest was the most frequent (31%) clinical manifestation of a disease followed by palpitations and syncopal episodes. The age of first symptoms' occurrence may vary from the early childhood to adulthood.

Resting ECG reveals short QT interval ≤ 320 ms (QTc ≤ 340 ms) and tall, peaked T waves in precordial leads with no, or very short, ST segment present (Fig. 15-4). In patients presenting with a short QT interval on the ECG, all factors potentially shortening QT intervals like hyperkalemia, hypercalcemia, acidosis, hyperthermia, and above all most frequently encountered, digitalis use should be ruled out in the first step of diagnosis. Significant shortening of atrial and ventricular refractory periods observed during EP study, together with increased dispersion of repolarization, is considered as an underlying substrate for malignant arrhythmias in SQTS patients. Atrial fibrillation as well as VF are inducible by programmed stimulation.

In respect to genetic testing, so far SQTS has been linked to three gain-of-function mutations influencing potassium channels and interfering with repolarization process (in KCNH2, KCNQ1, and KCNJ2 genes) and to two loss-of-function mutations in CACNB2b and CACN1C genes encoding subunits of cardiac L-type calcium channels.

Up to date, ICD implantation is the method of choice in patients with SQTS, the only treatment documented to prevent cardiac events in this group. However, a high rate of inappropriate ICD discharges due to oversensing of tall, closely coupled T waves was reported in SQTS patients. Several attempts have been made to use drugs prolonging QT interval as potential therapeutic options, but so far only quinidine was proven to prolong QT interval, normalize T wave morphology, improve QT adaptation to heart rate, prolong the ventricular refractory period, and prevent VF inducibility on EP study. Propafenone, even though did not normalize QT interval, clinically suppressed episodes of atrial fibrillation. Nevertheless, currently pharmacological treatment may be considered only as an adjunctive therapy.

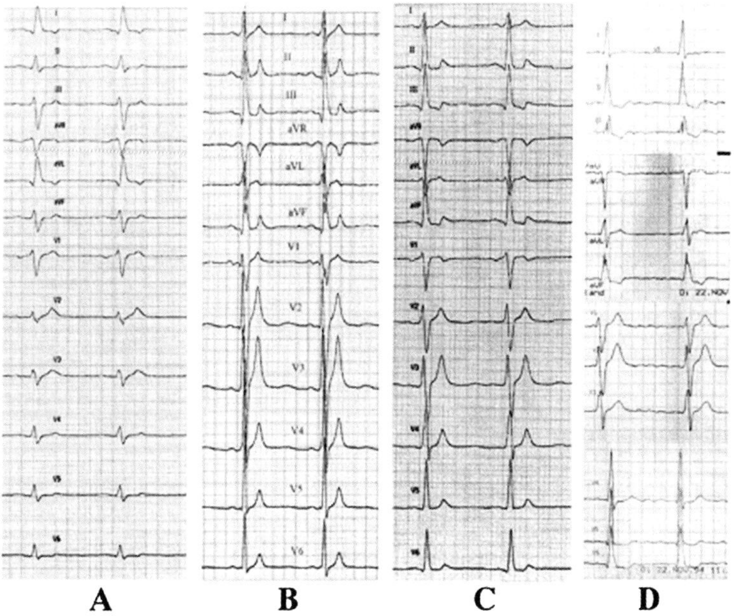

FIGURE 15-4. Exemplary ECGs of patients from one of the first families diagnosed with a short QT. A: Sinus rhythm, heart rate of 72 bpm, QT 270 ms; B: Sinus rhythm, heart rate 82 bpm, QT 260 ms; C: sinus rhythm, heart rate 75 bpm, QT 240 ms; D: ECG of a patient who died suddenly, atrial fibrillation, mean heart rate 85 bpm, QT 210 ms. (Reproduced from Gaita F, Giustetto C, Bianchi F, et al. Short QT syndrome: A familial cause of sudden death. Circulation. 2003;103:965–970, with permission.)

BRUGADA SYNDROME

Brugada syndrome is a genetically determined channelopathy, characterized by a typical pattern of ST segment elevation in right precordial leads resembling right bundle branch block and high risk of sudden death in patients with no evident underlying structural heart disease.

Three typical ECG patterns have been described in patients with Brugada syndrome. In Type 1, a coved ST-segment elevation greater or equal to 2 mm followed by a negative T wave is seen in more than one right precordial leads (V1 to V3). In type 2, saddleback configuration of ST-T segment is observed and ST is followed by a positive or biphasic T wave. Type 3 may show both coved or saddleback configuration, but ST-elevation is less or equal to 1 mm (Fig. 15-5). Prolongation of PR interval can also be observed in the ECG. Electrocardiographic changes in patients with Brugada syndrome are very dynamic, with possible day-to-day variation. In patients with concealed form or in those with ECG type 2 or 3, typical diagnostic ST changes can be unmasked by drugs, fever, or other triggering factors. Therefore, in patients suspected for Brugada syndrome but with ECG pattern type 2 or 3 provocation of characteristic ECG abnormalities with sodium channel blockers (ajmaline, flecainide, procainamide, and pilsicainide) and EP study to induce VT or VF should be performed to ascertain the diagnosis.

In patients with Brugada syndrome, the loss of function of sodium channel results in the imbalance between outward and inward positive currents during repolarization and consequently induces the heterogeneous loss of the action potential dome within

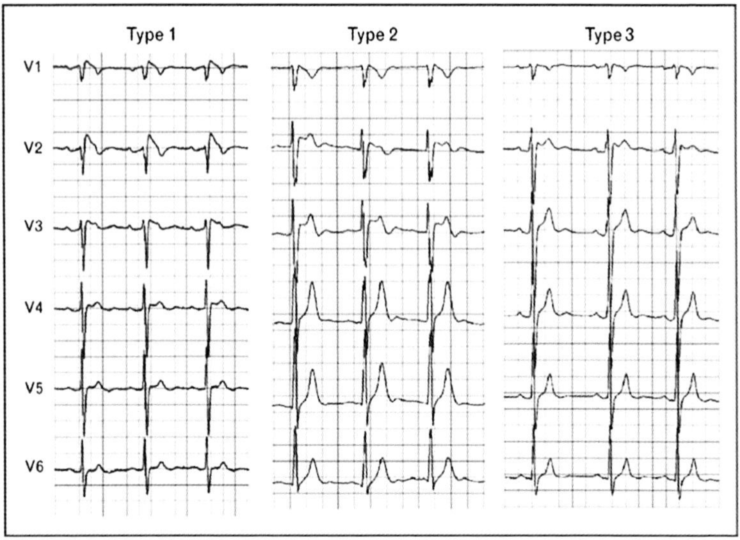

FIGURE 15-5. Typical for Brugada syndrome ECG patterns. Type 1 with a coved ST segment elevation of at least 2 mm followed by a negative T wave with little or no isoelectric separation; type 2 with a saddle-back pattern—ST elevation of at least 2 mm, followed by gradually descending ST segment elevation and a positive or biphasic T wave; and type 3—either cover or saddleback type with ST elevation of less than 1 mm. (Reproduced from Rossenbacker T, Priori SG. The Brugada syndrome. *Current Opinion Cardiol.* 2007;22:163–170, with permission.)

the phase 2 duration. Ventricular arrhythmias are therefore related to phase 2 reentry mechanism as a consequence of an increased dispersion of repolarization and refractoriness within epicardium and across the wall.

In order to recognize Brugada syndrome, and not only Brugada ECG pattern, spontaneous or induced ECG changes should be accompanied by clinical symptoms. There is a striking difference in prevalence of Brugada syndrome according to gender with 8:1 ratio between men and women. According to a consensus published in 2005, diagnosis of Brugada syndrome is confirmed only in patients who present with spontaneous or drug-induced type 1 ECG pattern and/or at least one of the following findings: documented VF or polymorphic VT, a family history of sudden cardiac death, coved (type 1) ECG in family members, EP inducibility of VT, syncope, or nocturnal agonal respiration.

Patients with a past history of cardiac arrest and those with clinical symptoms and spontaneous type 1 ECG pattern are considered as the higher risk group, while asymptomatic patients with only drug-induced ECG changes are considered as the "low risk" group. Genetic testing for the presence of SCN5A mutation only confirms diagnosis but does not contribute to risk stratification.

So far, only ICD therapy has been proven to be effective in patients with Brugada syndrome. Recommendations for ICD implantations in Brugada syndrome are shown in Figure 15-6 and in Table 15-4. Implantation of cardioverter-defibrillator is indicated as secondary prevention in patients with a documented history of cardiac arrest (class I) as well as in primary prevention in symptomatic patients with spontaneous type-1-ECG (class I) or drug-induced ECG changes (class IIA). It should also be recommended in asymptomatic patients with spontaneous type-1-ECG pattern and inducible VT/VF

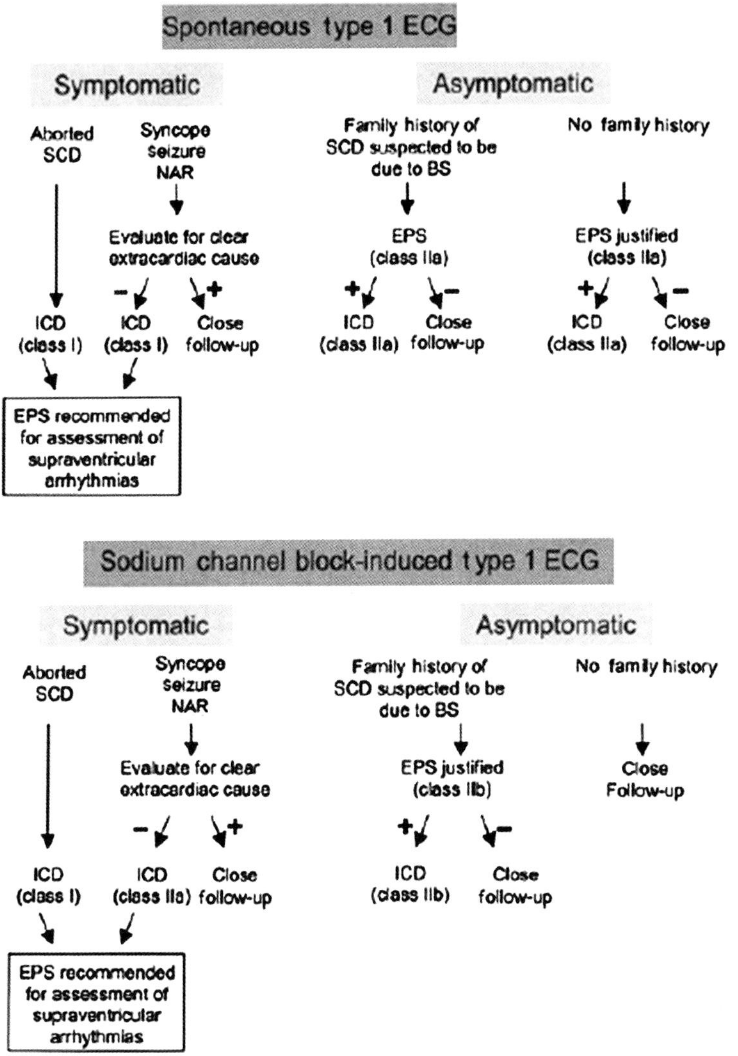

FIGURE 15-6. Indications for ICD implantation in patients with Brugada syndrome according to the Second Consensus Conference. (Reproduced from Antzelevitch C, Brugada P, Borggrefe M, et al. Brugada syndrome: Report of the second consensus conference. *Heart Rhythm.* 2005;2:429–440, with permission.)

(class IIa), or drug-induced type-1-ECG, family history of sudden death, and positive EP study (class IIB).

Regarding pharmacotherapy, quinidine has been the most extensively studied and proposed as the alternative for ICD treatment; however, no randomized data on effectiveness of this pharmacotherapy is available. Antiarhythmic drugs (sodium channel blockers from classes IA and IC, calcium antagonists, beta blockers), psychotropic drugs, first generation antihistaminics, alpha adrenergic agonists, and potassium channel opening drugs should be avoided.

CATECHOLAMINERGIC POLYMORPHIC VENTRICULAR TACHYCARDIA

Catecholaminergic polymorphic ventricular tachycardia (CPVT) is an inherited channelopathy associated with mutations in two genes: RYR2 encoding the cardiac ryanodine receptor channel (autosomal dominant form) and CASQ2 encoding calsequestrin, a calcium binding protein of sarcoplasmatic reticulum (autosomal recessive form). Genetic mutations result in abnormal calcium release from sarcoplasmatic reticulum and subsequent diastolic calcium overload.

From the clinical point of view, CPVT is characterized by exercise- or emotion-induced palpitations and/or syncopes in subjects with no structural heart disease. Most frequently, patients become symptomatic in early childhood, with the mean age of symptoms between 7 and 9 years old. High incidence of both supraventricular (predominantly atrial fibrillation) as well as ventricular arrhythmias is observed in patients with CPVT; however, bidirectional VT with alternating 180-degree-QRS axis on beat-to-beat basis is considered as the most typical ECG presentation of CPVT. This adrenergic-induced VT may be self-terminating but sometimes may degenerate into VF; therefore, cardiac arrest can be frequently found as the first manifestation of CPVT.

Unlike in previously described channelopathies, in case of CPVT resting ECG is non-contributory to diagnosis. Therefore, diagnostic process should include cardiac imaging

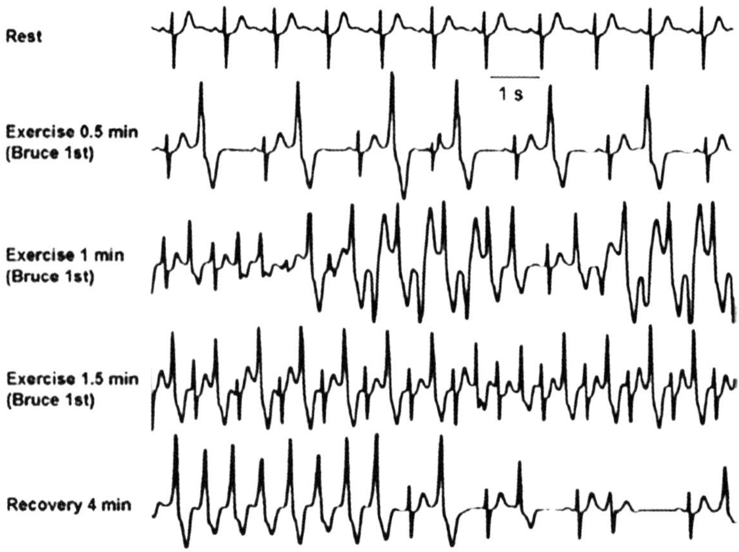

FIGURE 15-7. Exercise test in a patient with polymorphic VT and RyR2 mutation. Ventricular arrhythmias are observed with a progressive worsening during exercise. Typical bidirectional VT develops after 1 min exercise with a sinus rhythm of approximately 120 bpm. Arrhythmias rapidly recede during recovery. (Reproduced from Liu N, Ruan Y, Priori SG. Catecholaminergic polymorphic ventricular tachycardia. *Prog Cardiovasc Dis.* 2008;51:23–30, with permission.)

to rule out the presence of structural heart disease as well as ECG techniques to evaluate the relationship of arrhythmias with exercise or stress. Holter monitoring is useful to assess the arrhythmia presence during daily activities and under emotional stress, while exercise stress test helps to evaluate ventricular arrhythmias with increasing workload. Ventricular arrhythmia usually appears at the heart rate of 110 to 130 bmp and then aggravates both in number as well as in complexity with increasing heart rate with gradual progression from isolated premature beats to bigeminy, couplets, runs of nonsustained VT, and finally to a sustained bidirectional VT, not rarely degenerating into VF (Fig. 15-7). The mechanism of ventricular arrhythmias in patients with CPVT is explained by defective calcium handling as a result of underlying RYR2 and CASQ2 genes mutations. The excess of positive-ion calcium currents results in the depolarization of myocytes at the end of action potential creating delayed afterdepolarizations being potential trigger for arrhythmias. Experimental studies point that in CPVT ectopic beats arise from the epicardial region. CPVT is not inducible by programmed electrical stimulation.

Therapeutic approach in patients with CPVT includes beta-blockers titrated under control of exercise stress test, and ICD implantation in patients with a history of cardiac arrest, or in those in whom beta-blocker therapy is not sufficient to suppress arrhythmia. In addition, life-style modifications are needed aiming toward eliminating strenuous exercises which might trigger ventricular arrhythmias.

SUMMARY

It is expected that list of channelopathies will further grow with progressive improved understanding of genetic background of rare disorders leading to cardiac arrhythmias and sudden death. Sudden death associated with ECG pattern showing features of early repolarization with QRS notching (described by Haissaguerre) leads to newly identified channelopathy caused by abnormalities of the KCNJ8 gene encoding a subunit of yet another potassium channel K(ATP). Channelopathies should not be exclusively considered as ventricular diseases since atrial ion channels are involved in generation of atrial arrhythmias (e.g., the SCN5A sodium channel gene harboring mutations predisposing to atrial fibrillation), but this field is still in young stages of development.

KEY POINTS

1. The presence of channelopathies (LQTS, SQTS, Brugada syndrome, and CPVT) should be suspected in patients with no apparent structural heart disease who present with ventricular arrhythmias, unexplained syncope, cardiac arrest, or sudden death in family members.
2. History of syncope, family history of sudden death, and ECG findings usually lead to proper diagnosis. Careful evaluation of ECG changes, with particular attention paid to morphology of repolarization (ST segment and T wave), is essential. Genetic testing is especially valuable in LQTS in diagnosing borderline cases, in guiding the therapy, and in testing family members.
3. Patients with channelopathies with a recent history of syncope are at the highest risk of cardiac events or death.
4. High-risk patients with channelopathies are treated with ICDs as primary or secondary prevention of sudden death.
5. Initiation of treatment with drugs known to prolong QT interval (detailed list on www.qtdrugs.org) should be accompanied by a careful analysis of sequential ECGs with QT interval assessment to prevent occurrence of TdP.

SUGGESTED READINGS

Long QT Syndrome

Antzelevitch C, Shimizu W. Cellular mechanisms underlying the long QT syndrome. *Curr Opin Cardiol.* 2002;17:43–51.
Daubert JP, Zareba W, Rosero SZ, et al. Role of implantable cardioverter defibrillator therapy in patients with long QT syndrome. *Am Heart J.* 2007;153(suppl):53–58.
Goldenberg I, Moss AJ. Long QT syndrome. *J Am Coll Cardiol.* 2008;51:2291–2300.
Moss AJ, Robinson JL. Long QT syndrome. *Heart Dis Stroke.* 1992;1:309–314.
Moss AJ, Schwartz PJ, Crampton RS, et al. The long QT syndrome. Prospective longitudinal study of 328 families. *Circulation.* 1991;84:1136–1144.
Moss AJ, Zareba W, Hall WJ, et al. Effectiveness and limitations of beta-blocker therapy in congenital long-QT syndrome. *Circulation.* 2000;101:616–623.
Priori SG, Schwartz PJ, Napolitano C, et al. Risk stratification in the long-QT syndrome. *N Engl J Med.* 2003; 348:1866–1874.
Schwartz PJ, Moss AJ, Vincent GM, et al. Diagnostic criteria for the long QT syndrome: An update. *Circulation.* 1993;88:782–784.
Schwartz PJ, Priori SG, Spazzolini C, et al. Genotype-phenotype correlation in the long-QT syndrome: Gene-specific triggers for life-threatening arrhythmias. *Circulation.* 2001;103:89–95.
Zareba W. Genotype-specific patterns in long QT syndrome. *J Electrocardiol.* 2006;39:S101–S106.
Zareba W, Cygankiewicz I. Long QT syndrome and short QT syndrome. *Prog Cardiovasc Dis.* 2008;51: 264–278.

Short QT Syndrome

Gaita F, Giustetto C, Bianchi F, et al. Short QT syndrome: A familial cause of sudden death. *Circulation.* 2003;103:965–970.
Giustetto C, Di Monte F, Wolpert C, et al. Short QT syndrome: Clinical findings and diagnostic–therapeutic implications. *Eur Heart J.* 2006;27:2440–2447.
Schimpf R, Bauersfeld U, Gaita F, et al. Short QT syndrome: Successful prevention of sudden death in an adolescent by implantable cardioverter–defibrilator treatment for primary prophylaxis. *Heart Rhythm.* 2005;2:416–417.
Schimpf R, Borggrefe M, Wolpert C. Clinical and molecular genetics of the short QT syndrome. *Curr Opin Cardiol.* 2008;23:192–198.

Brugada Syndrome

Antzelevitch C, Brugada P, Borggrefe M, et al. Brugada syndrome: Report of the second consensus conference. *Heart Rhythm.* 2005;2:429–440.
Benito B, Brugada R, Brugada J, et al. Brugada syndrome. *Prog Cardiovasc Dis.* 2008;51:1–22.
Brugada P, Brugada J. Right bundle branch block, persistent ST segment elevation and sudden cardiac death: A distinct clinical and electrocardiographic syndrome. A multicenter report. *J Am Coll Cardiol.* 1992; 20:1391–1396.
Brugada R, Brugada P, Brugada J. Electrocardiogram interpretation and class I blocker challenge in Brugada syndrome. *J Electrocardiol.* 2006;39(4 suppl):S115–S118.

Catecholaminergic Polymorphic Ventricular Tachycardia

Liu N, Ruan Y, Priori SG. Catecholaminergic polymorphic ventricular tachycardia. *Prog Cardiovasc Dis.* 2008; 51:23–30.
Napolitano C, Priori SG. Diagnosis and treatment of catecholaminergic polymorphic ventricular tachycardia. *Heart Rhythm.* 2007;4:675–678.
Priori SG, Napolitano C, Memmi M, et al. Clinical and molecular characterization of patients with catecholaminergic polymorphic ventricular tachycardia. *Circulation.* 2002;106:69–74.

INDEX

Page numbers followed by "f" denote figures; those followed by "t" denote tables.

A

Activation mapping technique, 129–130, 130f
Adenosine-based tilt test, 165–167, 166f
Antiarrhythmic medications
  bolus and doses, 197t
  class IA drugs
    disopyramide, 198–199
    intravenous procainamide, 198
    quinidine, 198
  class IB drugs
    lidocaine, 199
    mexiletine, 199
    phenytoin, 199
  class IC drugs
    flecainide, 200
    propafenone, 200
  class II drugs, beta-blockers, 200–201, 201t
  class III drugs
    amiodarone, 202
    bretylium, 203
    dofetilide, 203
    dronedarone, 202
    ibutilide, 203
    sotalol, 202–203
    vernakalant, 203
  drugs classification, 195–196, 198, 196t
  pregnancy, therapy
    adverse effects, 207t–208t
    categories, definition, 206t
    uses, 206
  unclassified drugs
    adenosine, 204
    digoxin, 204–206
Arrhythmogenic right ventricular cardiomyopathy (ARVC)
  cardiac magnetic resonance (CMR) imaging, 87–88, 88f
  discretionary testing, 88–90
  ICD implantation, 92
  signal-averaged ECG (SAECG), 85
Atrial arrhythmias
  atrial fibrillation (*see* Atrial fibrillation (AF))
  atrial flutter (*see* Atrial flutter (AFL))
  atrial tachycardia (*see* Atrial tachycardia (AT))
Atrial fibrillation (AF)
  antithrombotic therapy, 45–47, 45t, 46f
  catheter ablation, 120–122
  catheter ablative therapy, 50–51, 51t
  classification, 40–41
  clinical presentation, 41
  diagnosis, 36
  epidemiology, 36–38, 37f, 38t
  initial evaluation, 41–42
  pathophysiology, 38, 39f, 40
  pharmacologic therapy, 48–50
  prognosis and complications, 42–44, 43f, 44f
  surgical ablative therapy, 50–51
  symptoms, 41
Atrial flutter (AFL)
  acute treatment, 56
  anticoagulation, 58
  catheter ablation, 118–120, 119f–121f
  clinical presentation
    complications, 53
    electrocardiogram, 52–53, 52f
    symptoms, 52
  complications, 53
  definition, 51
  diagnosis
    electrophysiological maneuvers, 55–56
    pharmacologic maneuvers, 54–55
  electrocardiogram, 52–53, 52f
  epidemiology, 52
  pathophysiology
    categorization, 54, 54f–55f
    mechanism, 53
    origin, 54
  symptoms, 52
  therapy
    acute treatment, 56
    anticoagulation, 58
    catheter ablation, 57f, 57–58
    long-term treatment, 57
Atrial tachycardia (AT)
  acute therapy, 60
  classification, 58, 59f, 59t
  definition, 58
  endocardial mapping, 62–63
  epidemiology, 58
  intracardial mapping, 62
  long-term pharmacologic therapy, 60–62, 61f
  macro reentrant AT, 63
  management, 60
  mapping
    3D mapping, AT ablation, 63
    endocardial mapping, 62
    intracardiac mapping, 62
  multifocal atrial tachycardia (MAT), 62
  prognosis, 59–60
Atrioventricular block (*see* Pacemaker implantation)
Atrioventricular nodal reentrant tachycardia (AVNRT)
  catheter ablation
    AV block, 21–22
    cryomapping and cryoablation, 22
    fast pathway ablation, 20
    fluoroscopic exposure reduction, 22
    magnetic guidance system, 22

Atrioventricular nodal reentrant tachycardia (AVNRT) (*Continued*)
recurrence, 21
remote navigation ablation system, 22
slow pathway ablation, 20–21, 21f
electrophysiology
atypical AVNRT, 15, 16f, 17, 19f
AV junction anatomy, 13, 13f
dual AV nodal pathways, 15, 16f
fast pathway, 13–15, 13f–16f
lower common pathway, 18
slow pathway, 13–17, 13f–16f
typical AVNRT, 15, 16f–18f
upper common pathway, 18
isoproterenol, 17
pharmacologic treatment
drug treatment, 20
vagal maneuvers, 18–20
Atrioventricular reentrant tachycardia (AVRT)
catheter-based ablation, 33–34
electrophysiology
antidromic AVRT, 27f–30f, 31
atrial fibrillation, 31
reentrant circuit, 28f
orthodromic AVRT, 28, 28f
pharmacologic treatment, 32–33
risk stratification, 31–32

B

Beta-blockers (*see* Antiarrhythmic medications)
Bradycardia
atrioventricular block (AVB)
endocavitary recording, 6, 8f
intra/infra-hisian block, 6–8, 6f–7f
nodal block, 5, 7f
provocative test, predictive value, 7
types, 5, 6f–7f
sinoatrial block
corrected sinus node recovery time (CSNRT), 4f, 3–4
first-degree block, 2
second-degree block, 2, 3f
sinoatrial conduction time (SACT), 4, 5f
sinus arrest, 2
third-degree block, 4f
sinus rhythm
definition, 1
electrical activation, 2f
Brugada syndrome, 116, 116f, 146t, 219–221, 220f, 221f

C

Cardiac arrest
cardiac magnetic resonance (CMR) imaging, 87–88, 88f
discretionary testing, 88–90, 89f
exercise testing, 85, 87f
signal-averaged ECG (SAECG), 85
survivors
cardiac function assessment, 84–85
coronary angiography, 85, 86f
investigation strategy, 83–84, 83f
resting electrocardiogram, 84, 84f
Cardiac mapping system
anatomic ablation, 128–129
body surface mapping, 128
contact mapping, 128
electroanatomic mapping system, 129
fluoroscopic imaging, 129
focal mechanisms, 128
intracardiac positioning system, 129
techniques, 135t
activation mapping, 129–130, 130f
entrainment mapping, 131–133, 132f
pace mapping, 130–131, 131f
substrate mapping, 133–134, 133f–134f
tools, 129
reentrant arrhythmias, 128–129
Cardiac resynchronization therapy (CRT)
clinical trial data, 151–152
electromechanical events, 151
indications, 152
Cardiac rhythm management
internal cardioverter-defibrillator (ICD) implantation
primary prevention, 148–151, 149t
secondary prevention trials, 146, 148, 147t
types, 146, 146t
pacemaker implantation
atrioventricular block, 144–145
hypertrophic obstructive cardiomyopathy, 145
neuromuscular disorders, 145
sinus node dysfunction (SND), 142–144
sleep apnea syndrome, 145
physiologic pacing system
AV synchronous pacing, 138
dual chamber and VVI implantable defibrillator (DAVID) trial, 138
indications, 142t
managed ventricular pacing, 138, 141f
MOST data, 138
pacing and mode selection, 138, 139t–140t
single chamber ventricular based pacemaker, 141
ventricular pacing, 137–138, 138t
Cardiac syncope
arrhythmias, 77–79, 78f, 79f
autonomic dysfunction
carotid sinus hypersensitivity, 75
chronic orthostatic intolerance, 75
tilt table testing, 75–76, 76f
vasovagal syncope, 76–77
differential diagnosis, 74f, 74–75
disorders, 74
Cardioverter defibrillators, 108
Carotid sinus hypersensitivity, 75
Carto electroanatomic mapping system, 101–102, 101f, 102f
Catecholaminergic polymorphic ventricular tachycardia (CPVT), 216t, 222–223, 222f
discretionary testing, 89, 89f
exercise testing, 85
ICD implantation, 92
initial investigation strategy, 83
surgical ablation, 93

Catheter ablation (*see also* Cardiac mapping system)
biophysics, 126, 126f–127f
catheter mapping, 127–128
energy sources, 126–127
historical development, 125–126
Channelopathies
action potential and membrane currents, 210, 211f
Brugada syndrome, 216t, 219–222 220f, 221f
catecholaminergic polymorphic ventricular tachycardia (CPVT), 216t, 222–223, 222f
long QT syndrome (LQTS)
Bazett-corrected values, 213t
clinical pathology, 210
diagnosis, 211, 213–214, 213t, 214f, 215t
drug-induced prolongation and TdP, 216–217, 218t
genetic types and ion channels, 212t
risk stratification and management, 214–216, 216t
short QT syndrome (SQTS), 217–218
Chronic orthostatic intolerance, 75
Corrected sinus node recovery time (CSNRT), 4f, 3–4
Cryoablation, 100, 126–127

D
Device functional information
basic programmed data, 170–171, 171f–172f
battery status, 171, 173f
high voltage charge circuit, 172, 173f
lead status, 172–174, 174f–176f

E
Effective refractory period (ERP), 31–32
Electrical cardioversion
biphasic waveforms, 162, 164, 163f, 164f
shock waveforms, 162, 163f, 164
Electrophysiology
ablation, energy sources
cryoablation, 100
irrigation system, 100
radiofrequency generators, 99–100
arrhythmias, catheter ablation
atrial fibrillation, 120-121, 122f
atrial flutter, 118–119, 119f–121f
ventricular arrhythmias, 122–123, 123f
Brugada syndrome, 116
cardioverter defibrillators, 108
catheters, 97–98, 98f–99f
echocardiography
intracardiac ultrasound (ICUS) imaging, 105–106, 106f
transthoracic echocardiography (TTE), 104
fluoroscopy, 99
multichannel physiologic recorders, 95, 96f, 97
paroxysmal supraventricular tachycardia (PSVT)
ATs, 113
AVNRT, 111, 111f–112f
orthodromic reciprocating tachycardia (ORT), 111, 113
supraventricular tachycardia (SVT), 111
remote navigation systems, 107–108
risk stratification
limitations, 115
structural disease, 113–114
stimulators, 97
syncope
intra-hisian block, 117, 117f
type II AV block, 118, 118f
vasodepressor syncope, 118
three-dimensional mapping systems
carto electroanatomic mapping, 101–102, 101f–102f
impedance-based mapping systems, 102
noncontact mapping, 102, 104, 103f
ventricular stimulation, 115–116, 115f
Entrainment mapping technique, 131–133, 132f

G
Gas gauge, 171, 173f

H
Heart rate turbulence (HRT), 159, 161, 162f
Heart rate variability
chronic heart failure, 158, 159f
frequency-domain analysis, 158
ICD implantation, 158–159
respiratory sinus arrhythmia (RSA), 157
sudden arrhythmic death, 157
time-domain analysis, 158
Holter monitor, 154, 155t

I
Idiopathic monomorphic ventricular tachycardia, 71
Impedance-based mapping systems, 102
Implantable cardioverter-defibrillators (ICDs), 215–216, 216t (*see also* Channelopathies)
atrial fibrillation with fast pacing rate, 182–183
device functional information
basic programmed data, 170–171, 171f–172f
battery status, 171, 173f
high voltage charge circuit, 172, 173f
lead status, 174, 176, 177f–178f
failure to pace, 183
implantation, indications
primary prevention ICD, 148, 149t, 150–151
secondary prevention trials, 146, 147t, 148
types, 146, 146t
inappropriate shocks, 183
loss of capture, 183
lung wetness, 183–184, 184f
Intracardiac ultrasound (ICUS) imaging, 105–106, 105f, 106f

L

Long QT syndrome (LQTS)
  acute management, 90
  Bazett-corrected values, 213t
  clinical pathology, 210
  diagnosis, 211, 213–214, 213t, 214f, 215t
  discretionary testing, 89
  drug-induced prolongation and TdP, 216–217, 218t
  exercise testing, 85, 87f
  genetic types and ion channels, 212t
  ICD implantation, 92
  initial investigation strategy, 83–84, 83f
  medical therapy, 91
  resting electrocardiogram, 84, 84f
  risk stratification and management, 214–216 216t
  surgical ablation, 93

M

Microvolt T wave alternans (MTWA), 159, 160t, 161f
Mobile cardiac outpatient telemetry monitoring system, 155t, 156
  heart rate variability
    chronic heart failure, 158, 159f
    frequency-domain analysis, 158
    ICD implantation, 158–159
    respiratory sinus arrhythmia (RSA), 157
    sudden arrhythmic death, 157–158
    time-domain analysis, 158
  signal-averaged ECG (SAECG), 156–157, 157f
  T wave alternans (TWA) test, 159, 160t, 161f
Mobitz sinoatrial block, 2, 3f
Monomorphic ventricular tachycardia (MMVT) (*see also* Ventricular tachycardia (VT))
  idiopathic monomorphic VT, ablation, 71
  mechanism, 66–67, 66f
  structural heart disease, ablation
    entrainment mapping, 68–71, 69f, 70f
    scar-related sustained monomorphic tachycardia, 68
Multichannel physiologic recorders, 95, 96f, 97

N

Noncardiac syncope, 74f, 79
Noncontact mapping system, 102–104, 103f
Noninvasive monitoring tools
  Holter monitor, 154
  mobile cardiac outpatient telemetry monitoring system, 155t, 156
    heart rate variability, 157–159, 159f
    signal-averaged ECG (SAECG), 156–157, 157f
    T wave alternans (TWA) test, 159, 160t, 161f
  transtelephonic electrocardiographic monitoring, 154, 156

O

Outflow tract tachycardias, 68

P

Pace mapping technique, 130–131, 131f
Pacemaker implantation
  atrioventricular block
    acute myocardial infarction (AMI), 145
    chronic bifascicular block, 145
    complete heart block, 144
    first degree AV block, 144
    infiltrative disease, 145
    second degree AV block, 144
  hypertrophic obstructive cardiomyopathy, 145
  neuromuscular disorders, 145
  sinus node dysfunction (SND)
    bradycardia, 142–143
    paroxysmal AF, 143–144
    syncope, 142
  sleep apnea syndrome, 145
Paroxysmal supraventricular tachycardia (PSVT)
  atrioventricular nodal reentrant tachycardia (AVNRT)
    catheter ablation, 20–22, 21f
    electrophysiology, 13–18
    pharmacologic treatment, 18–20
  clinical presentation, 11–12, 11f, 12t
  electrophysiology
    ATs, 113
    AVNRT, 111, 111f–112f
    orthodromic reciprocating tachycardia (ORT), 111, 113
    supraventricular tachycardia (SVT), 111
  epidemiology, 10–11
  Wolff-Parkinson-White (WPW) syndrome
    catheter-based ablation, 33–34
    electrophysiology, 23–31
    epidemiology, 22–23
    pharmacologic treatment, 32–33
    risk stratification, 31–32
Patient rhythm diagnostics, 174, 176, 177f–178f
Physiologic pacing system
  AV synchronous pacing, 138
  dual chamber and VVI implantable defibrillator (DAVID) trial, 138
  indications, 142t
  managed ventricular pacing, 138, 141f
  MOST data, 138
  pacing and mode selection, 138, 139t–140t
  single chamber ventricular based pacemaker, 141
  ventricular pacing, 137–138, 138t
Polymorphic wide complex tachycardia (PM WCT), 191–192, 192f
Postural orthostatic tachycardia syndrome (*see* Chronic orthostatic intolerance)
Pulmonary artery diastolic pressure (ePAD), 184

R

Radiofrequency (RF) ablation, 125–126, 126f
Remote magnetic navigation (RMS) system, 107
Rhythm-specific information, 178, 179f–181f, 181

S

Scar-related sustained monomorphic tachycardia, 68
SELF clinical pathway, 80f, 80–81
Shock waveforms, 161, 163f
Short QT syndrome (SQTS), 217, 218
Signal-averaged ECG (SAECG), 85, 156–157, 157f
Sinoatrial conduction time (SACT), 4
Sinus bradycardia, 2Sinus node dysfunction (SND) (*see* Pacemaker implantation)
Substrate mapping technique, 133–134, 133f–134f
Sudden cardiac death (SCD)
  acute management, 90-91
  cardiac arrest
    cardiac function assessment, 84–85
    cardiac magnetic resonance (CMR) imaging, 87–88, 88f
    coronary angiography, 85, 86f
    diagnostic algorithm, 83f, 84
    discretionary testing, 88–90, 89f
    exercise testing, 85, 87f
    resting electrocardiogram, 84, 84f
    signal-averaged ECG (SAECG), 85
  clinical causes, 82–83
  genetics, 90
  primary prevention
    ICD implantation, 91–92
    medical therapy, 91
  secondary prevention
    catheter ablation, 93
    ICD implantation, 92
    medical therapy, 92–93
  treatment, 90
Supraventricular tachycardia (SVT)
  atrioventricular nodal reentrant tachycardia (AVNRT)
    catheter ablation, 20–22, 21f
    electrophysiology, 13–18
    pharmacologic treatment, 18–20
  clinical presentation, 11–12, 11f, 12t
  epidemiology, 10–11
  Wolff-Parkinson-White (WPW) syndrome
    catheter-based ablation, 33–34
    electrophysiology, 22–31
    epidemiology, 22–23
    pharmacologic treatment, 32–33
    risk stratification, 31–32
Syncope
  cardiac syncope
    arrhythmias, 77–79, 78f, 79f
    autonomic dysfunction, 75–77, 76f
    differential diagnosis, 74f, 74
    disorders, 74
  diagnostic evaluation, 81
  electrophysiology
    intra-hisian block, 117, 117f
    type II AV block, 118, 118f
  noncardiac syncope, 74f, 79
  SELF clinical pathway, 80f, 80–81

T

T wave alternans (TWA) test, 159, 160t, 161f
Tilt table test
  adenosine-based tilt test, 166f, 167
  isoproterenol, 167
  limitation, 167
Torsade de pointes (TdP) (*see* Long QT syndrome (LQTS))
Transtelephonic electrocardiographic monitoring system, 154, 156
Transthoracic echocardiography (TTE), 104
Transvenous pacing
  catheter packaging, 165
  ECG guidance, 165
  indications, 164, 165t
  venous access route, 164

V

Vasovagal syncope, 76–77
Ventricular tachycardia (VT)
  ECG localization, 67f, 67–68
  idiopathic monomorphic VT, ablation, 71
  LV fascicular VT, 72–73
  mapping, 72, 72f
  mechanism, 66f, 66–67
  outflow tract tachycardia, 71
  preablation assessment, 65
  structural heart disease, ablation
    entrainment mapping, 68, 69f, 70f, 70–71
    scar-related sustained monomorphic tachycardia, 68
    substrate mapping, 71

W

Wenckebach sinoatrial block, 2, 5f
Wide complex tachycardia (WCT)
  management, 192–193, 193f
  polymorphic (PM), 191–192, 192f
  uniform-morphology, diagnostic possibilities, 186–191, 187t, 188t, 189f–191f
  ventricular *vs.* supraventricular, 187–191, 188t, 189f–191f
Wolff-Parkinson-White (WPW) syndrome
  accessory pathway (AP), electrophysiology, 23–31
    atrial fibrillation, 31
    ECG-based AP localization algorithms, 24, 24f–27f
    locations, 23, 23f
    types, 23
  catheter-based ablation, 33–34
  epidemiology, 22–23
  risk stratification, 31–32